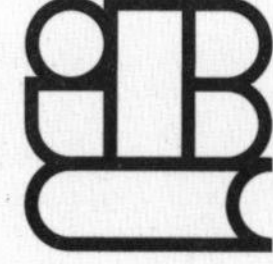

D1205686

The Future of Primary Care

Jonathan Showstack

Arlyss Anderson Rothman

Susan B. Hassmiller

Editors

The Future of Primary Care

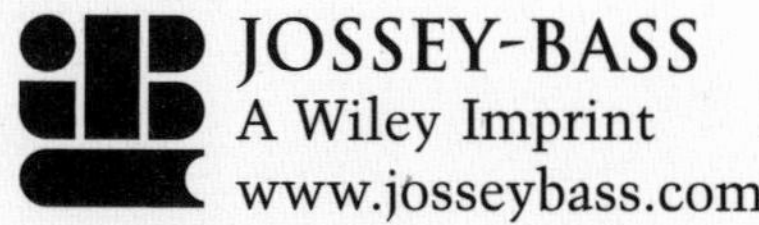
JOSSEY-BASS
A Wiley Imprint
www.josseybass.com

Published by Jossey-Bass
A Wiley Imprint
989 Market Street, San Francisco, CA 94103-1741 www.josseybass.com

Jossey-Bass books and products are available through most bookstores. To contact Jossey-Bass directly call our Customer Care Department within the U.S. at 800-956-7739, outside the U.S. at 317-572-3986, or fax 317-572-4002.

Jossey-Bass also publishes its books in a variety of electronic formats. Some content that appears in print may not be available in electronic books.

Library of Congress Cataloging-in-Publication Data

The future of primary care / [edited] by Jonathan Showstack, Arlyss Anderson Rothman, Susan B. Hassmiller.— 1st ed.
p. cm.
Includes bibliographical references and index.
ISBN 0-7879-7243-6 (alk. paper)
1. Primary care (Medicine) 2. Primary care (Medicine)—Forecasting.
[DNLM: 1. Primary Health Care—trends. W 84.6 F996 2004]
I. Showstack, Jonathan, 1946– II. Rothman, Arlyss Anderson, 1948-
III. Hassmiller, Susan B., 1954-
RC48.F88 2004
610'.23'73—dc22
2003020016

Printed in the United States of America
FIRST EDITION
PB Printing 10 9 8 7 6 5 4 3 2 1

Contents

Preface

The term *primary care* means different things to different people. Many of us have championed primary care because of its theoretical and practical contributions to the health of persons and populations. Despite the rise of "scientific medicine" and specialization, the concept of primary care has achieved an important place in the delivery of health services. Over the past century, primary care has developed from the idea of a family doctor who tended to the medical, and at times the emotional and social, needs of his patients to a new and much richer and idealized concept that encompasses prevention, continuity of care, health maintenance, and death with dignity. The renaissance of primary care that began in the 1970s, however, has begun to wane. Today a number of organizational, economic, and social forces are presenting new challenges to primary care. How those challenges are addressed will determine, in large part, the future of primary care and the role of primary care in addressing the health needs of our population.

The attributes of first contact, continuous, and comprehensive care make primary care an excellent entry point to and coordinator of care. These same characteristics, however, also make primary care an ideal gatekeeper for managed care and other systems that wish to control access to and use of services. The success of so-called boutique providers who guarantee access, a continuous relationship with a primary care physician, and personalized referral to a specialist in return for a retainer fee (for those who can afford it) demonstrates another aspect of the attractiveness of primary care amid a rising tide of consumerism and so-called market-driven medicine.

Almost uniquely among health care specialties, primary care providers have been willing, even eager, to include within their responsibilities a variety of functions that are not strictly medical in nature and go well beyond a provider's practice site. The use of a team of providers with varied expertise is a logical extension of this broadening of the definition of the role of primary care. This expansion of responsibility also begs the question, however, of whether primary care has become too complex, taken on too much, promised too much to too many. Must a primary care provider care for all, be up-to-date on all of the latest discoveries and treatments, be an expert diagnostician, and have the patience to care for persons with chronic illness, the compassion to care for those at the end of life, the sophistication to recognize behavioral and social problems, the communication skills to encourage patient behavior change? Have we raised the bar too high, put too much responsibility on the shoulders of primary care?

In response to concerns about the future of primary care, the Robert Wood Johnson Foundation sponsored a small invited meeting of leaders in primary care and other health sectors to discuss the current and future challenges to primary care and to develop new and innovative ideas about how primary care might meet the needs of our population, both now and in the future. Forty-five persons attended the meeting, organized by a team at the University of California, San Francisco, that worked with an advisory committee and foundation staff to define the meeting's goals, objectives, and content.

Held in early October 2001 in Glen Cove, New York, the goal of The Future of Primary Care meeting was to identify a set of normative ideas and principles to help in future discussions about the definition and creation of a health care system that will address the future needs of our population. The premise of the meeting was that primary care is at a crossroads. Especially as changes occur in our population and in the financing and organization of the health care system, the future of primary care should not be taken for granted. Rather, primary care must be able to justify its place in a system where specialist physicians and nurses are increasingly providing principal care and where patients often choose to go to nontraditional settings for their care. An objective of the meeting was to question the current definitions and assumptions associated with primary care and examine whether they are still relevant, either in today's or a redesigned health care system.

The Glen Cove meeting was not a consensus conference. No votes were taken, and there were lively discussions and debates about a wide variety of ideas and issues. The discussions focused on the identification and development of ideas that could describe and help define normative systems of care. The central question was, "What principles can be identified for the organization and delivery of care to address the needs of our future population?" Rather than focusing on adjusting current financing and workforce policies to today's fragmented and often dysfunctional health care system, the goal was to start a dialogue on how primary care *should* be delivered. The principles and ideas identified could then be used in the construction of new primary care systems, with finance and workforce policies created to support the development and use of the new systems.

As preparation for the meeting, fifteen papers were commissioned to provide background for the discussions. They described the current state of primary care, the components of primary care, and provided ideas about how primary care might be reconstructed. Revised versions of four of these papers were published as part of a supplement focusing on the future of primary care in the February 4, 2003, issue of *Annals of Internal Medicine.* We present these papers in their entirety here, as well as ideas and recommendations that emanated from the meeting regarding the future of primary care. It is our hope that this book will stimulate additional thought and discussion about the current conditions and future of primary care.

ACKNOWLEDGMENTS

We thank the Robert Wood Johnson Foundation for its continuing commitment to primary care and for providing support for the development of this book. We also thank Elizabeth Hirose for administrative and editorial support.

December 2003

Jonathan Showstack
San Francisco, California

Arlyss Anderson Rothman
Orinda, California

Susan B. Hassmiller
Princeton, New Jersey

Editors

Dedicated to primary care providers
and their tireless efforts to ensure
the best care possible for their patients

The Authors

Jonathan Showstack, Ph.D., M.P.H., is professor of medicine and health policy in the Division of General Internal Medicine, Department of Medicine, and the Institute for Health Policy Studies, School of Medicine, University of California, San Francisco. He earned a doctorate in sociology from the University of California, San Francisco, and a master's degree in health administration and planning from the University of California, Berkeley. His research focuses on evaluating the relationships among organizational characteristics, costs, clinical outcomes, and patient satisfaction; the impact of policies related to undergraduate and graduate health professions education; strategic planning in health care organizations; and the assessment of medical interventions and technologies.

Arlyss Anderson Rothman, Ph.D., M.H.S., R.N.-C.S., F.N.P., is assistant professor in the School of Nursing, Department of Family Health Care Nursing, at the University of California, San Francisco. She has a doctorate in organizational theory and health services delivery and a master's degree in health services; she is also trained and practices as a family nurse practitioner. Dr. Anderson Rothman has studied nurse practitioner practice in California, the future of medical education in California, interdisciplinary health care teams in ambulatory care, residents' attitudes toward fellowship training, the future of primary care in the United States, and the need for nurse management training programs.

Susan B. Hassmiller, R.N., Ph.D., F.A.A.N., is a senior program officer at the Robert Wood Johnson Foundation (RWJF). Her work focuses on public health, primary care, prevention, and the nursing shortage. Her career has been dedicated to the care of vulnerable populations and prevention. Before joining RWJF in September 1997, she was the executive director of the U.S. Public Health Service Primary Care Policy Fellowship and other national and international primary care initiatives at the

Health Resources and Services Administration. She received the doctorate in nursing administration and health policy from George Mason University in Fairfax, Virginia; master's degrees in health education from Florida State University and community health nursing from the University of Nebraska Medical Center in Omaha; and a bachelor's degree from Florida State University. She is a fellow in the American Academy of Nursing and a member of the National Board of Governors for the American Red Cross.

Helen Burstin, M.D., M.P.H., is the director of the Center for Primary Care, Prevention and Clinical Partnerships at the Agency for Healthcare Research and Quality (AHRQ). Prior to her appointment at AHRQ, she was an assistant professor at Harvard Medical School and director of quality measurement at Brigham and Women's Hospital in Boston. Burstin is a graduate of the State University of New York at Upstate College of Medicine and the Harvard School of Public Health. She performed a residency in primary care internal medicine at Boston City Hospital and a fellowship in general internal medicine at Brigham and Women's Hospital and Harvard Medical School and is board certified in internal medicine. She is a member of the editorial board of the *Journal of General Internal Medicine.* Burstin is president of the American Medical Student Association Foundation and a member of the board of directors of La Clinica del Pueblo, a free Latino clinic in Washington, D.C., where she is a volunteer staff physician.

Christine Cassel, M.D., M.A.C.P., became president and CEO of the American Board of Internal Medicine (ABIM) and ABIM Foundation in Philadelphia in July 2003 after serving as dean of the School of Medicine and vice president for medical affairs at Oregon Health and Science University in Portland, Oregon. She is a leading expert in geriatric medicine, medical ethics, and quality of care. Among many professional associations, Cassel is president of the American Federation for Aging Research; chair of the board of the Greenwall Foundation, which supports work in bioethics; member of the Advisory Committee to the director at the National Institutes of Health; and member of the Governing Council of the Institute of Medicine. Cassel was formerly chair of the Department of Geriatrics and Adult Development and professor of geriatrics and medicine at Mount Sinai School of Medicine in New York City. During ten years at the University of Chicago, Pritzker School of Medicine, she was chief of the Section of General Internal Medicine, professor of geriatrics and medicine, site director of the Robert Wood Johnson Clinical Scholars Program, and director of the Center for Health Policy Research. She received her medical degree from the University of Massachusetts and completed her residency training in internal medicine at Children's Hospital and the University of California, San Francisco, with subsequent fellowships in bioethics and geriatrics at San Francisco and Portland, Oregon. She is nationally prominent as chief editor of a seminal textbook, *Geriatric Medicine,* which recently appeared in its fourth edition.

Tina L. Cheng, M.D., M.P.H., is chief of general pediatrics and adolescent medicine at Johns Hopkins University School of Medicine with a joint appointment in the Bloomberg School of Public Health. She received her B.A. and M.D. from Brown University's Program in Medicine and an M.P.H. in epidemiology from the University of California, Berkeley. She completed residencies in pediatrics and preventive medicine at the University of California, San Francisco, and Berkeley and fellowship training in general academic pediatrics at the University of Massachusetts. Cheng has been active in clinical care, research, advocacy, and teaching of medical students, residents, fellows, and public health students. Her clinical and research interests are in child and adolescent injury and violence prevention, teen pregnancy and parenting, community-based research, and access to care. She is a founder of the Generations Program, a comprehensive program for teen parents and their children, and the DC Secondary Prevention Coalition, a community coalition serving the needs of young families. A previous Robert Wood Johnson Foundation Generalist Faculty Scholar, her current work involves the design and evaluation of community-based interventions addressing violence and pregnancy prevention.

Carolyn Clancy, M.D., is the director of the Agency for Healthcare Research and Quality (AHRQ). Prior to this appointment, Clancy had served as AHRQ's acting director and as director of AHRQ's Centers for Outcomes and Effectiveness Research (1997–2002) and Primary Care Research (1993–1998). A general internist and health services researcher, Clancy is a graduate of Boston College and the University of Massachusetts Medical School. Following clinical training in internal medicine, she was a Henry J. Kaiser Family Foundation fellow at the University of Pennsylvania. Clancy's major research interests include women's health, primary care, access to care, and the impact of financial incentives on physicians' decisions. She has published widely in peer-reviewed journals and has edited or contributed to six books.

Beth Demel, M.P.A., has over ten years of health policy research experience. She is currently a health communications consultant based in New York City. Demel previously held health policy analyst positions with the Brookdale Department of Geriatrics at Mount Sinai School of Medicine and the Medicare Rights Center. She has authored and edited numerous health policy and medical publications. Her research has primarily focused on Medicare, geriatrics, palliative care, and public health education and policy. She has a master's degree from Columbia University School of International and Public Affairs.

Larry A. Green, M.D., is the founding director of the Robert Graham Center: Policy Studies in Family Practice and Primary Care in Washington, D.C. He completed his residency in family medicine at the University of Rochester and Highland Hospital and entered practice in Arkansas in the National Health Services Corps, after which he joined the faculty at the University of Colorado. Green was the Woodward-Chisholm Chairman of the Department of Family Medicine at the University of Colorado for fourteen years. He continues to serve on the faculty of the University of Colorado, where he is professor of family medicine, and as director of the National Program Office for Prescription for Health, sponsored by the Robert Wood Johnson Foundation and the Agency for Healthcare Research and Quality. Much of Green's career has been focused on developing practice-based, primary care research networks. He practices as a certified Diplomate of the American Board of Family Practice. He is a member of the American Academy of Family Physicians, the Society of Teachers of Family Medicine, the World Organization of Family Doctors, and the North America Primary Care Research Group. He received his M.D. from Baylor College of Medicine, Houston, Texas.

Harry R. Kimball, M.D., M.A.C.P., served as president and chief executive officer of the American Board of Internal Medicine (ABIM) and the ABIM Foundation from 1991 to 2003. He was elected to the ABIM board of directors in 1983 and served as chair in 1989–1990. Kimball received his medical degree from Washington University School of Medicine in St. Louis and completed residency training in internal medicine at the University of Washington School of Medicine in Seattle. He served seven years at the National Institute of Allergy and Infectious Diseases and fourteen years in the clinical practice of internal medicine and infectious diseases in rural Washington State. Kimball was professor of medicine at Tufts University and chief of general internal medicine at the New England Medical Center in Boston. He is currently professor of medicine at the University of Pennsylvania, master of the American College of Physicians, fellow of the Royal College of Physicians (London), and distinguished fellow of the European Federation of Internal Medicine and holds an honorary degree of doctor of science by Jefferson Medical College of the Thomas Jefferson University for his contributions to medical education.

Jonathan D. Klein, M.D., M.P.H., is an associate professor of pediatrics and of preventive and community medicine at the University of Rochester School of Medicine. An expert in adolescent medicine and in child and adolescent health services research, his research focuses on adolescents and access to care and on quality improvement of primary care services for children and youth. He has received degrees from Brandeis University, New Jersey Medical School, and the Harvard School of Public Health, and he trained in pediatrics at Boston Floating Hospital/New England Medical Center and in the Robert Wood Johnson Clinical Scholars Program at the University of North Carolina at Chapel Hill. Klein chairs the American Academy of Pediatrics Committee on Adolescence and is a member of the U.S. Preventive Services Task Force. From 1999 to 2002, he was founding chair of the American Academy of Pediatrics Center for Child Health Research Tobacco Consortium.

Eric B. Larson, M.D., M.P.H., is director of the Center for Health Studies, Group Health Cooperative. A graduate of Harvard Medical School, he trained in internal medicine at Beth Israel Hospital in Boston, completed a Robert Wood Johnson Clinical Scholar fellowship and a master's degree at the University of Washington, and then served as chief resident of University Hospital in Seattle. From 1989 to 2002, Larson was the medical director of University of Washington Medical Center and associate dean for clinical affairs. His research spans a range of general medicine topics and has focused on aging and dementia topics, including a long-running study of aging and cognitive change. He has served as president of the Society of General Internal Medicine, chair of the Office of Technology Assessment/Department of Health and Human Services Advisory Panel on Alzheimer's Disease and Related Disorders, and is currently chair elect of the board of regents, American College of Physicians.

Bernard Lo, M.D., is professor of medicine and director of the Program in Medical Ethics at the University of California, San Francisco. He directs the Greenwall Faculty Scholars Program in Bioethics and formerly was the director of the Robert Wood Johnson Foundation initiative on Strengthening the Doctor-Patient Relationship in a Changing Health Care Environment. Lo's work focuses on ethical issues in human subjects research and ethical issues in end-of-life care. He chaired the End of Life Committee of the American College of Physicians–American Society of Internal Medicine, which developed consensus recommendations for clinical care near the end of life. Lo has written extensively on decisions about life-sustaining interventions, decision making for incompetent patients, physician-assisted suicide, ethical issues regarding human immunodeficiency virus infection, stem cell research, and human cloning. He is the author of *Resolving Ethical Dilemmas: A Guide for Clinicians.* He is also a practicing general internist who teaches clinical medicine to residents and medical students.

Nicole Lurie, M.D., M.S.P.H., is a senior natural scientist and the Paul O' Neill Alcoa Professor of Health Policy at the RAND Corporation. Prior to that, she was professor of medicine and public health at the University of Minnesota and medical adviser to the commissioner at the Minnesota Department of Health. From 1998 to 2001, she was principal deputy assistant secretary of health in the U.S. Department of Health and Human Services. Lurie attended college and medical school at the University of Pennsylvania and completed her residency and M.S.P.H. at the University of California, Los Angeles, where she was also a Robert Wood Johnson Foundation Clinical Scholar. Her academic work focuses on health services research and health policy, primarily in the areas of access to and quality of care, managed care, mental health, prevention, and health disparities. She serves as senior editor for *Health Services Research.* She was president of the Society of General Internal Medicine and is on the board of directors for the Academy of Health Services Research. She is the recipient of numerous awards, including the AHSR Young Investigator Award, the Nellie Westerman Prize for Research in Ethics, and the Heroine in Health Care Award, and she is a member of the Institute of Medicine.

Gordon T. Moore, M.D., M.P.H., is a professor in the Department of Ambulatory Care and Prevention at Harvard Medical School. His academic work has been in health care policy, health system design, clinical process improvement, and designing and evaluating educational programs for medical students, residents, and other health professionals. Moore now directs Partnerships for Quality Education, a national initiative funded by the Robert Wood Johnson Foundation to train doctors in the skills of managing care. In his nonacademic work, Moore has been an administrator and leader in managed care, a strategic consultant to health insurers in the United States and Europe, and a teacher and consultant to doctors in hospitals, medical schools, and integrated delivery systems settings.

Mary O'Neil Mundinger, R.N., Dr.P.H., is the Centennial Professor in Health Policy and dean of the Columbia University School of Nursing. She is a member of the Institute of Medicine of the National Academy of Sciences, the American Academy of Nursing, and the New York Academy of Medicine. Mundinger is the founder of Columbia Advanced Practice Nurse Associates, the first nursing school faculty practice where nurse practitioners hold commercial managed care contracts and are compensated at the same rate as primary care physicians. In 1998, she was named Nurse Practitioner of the Year by *The Nurse Practitioner: The American Journal of Primary Health Care.* Mundinger holds a B.S. cum laude from the University of Michigan and a doctorate in public health from Columbia University School of Public Health. In 1996, she was awarded a doctor of human letters (honorary) from Hamilton College. She is a noted health policy expert, primarily known for her work on workforce issues and primary care. Author of *Home Care Controversy: Too Little, Too Late, Too Costly* (1983) and *Autonomy in Nursing* (1980), she has led Columbia's nursing school since 1986.

Harold A. Pincus, M.D., professor and executive vice chairman of the University of Pittsburgh School of Medicine's Department of Psychiatry, is also senior scientist and director of the RAND Health Institute in Pittsburgh and director of the Robert Wood Johnson Foundation's National Program on Depression in Primary Care: Linking Clinical and Systems Strategies. Previously, he was the American Psychiatric Association's (APA) deputy medical director and founding director of the APA's Office of Research; special assistant to the director of the National Institute of Mental Health; and an RWJF Clinical Scholar. Pincus was vice chair of the task force on the fourth edition of the *Diagnostic and Statistical Manual of Mental Disorders*, has been appointed to editorial boards of nine major scientific journals, and served as consultant to a variety of federal agencies and private organizations, including the U.S. Secret Service, the World Health Organization, and the Institute of Medicine.

Pincus has edited or coauthored 15 books and over 250 scientific publications in health and science policy, research career development, and the diagnosis and treatment of mental disorders. His current research interests focus on relationships among mental health, substance abuse, and general medical care, developing and empirically testing models of those relationships to improve patient outcomes. He received the William C. Menninger Memorial Award of the American College of Physicians, the Health Services Research Senior Scholar Award of the APA, and Columbia University's Emily Mumford Medal.

Dana Gelb Safran, Sc.D., is director of the Health Institute at Tufts–New England Medical Center and associate professor in the Department of Medicine, Tufts University School of Medicine. Her empirical research has emphasized the measurement of primary care quality, with a focus on patients' experiences of care and outcomes. She received her master's and doctoral degrees in health policy from the Harvard School of Public Health. Safran has led numerous state and national studies that have examined differences in primary care performance under the leading models of health insurance in the United States and that identify the influence of doctor-patient relationship quality on outcomes. The measurement approach that she pioneered is currently being applied in numerous demonstration projects nationwide that are testing the feasibility and value of adding measures of doctor-patient relationship quality to the nation's portfolio of health care quality measures. Since 1998, Safran's national studies of Medicare beneficiaries' access to care, quality, and health outcomes have contributed to policy discussions concerning the performance of Medicare health maintenance organizations and the debate about prescription drug coverage.

Lewis Sandy, M.D., M.B.A., is executive vice president of United Healthcare in Edina, Minnesota. From 1997 to 2003, he was executive vice president at the Robert Wood Johnson Foundation (RWJF) overseeing grantmaking programs, strategic planning, and foundation operations. Under his leadership, RWJF developed grant programs to help low-income children obtain health insurance coverage, train physicians in palliative care, and support obstetricians and managed care organizations in implementing approaches to smoking cessation. A practicing internist, he received his B.S. and M.D. degrees from the University of Michigan and performed a residency in internal medicine at the Beth Israel Hospital in Boston, Massachusetts. He earned an M.B.A. from Stanford University, where he was an Arjay Miller Scholar and a Henry J. Kaiser Family Foundation Health Management Fellow and was a Robert Wood Johnson Clinical Scholar at the University of California, San Francisco. Prior to joining RWJF in 1991, he was a health center medical director at Harvard Community Health Plan in Boston. Sandy is a fellow of the American College of Physicians and serves on a number of advisory committees, including the Clinical Research Roundtable of the Institute of Medicine, the University of Michigan's Center on Medical History, the Tufts Managed Care Institute, and the Health Sector Assembly.

Steven Schroeder, M.D., is Distinguished Professor of Health and Health Care, Division of General Internal Medicine, Department of Medicine, University of California, San Francisco (UCSF), where he also heads the Smoking Cessation Leadership Center. Between 1990 and 2002, he was president and CEO of the Robert Wood Johnson Foundation. He graduated from Harvard Medical School and trained in internal medicine at the Harvard Medical Service of Boston City Hospital and in epidemiology as an epidemiology intelligence service officer at the Centers for Disease Control. In 1980, he founded the Division of General Internal Medicine at UCSF. Schroeder has published extensively in the fields of clinical medicine, health care financing and organization, prevention, public health, and the health care workforce. He serves on the Council of the Institute of Medicine and has six honorary doctoral degrees and numerous awards.

Barbara Starfield, M.D., M.P.H., is University Distinguished Professor with appointments in the Departments of Health Policy and Management and Pediatrics at the Johns Hopkins University Schools of Public Health and Medicine. Starfield received her B.A. degree from Swarthmore College, her M.D. degree from the State University of New York (Health Sciences Center in Brooklyn), and her M.P.H. degree from the Johns Hopkins University. She is a fellow of the American Academy of Pediatrics and a member of the Institute of Medicine.

Starfield is the director of the Johns Hopkins University Primary Care Policy Center. Her work focuses on understanding the impact of health services on health, especially with regard to the relative contributions of primary care and specialty care on reducing inequities in health, and on the relationship between clinical care and services to populations. Of particular note are her contributions in the areas of primary care, quality of care, health status assessment (particularly for children), and case-mix assessment and adjustment. She is the recipient of numerous national awards, including the first Pew Primary Care Research Award (1994), the Distinguished Investigator Award of the Association for Health Services Research (1995), and the American Public Health Association's Martha May Eliot Award (1995). She was the cofounder and first president of the International Society for Equity in Health, a scientific society devoted to contributing knowledge to assist in the furtherance of equity in the distribution of health.

Edward H. Wagner, M.D., M.P.H., F.A.C.P., is a general internist and epidemiologist and director of the W. A. MacColl Institute for Healthcare Innovation at the Center for Health Studies (CHS), Group Health Cooperative of Puget Sound. He served as director of the CHS at Group Health Cooperative from 1983 to 1998. The MacColl Institute for Healthcare Innovation is concerned with developing and evaluating health care innovations to serve the needs of the chronically ill. Wagner is principal investigator of the Cancer Research Network, a National Cancer Institute–funded consortium of eleven health maintenance organizations that are conducting collaborative cancer effectiveness research. He is professor of health services at the University of Washington School of Public Health and Community Medicine and serves on the editorial boards of *Health Services Research,* the *Journal of Clinical Epidemiology,* and *BMJ-USA*. Wagner is director of Improving Chronic Illness Care, a national program of the Robert Wood Johnson Foundation.

Michael Weitzman, M.D., is executive director of the American Academy of Pediatrics' Center for Child Health Research and professor and associate chairman of pediatrics at the University of Rochester School of Medicine and Dentistry; he was formerly director of the Division of General Pediatrics and pediatrician-in-chief at Rochester General Hospital. He has served as director of maternal and child health for the City of Boston and director of general pediatrics and the fellowship training program in academic general pediatrics at Boston City Hospital and Boston University School of Medicine. Weitzman has conducted research and written extensively on such diverse issues as childhood lead poisoning, chronic illness, exposure to cigarette smoke, breast feeding, excessive school absences, the academic benefits of the School Breakfast Program, and the epidemiology of children's mental health problems, health risk behaviors, school failure, and asthma. He was the 1997 recipient of the Ambulatory Pediatrics Association's Research Award for the Fellowship Training Program in Academic General Pediatrics, which he has directed for the past ten years.

PART ONE

Primary Care at a Crossroads

The chapters in this part address current dilemmas and threats to primary care from both the clinician's and the patient's perspectives. In Chapter One, Gordon Moore describes the basic dilemmas facing primary care today and discusses the effect of market forces on this level of the system. Although the clinician may be feeling many of these pressures, Moore describes other forces within the system that threaten the well-being of primary care. Dana Gelb Safran examines in Chapter Two the patient's view of and experience with primary care, with some surprising results and thought-provoking ideas. In Chapter Three, Bernard Lo focuses on the effect of the self-care and alternative care movements and the importance of improved information technologies in providing high-quality care.

CHAPTER ONE

Primary Care in Crisis

Current Pressures and Threats to Primary Care as We Know It

Gordon T. Moore

Primary care, or general practice as it was known then, was the dominant mode of delivery of medical care in the first half of the twentieth century. The romantic ideal of the doctor was the local general practitioner (GP), available twenty-four hours a day, healing the sick, aiding the needy, scion of his (usually, since there were few women in the field) community, avuncular, and friend of his patients in good and bad times.

This image faded in the second half of the century, largely displaced as a result of the stunning clinical successes of scientific medicine and specialization. The idealized doctor became the white-jacketed expert, explaining the latest medical advance on the network news and performing medical miracles. Primary care became the poor cousin, still part of the family but rather looked down on by scientists and specialists, as well as the public at large.

To be sure, the organizations that sponsored general practice in a response to its weakening position in the 1970s—the Royal College of General Practice in England and the newly minted American specialty of family medicine—endeavored to redesign general practice, emphasizing longer and more rigorous preparation, continuing education, and periodic assessment of competency. With this emphasis, generalists had some success in positioning themselves as the primary provider, offering continuity and breadth of service and serving as the point of entry into the medical care system. In Europe, this model of primary care first and specialist care only on referral became enshrined in public systems; in the United States, our pluralistic system did not carve out a politically determined role for generalists, and the market still determines who provides the care and how much is paid for the services.

In the United States, by and large, specialists took the upper hand in this market in the last half of the twentieth century. The primary care fields have suffered, usually receiving lower reimbursement and income than their subspecialty colleagues and garnering less prestige and influence in academic centers and elsewhere. The call in the 1970s for more primary care and the replacement of general practice by the more rigorous and revitalized field of family medicine raised hopes that generalism would regain ascendancy. But technical specialism continued its domination of market share of medical graduates.

This progressive loss of influence seemed to have halted in the 1990s when managed care rediscovered primary care. The argument emerged that primary care would be the health care system's gatekeeper for quality and costs, assessing the need for referral and caring for much of what otherwise would be sent to specialists, who would cost more yet offer no better outcomes. Although this model was attractive to managed care and to many in primary care, it fell afoul of the medical, media, and ultimately public and political backlash against managed care. Linking primary care to managed care led to a significant setback for the field. Many experts lamented that "primary care's time has finally come and gone."

Many feel that such setbacks are temporary, while others see dark storm clouds gathering over the prospects of primary care for the future. This chapter, which explores the emerging threats to primary care and its strength, has two aims. The first is to convince those who remain optimistic about future prospects for the primary care model as it currently exists that there are indeed serious, even potentially fatal, threats if primary care does not change. The second is to help those who already perceive primary care to be threatened and deeply troubled to move quickly through the Kübler-Ross sequence of initial reaction to loss—denial, anger, and depression—to the stages of acceptance and renewal. For this group, I hope this chapter will identify core assets of primary care generalism that will make it possible for the field to think strategically and emerge strongly positioned for the future. It is out of such a review that adaptation and change, a need that is a constant in today's environment, will come.

IS OUR MODEL OF PRIMARY CARE TRULY UNDER THREAT?

Multiple factors bear on the relative success or failure of primary care in the future. To start, perhaps we need to define the terms of success, the dependent variable that we should be following to determine if the forces buffeting primary care are leading to adverse effects. For this chapter, I define success in primary care in both health and economic terms. Success for primary care would be a growing influence of primary care on improving the health of Americans—an influence that is recognized by a growing share of resources and a growing number of practitioners choosing this area. If successful, primary care would be valued by the public, manifested by rising income and increasing esteem for practitioners, a growing number of jobs, and an enlarging pool seeking primary care training in order to be eligible for such desirable work.

The sum of, and interactions between, serious threats to primary care leave me doubtful about the ability of the field to survive in its current form. The factors that I review are eroding rather than enhancing the future success of primary care. They constitute threats from both outside and within the four professional fields that provide primary care: family medicine, primary care internal medicine and pediatrics, and advanced practice nursing.

Oversupply

Primary care is most immediately vulnerable to a glut of practitioners. For years, medical education, including primary care, has been unable to rationalize its supply. Medical student numbers continue to outpace national population growth. The addition of foreign medical graduates to the residency pool further swells the numbers of graduating doctors seeking work. Lately, advanced practice nursing has been the most rapidly growing of the primary care specialties. Nurses and physician assistants continue to enlarge the primary care pool.

An increased supply might not be a problem if there were the money to support all those who wish to work. However, as we shall see, the growth of clinicians in primary care is probably outstripping the resources available for the kinds of services provided today by primary care.

Competition

With growing numbers of primary care providers competing for limited resources, competition is inevitable. Claims of superiority of each field are rife. This debate creates an environment in which the public can only be confused and where the claims and counterclaims serve to convince politicians and the public that they would be foolish to promote primary care if the providers themselves cannot agree on what it is and who should do it. Primary care doctors compete with each other's specialties and nurses with all of them.

The oversupply of manpower is substantially distorting the medical care hierarchy. The vast and growing ranks of specialists swell the number of doctors who can argue that they can provide primary care. The high at the top of this hierarchy—medical subspecialists—are able to move down into primary care services. In urban areas, they do so by taking over primary and principal care of patients, displacing primary care clinicians. In rural communities, specialists migrating from oversupplied cities compete in their specialized areas with generalists who formerly performed such services. In time, many of the specialists, especially in medicine and obstetrics and gynecology, will draw primary care patients as well. Finally, the growth of hospitalists—generalists working full time to manage the care of hospitalized patients—represents a serious threat to primary care doctors, much of whose income formerly was generated by the hospital care that they delivered.

Substitution

Another threat to primary care is that nonmedical alternatives could substitute for primary care. Three examples of these are the Internet, alternative medicine, and pharmacists and drug companies.

The Internet is a rapidly growing source of medical information that could substitute for primary care. While varying in quality, the Internet is an awesomely rich source of self-help. For many patients, the Internet is the first resource they consult when they are ill. It can only expand and improve as technology becomes more interactive and more capable of sophisticated decision support. Available anywhere, at any time, and for little, if any, money, the Internet has the capability to deeply erode the business of primary caretakers.

Other health care fields are also competing for primary care. Alternative medicine is growing rapidly and surely must siphon off resources that could otherwise support primary care.

Another substitution is pharmacists, pharmacies, and drug companies. Drugstores are increasingly integrating vertically into doctors' territory, and the closest opportunity for them is primary care. Traditionally, pharmacists have always been a source of medical advice. However, technology is making it more and more possible for them to disintermediate primary care. Pregnancy testing, HIV test kits, and quick throat cultures are examples of technology that makes it easy for a pharmacy to take over functions previously delivered by clinicians. This threat plays out further as drugs are removed from prescription status and become available over the counter. The pharmacist, perhaps backed up with decision support tools, becomes a lay primary care provider. Drug companies, anxious to push their products, are likely to target pharmacists as a group that is more amenable to influence than are doctors or nurses. Already, some of the larger drugstore chains, responding to a growing number of customers lacking health insurance and needing low-cost alternatives to doctor care, are offering clinical services backed up by nurses or by doctors available by telephone.

Consumer Trends

Playing into and reinforcing these trends is rising consumerism. The American consumer is better educated about health, has more accessibility to health information, and is more determined to have control over personal health care than ever before. Moreover, the public loves technology and subscribes to the notion that modern medicine can cure almost anything. These trends are growing, and their influence will be augmented by the aging of the baby boomers into the older years of high medical use. These consumers are sophisticated, informed, and assertive. They want to be in control. They will get what they want or go elsewhere. By and large, this group is quite capable of challenging the competence and sophistication of their care, of demanding and getting what they want, of finding information and care over the Internet, or of choosing a specialist over a generalist provider of care. In this model, the consumer will constitute a growing challenge to the taken-for-granted position of primary care in the health care system.

Population Models of Care

The often poor performance of traditional medical care in conditions such as diabetes or asthma has led to the growth of population approaches that often remove the patient from the care of an individual primary care provider. Examples of such approaches, called chronic illness management, include systematic programs to manage diabetes, asthma, congestive heart failure, and depression. In each category, patients with these conditions are identified, and systems are developed to improve their care. Many, if not most, chronic illness programs enroll these patients in an alternative, specialized system that is built to provide condition-specific care. Patients are often then lost to their primary care providers, although lip-service is paid to maintaining primary care continuity.

Even when the patient remains with the primary provider, chronic disease management can reduce the demand for primary care services. If patients improve, they may need less primary care. The use of guidelines, reminders, and patient self-education reduces dependence on clinicians and transfers the care to the patients themselves.

Such systems are a response to a failure of the primary care provider to achieve consistently excellent care and results. Some of these systems are designed to help the primary provider improve care. But if care does not reach agreed-on standards, both patients and insurers are likely to turn increasingly to such parallel, and ultimately competitive, methods of care for bread-and-butter chronic conditions that constitute much of the work of primary care.

Insurance Trends

Recent trends in insurance are threatening the future success of primary care. Aging of the population, growth of new technologies, and burgeoning use of expensive drugs are pushing medical care costs rapidly upward. These trends are converging in a way that will reduce the insurance funding available to pay for primary care services.

Changes in payment for primary care are a result of purchasers' and insurers' adaptations to rapid escalation in the costs of medical care. Employers and governments are resisting paying for these increases. In the face of rising costs and higher premiums, companies have responded by capping their expense and passing the increases on to those who are insured. They are doing so by contributing a fixed amount, and decreasing proportion, of rising premiums. Faced with an expanding bite from their wages, employees are increasingly "going bare." Those who choose to go without insurance because they are not willing to pay their share of the premium are usually young and at low risk of needing to use the insurance. Those who choose to pay and remain in the insurance pool are a more at-risk pool. This so-called adverse selection leads to a self-reinforcing problem: costs escalate, low-risk people leave the pool, and premiums thus escalate even more rapidly, creating an insurance death spiral.

In response to this problem, insurers try many ways to keep costs down and retain low-risk insured patients in the pool. The approaches include high deductibles, substantial increases in copayments, and benefit limitations. The last are usually restrictions in less costly items and primary care; the insurers reason that those who are insured are better able to pay for these out of pocket than for high-cost or even catastrophic hospital or specialty care. Thus, potential users are faced with either no coverage or the need to pay a high proportion of an office visit. Both situations have been shown to reduce care-seeking behavior of patients.

In this spreading model, patients will eventually be paying for much or all of the costs of most primary care. We will regress toward the health insurance system present in the 1960s when comprehensive insurance first emerged in response to policies that covered only hospital and emergency care. Many will seek less expensive alternatives or forgo care altogether. Some, if their insurance covers it, will immediately seek specialist or emergency room care. Primary care may become largely a retail, self-pay operation rather than insured, and the amount of money thus available to support it will compete with other uses of disposable income and inevitably decrease.

Threats from Within Medicine

Primary care recruitment is waning, after rising for several years. Although this may be an appropriate market response to a field that is oversupplied with practitioners, the consequences of such a change may be inimical to the future of primary care. The threat is that those attracted to primary care may be less competent. Ultimately, the less the public believes that primary care can deliver excellence, the more likely they are to go elsewhere.

This threat has long been incipient. There is an intellectual snobbery about primary care that is active at the level of medical school and residency. The view is that primary care is not at the cutting edge, not intellectually rigorous, and not scientifically challenging. If lower status, then primary care will attract less competent practitioners who will be paid less. At the same time, primary care is difficult, and burnout is prevalent already. Working alone in complicated and ambiguous clinical situations is stressful, lonely, anxiety provoking, and exposed to litigation. The danger from these circumstances is that primary care may come to be seen as the bush leagues of medical care, a condition that will make it increasingly difficult for the field to change what it does to a higher value-added positioning in the medical care system of the future.

Aging of the Primary Care Product

Weaving through the specific threats already described runs an even more serious leitmotif: that primary care is an aging product that is no longer providing what patients want and need. I examine this in more detail in the next section, but the progressive erosion of primary care in the medical marketplace is a worrying sign that our publics may want something different from what we have been providing. Products have life cycles. Companies, for example, are quick to initiate efforts to understand why one of their commercial products is beginning to lose ground. Is it an aging product in its final phases, are there competitors providing something better, is the market saturated, has the product priced itself out of its market, or has quality declined? As noted above, some of the changes experienced by purchasers, insurers, and the public have shifted the ground under primary care. I believe there are strong signals that we are no longer fully meeting the needs or demands of those whose business we must have.

THE NIGHTMARE SCENARIO

These factors in some combination can reinforce each other to create a death spiral for primary care. A widening gap between what we provide and the public wants, decreasing resources, eroding incomes for doctors and nurses, weakening recruitment of top-notch clinicians, diminishing work opportunity, and falling prestige will surely lead to a troubled sector. Such circumstances will lead to increased interprofessional sniping and further erosion of the public's confidence in primary care.

If these circumstances occur, fewer qualified applicants will choose to enter primary care, leading to even greater numbers of specialists and further erosion of primary care from that sector. A demoralized field will attract fewer humanistically oriented students to apply to medicine. Primary care wars could result from competition among its constituent professionals. At some point, these problems become self-reinforcing and irreversible.

ACCEPTANCE AND RENEWAL: FROM PROBLEM TO OPPORTUNITY

What process might counter this trend? In response to a changing marketplace, political uncertainty, and shifting consumer expectations, primary care will need to reinvent itself. Other industries have done so successfully. What is needed is strategic planning to develop primary care as a new product in the medical marketplace.

Fortunately, after the initial shocks attendant on loss, acceptance and renewal eventually begin. In this section, I set the stage for this renewal process.

What Do Our Publics Want?

Government and corporate funders of health care want more cost-effectiveness of the health care system but not at the expense of consumer anger and disillusionment directed toward them. These objectives have not changed over several decades, but are likely to become more intense in the future. In the face of rising costs, it is clear that their strategy is to pass these on to the consumer rather than raising the financial contribution of either government or businesses to health insurance. In this process, they want a system that they can trust to do things right, to do the right things, and to be accountable and ethical.

Consumers, or patients, are facing wrenching changes in perspective and reality about health care in the future. For decades, they have wanted insurance that provides comprehensive, high-quality care and includes freedom of choice of doctors and hospitals. They want the latest technology that they hear about in the media. Consumers also want, and expect, good service that is timely and convenient. They have come to view these elements as their basic right. Moreover, most Americans feel they are owed this and that their insurance costs are a benefit paid for by others rather than themselves. Politicians, burned by efforts in the past to address health concerns, are wary of disabusing the public of these views.

The future holds some painful realities for American health care consumers, although there is also good news. New scientific advances are making medical care better, for example. The bad news is that these advances, combined with the aging of the population, will drive up costs at double-digit levels. The payers are responding by passing these increases on to patients, who increasingly will find their coverage eroded. Most will discover that their insurance is coming to resemble catastrophic hospital and emergency insurance coverage, the predominant form in the 1960s. More of the office care and prevention and, ultimately, some of the elegant diagnostic and treatment improvements will be paid directly by the consumer.

I believe that the loss of health insurance as the middle classes have come to know it will create a bloody battle in one of our next several elections. Realistically, however, the options of governments, businesses, or the large insurers to respond are limited. The only degrees of freedom will come by helping, or forcing, the public to face some of the fundamental realities of health care: that more high-tech care is less cost-effective than preventive medicine and public health efforts to achieve healthy behaviors; that the right to sue more often generates extra costs borne by the system than improved quality, adequate retribution money, or personal satisfaction; that free choice of providers and hospitals can be available only to those willing to pay the extra cost of such a system; and that high-cost miracle care cannot be extended to everyone at a cost that the public can support.

The consequence of this discussion cannot be known. However, we can be sure that what emerges will be health insurance and care systems quite different from today's.

We also can make a good bet that there will some important changes for the better. Consumers will want to take matters into their own hands, especially once they realize that it is their money that is paying for their medical care. Consumer knowledge and influence and assertiveness will grow. The Internet will play a greater role in providing information and even care. As more care is paid for by users, they will need advice they trust about how, when, and even whether they should pay for a recommended test, treatment, or procedure. And health systems that accept insurance risks will recognize the importance of measuring outcomes, reengineering their clinical care processes, and delivering results that meet or exceed prospectively understood and agreed levels of cost, quality, service, and coverage.

What Does Primary Care Bring to the Table in Such Circumstances?

Despite its sometimes confusing richness and complexity, primary care comprises a definable set of core capacities, best revealed by deconstructing primary care as it is carried out by its adherents. Such an effort reinforces the view that primary care's strengths come from its placement close to the patient, its generalism, and the dominant disciplinary strengths of its constituent specialties.

Primary care is, by definition, close to the patient in place and over time. This creates the capacity of primary care to see the patient's problems in the rich context of family, community, and work and against the backdrop of life events and developmental stages. Primary care has unique capacity to know the patient and the illness, not merely the disease. Furthermore, the continuous and prolonged rather than episodic and brief relationship between primary care and patients generates mutual understanding and trust. Of all the attributes of primary care valued by patients, continuity ranks the highest.

Second, primary care clinicians are broad in their medical and health perspectives. They are trained as generalists, specializing, as family medicine says so well, "in all of you." Generalist training prepares a clinician to sort out ill-formed problems. In other words, no other health providers should be able to improve on the ability of primary care to sort through problems and symptoms, manage ambiguous circumstances, and adapt and shape care to the needs at hand. This creates the unique capacity to triage diverse problems and manage the care appropriately.

Primary care also draws on the core strengths of each of its four constituent disciplinary fields: family medicine, pediatrics, internal medicine, and nursing. From family medicine comes two core attributes: breadth and adaptability. Family medicine graduates have a breadth of knowledge and skills in clinical medicine. The training creates adaptability—the capacity of flexibility and inventiveness in providing whatever is needed, creating the capability to be the most cost-effective single care provider and to manage and coordinate care in the most effective fashion. From pediatrics, primary care draws disciplinary strength in human development, prevention, and health behavior modification. Nursing contributes its patient-centered, community, social, and cultural orientation. Internal medicine contributes rigorous clinical decision making based on pathophysiology and its strength in critical thinking, research-based evidence, and the decision sciences. Of course, none of these fields has an exclusive on these attributes, but each has its relative strengths that can be drawn on to create a diverse mix of competencies out of which to fashion the new primary care.

Finally, primary care is the health professionals' equivalent of the stem cell—a clinician capable of developing into multiple areas of competency based on the need. This characteristic is uniquely suited to the uncertainty of today's environment. Whatever the future might bring in health care delivery, primary care clinicians will be the quickest to respond and adapt and to provide the clinical skills needed to make the new system work well.

By fitting the most likely characteristics of the new health system with the core strengths of primary care, one can speculate about models that serve our publics well and in which the new primary care might make unique contributions. I believe that in the new era, the public will need an efficient, cost-effective system that can deliver the most health for whatever resource is available and to do it in a way that serves patients respectfully and attentively. In my view, this system will need to be effective in several basic areas: to do its work in the most efficient way possible; to continuously evaluate and redesign itself; to coordinate, integrate, and manage the clinical processes of care; to be patient centered and sensitive to patients' needs; and to be parsimonious, that is, doing only those things that can be justified and defended on rational and, where possible, evidence-based grounds. Patients will be paying for much care out of pocket, so they will need a sophisticated and trusted adviser who can help them make the best decisions. And they will need a system that continuously educates and prepares them to care for themselves.

In such a system, primary care could play a major role. Primary care clinicians could provide immediate and convenient access to care, sort out the problems, deliver much of the care, refer accurately, and coordinate and integrate subspecialty care. Primary care could provide trust-enhancing continuity. Primary care clinicians could partner with patients as an expert coach in shared decision making. And they could manage resources so that all available funding is used optimally to achieve the health outcomes targeted for the patients under their care. To do so, primary care will expand beyond its more restricted role as a provider of medical care to become engaged with the analysis of population needs and the provision of public health types of interventions for risk groups, communities, and other populations.

Primary care will probably not be a unified field in the future. Consumers will have more options and will have to make more choices. In our typical American way, the new system will probably be pluralistic and market based, until the public makes its choices and sorts out the models on offer. Since one of its strengths is its adaptability, primary care will be plugging gaps in many different settings doing many different things. But these activities should be built around a core concept of functioning that blends some of the elements mentioned above. In Table 1.1, I have provided a dozen examples of ways in which primary care might move in the future, contrasting the new activity with the way that we think about the provision today.

AN AWAKENING?

There is no easy prescription for what primary care should become. Nevertheless, we must agree to begin a strategic process that starts us moving in the right direction.

Today	Tomorrow
Order services; others pay	Responsible for managing the budget
Personal medical care only	Include personal and population prevention and health promotion
The professional controls	Patient controls; clinician is trusted adviser
Defined roles and autonomy	Team player
Deliver primary care and refer to specialist	Coordinate all care
Work in office and hospital	Where the problem is handled best
Produce patient visits	Produce health outcomes
Expert-based practice	Knowledge-based practice
Do everything possible	Do only what evidence suggests will help the patient
Organize systems around doctor's time	Accommodate systems to patient's time
React to external profiling	Generate the data and constantly improve
Paid for process	Paid for results

Table 1.1. Ways That Primary Care Can Add Value in the Future.

What we know is that things will need to change. We know that the process must fearlessly identify primary care's strengths and real weaknesses. We must lay our internal competitive issues on the table where they can be discussed, and stop covering them over where they remain disabling but undiscussable.

Primary care will need to add real value in the new health care system. Such change will not come by doing things the way we have in the past. Rather, it will occur when primary care identifies how it can add unique value in the value chain of medicine. This will require an unemotional strategic analysis of strengths, weaknesses, opportunities, and threats. We must be prepared to deconstruct the historic functions of primary care, looking for clues about where the new generalist can add value.

This process will not be easy. Old enmities must be set aside. Hidden assumptions will need to be revealed. Hard-nosed realism must replace romantic idealism, while we seek to hold on to the idealistic elements of primary care. Political correctness must give way to open discussions of what might work and what will not. If this process, painful as it might be, is not undertaken, the future of primary care as we know it is deeply under threat.

CHAPTER TWO

Primary Care Performance

Views from the Patient

Dana Gelb Safran

From the earliest definitions of the term *primary care* to the most recent, all have stressed that primary care is predicated on a sustained relationship between patients and the clinicians who care for them (Institute of Medicine, 1978; Donaldson, Yordy, Lohr, and Vanselow, 1996; Millis, 1996; Alpert and Charney, 1973; Starfield, 1992). Most definitions have not delineated particular clinical disciplines to which primary care belongs (or those to which it does not) and have indicated that the primary care provider can be a single clinician or a team. In other words, formal definitions of primary care over the past three decades have defined it based on characteristics of the care itself, and not the characteristics of the care providers, their settings, or their practice configuration.

Beyond the requirement for sustained clinician-patient relationships, primary care has been defined as encompassing the following essential elements: accessibility, continuity, integration, a whole-person orientation, comprehensiveness, and clinical management (Institute of Medicine, 1978; Donaldson, Yordy, Lohr, and Vanselow, 1996; Millis, 1996; Alpert and Charney, 1973; Starfield, 1992). Drawing inferences from information obtained from adults nationwide, this chapter examines the current status of primary care relationships in the United States, identifies key strengths and limitations as experienced and reported by patients, and proposes possible directions for improving primary care performance and outcomes.

THE STATUS OF PRIMARY CARE RELATIONSHIPS: WHAT PATIENTS TELL US

Having a Primary Physician

There are no administrative data systems that track the percentage of Americans with a primary care provider. However, numerous national surveys give insight into this issue. Most recently, the 1996 Medical Expenditure Panel Survey (MEPS), administered to a national probability sample of U.S. households, reported that 77 percent of Americans in all age groups have a "usual primary care provider" (Weinick and Drilea, 1998). MEPS defines this as having a particular health professional or site to whom the individual goes under each of four circumstances: when sick or needing health-related advice, with a new health problem, to obtain preventive care such as general checkups and immunizations, and to obtain a referral to other health professionals. These criteria, particularly the fourth one, may lead MEPS to underestimate the percentage of Americans with a regular source of primary care. Approximately half of Americans with employer-sponsored insurance and 56 percent of publicly insured Americans have insurance arrangements that do not require referrals for specialty care or other health services (Health Care Financing Administration, 2001a, 2001b, 2001c; American Association of Health Plans, 1999).

Nonetheless, the 1996 MEPS estimates are fairly consistent with those observed in the 1987 National Medical Expenditure Survey (predecessor to MEPS), where 82 percent of Americans reported having a "usual source of care" (Agency for Health Care Policy and Research, 1998). Similarly, 80 percent of adults completing the 1994 General Social Survey (GSS), administered to a national probability sample of U.S. households, reported having a particular physician whom they considered to be their "regular personal doctor." And in 1975, when the concept of primary care was first being formalized in the United States, 88 percent of U.S. adults reported having a "regular source" of care, with 78 percent naming a particular physician and 10 percent considering an institution or several doctors to be their regular source of care (Aiken and others, 1979).

Thus, it appears that over the past two decades, despite marked changes in the U.S. health care delivery systems and, in particular, the emergence of managed care arrangements that emphasize the role of the primary care physician, there has been little change (possibly a slight decline) in the percentage of Americans who report having a regular source of care. Moreover, the vast majority of Americans appear to consider their regular source of care to be a particular named physician, not a site or group. This has extremely important implications, which we will come back to in depth, for the future of primary care.

With regard to the clinical background and specialty of primary care providers, research to date suggests that the majority of Americans rely on generalist physicians for their primary care, but that a substantial minority rely on specialists. There are no national estimates indicating the percentage of Americans who consider their primary provider to be a nurse practitioner or other nonphysician. In 1979, Aiken and others reported that among adults who identified a primary physician, 20 percent named a specialist and 80 percent named a generalist physician. This finding stimulated discussion and debate, which has grown heated in recent years, as to whether specialists represent a hidden network of primary care providers in the United States. In 1996, our study of primary care in Massachusetts found that 87 percent of patients identifying a "regular personal doctor" named a generalist physician, while 13 percent named a specialist (Safran and others, 1998a). Rosenblatt and others (1998) illuminated this issue in a study of 373,505 patients receiving ambulatory care in Washington State. The authors concluded that specialists continue to play a central and sustained role in many patients' care. In fact, 15 percent of patients received care exclusively from specialists over the two-year observation period, suggesting that they may have been serving as patients' primary (or only) physicians. However, the authors point out that it remains unclear whether specialists who serve as a patient's primary physician are providing primary care—in particular, whether they meet requirements for comprehensiveness of care—or whether they are attending to a narrow set of issues within their clinical expertise. There is little empirical data to inform this issue from the perspective of the clinical services provided. Information from patients suggests that those who rely on generalists versus specialists perceive no performance differences on defining elements of primary care, including access, continuity, preventive risk counseling, interpersonal treatment, communication, and whole-person care (Smith and Buesching, 1986; Safran, Tarlov, and Rogers, 1994; Safran and Taira, 1999).

Primary Care Experiences Reported by Patients, 1986–2000

With this picture of primary care arrangements in the United States and the understanding that these have been remarkably stable despite dramatic changes in the organization and financing of health care, it is useful to learn about the primary care experiences reported by patients. What are the relative strengths and weaknesses of primary care delivery in the United States from the patient's viewpoint? To what extent do patients' primary care experiences differ under different delivery system arrangements and in different areas of the country? To what extent do patients perceive the quality of primary care to be changing? What accounts for the changes?

To address these issues, we summarize what we have learned over the past decade through fielding the Primary Care Assessment Survey (PCAS) in several large-scale research studies in diverse segments of the adult population and in diverse areas of the country. The PCAS is a validated patient-completed questionnaire that measures the defining characteristics of primary care as posited by the Institute of Medicine Committee on the Future of Primary Care and others who offered earlier definitions of the term (Smith and Bueshing, 1986). The PCAS measures seven features of primary care through eleven summary scales: access (financial and organizational), continuity (relationship duration, visit based), comprehensiveness (whole-person knowledge of the patient, preventive risk counseling), integration of care, quality of the clinician-patient interaction (clinician-patient communication, thoroughness of physical examinations), interpersonal treatment, and patient trust. All concepts are measured in the context of a specific clinician-patient primary care relationship and reference the entirety of that relationship (that is, they are not visit specific). This is consistent with the IOM definition and others (Institute of Medicine, 1978; Donaldson, Yordy, Lohr, and Vanselow, 1996; Millis, 1996; Alpert and Charney, 1973; Starfield, 1992), which emphasize that primary care is founded on sustained clinician-patient relationships.

The fundamental importance of sustained, whole-person-oriented care from the point of view of full-time primary care physicians is well illustrated by these quotations from doctors interviewed in 1994 as part of a study on the definition and meaning of primary care:

> Well, continuous care is the notion. Maybe that's a better word than *ongoing*. But the whole idea is that it's not episodic around the prob-

lem. The commitment is long-term. Which enables you to use time. One of the biggest differences between primary care and a specialist is that a specialist is asked to answer a question at a point in time. And they, therefore, have a certain pressure to do everything they know how to do to answer that question at that point in time. A primary care physician has the luxury of following things over time, letting time be a diagnostic help, rather than an impediment and a challenge. It's a big, big difference and an important one [Safran, 1994, p. 4].

The other piece of continuous care is that it's a commitment to the patient that you are going to be there tomorrow and the next day. That what you do now is going to be building for everything you're going to be doing in the future [Safran, 1994, p. 4].

Other men and women are responsible for different parts and pieces and different areas, but there must be, there has to be, there should be one person responsible for the whole picture. Who has the ability, cognitively and emotionally, to put it all together and to put the different recommendations into a context of that patient's life [Safran, 1994, p. 4].

Being someone's primary care doctor is like a marriage [Safran, 1994, p. 4].

How much do I need to know? The more I know about what's going on in a patient's life, the more likely I am to be able to help that patient [Safran, 1994, p. 4].

I think the way you get that [whole-person relationship] is by really trying to understand who the patient is. And again, understanding who the patient is will be much more than just a review of the organ systems [Safran, 1994, p. 4].

It's not enough just to have a very strong medical knowledge of physiology and anatomy. You've got to understand the psychosocial. And I think for primary care, that's an important part of training. Because you can miss a lot of issues and not understand them unless you're very sensitive to psychosocial issues of the person, and the person in their family and their community. . . . So it's not by organ system or age. We have a general knowledge of who the person is [Safran, 1994, p. 4].

> I think to be a primary care physician, you just have to look beyond a person's organ systems. It shouldn't be, you know, from the chin to the knees [Safran, 1994, p. 4].

SUSTAINED PARTNERSHIPS PROVIDING WHOLE-PERSON CARE: HOW ARE WE DOING?

Despite these compelling testimonials from clinicians who provide primary care, data from patients suggest that whole-person care is a weak link in primary care performance. The PCAS measure of physicians' whole-person knowledge of their patients consistently ranks lowest among five measures of interpersonal care. Table 2.1 illustrates the observed performance with regard to whole-person care, showing item-level results for several of the PCAS questions on this topic. The data derive from two longitudinal studies in which the PCAS was administered: (1) a study of adults employed by the Commonwealth of Massachusetts and enrolled in any of twelve health plans offered to state workers and (2) a study of Medicare beneficiaries sampled from both the traditional (fee-for-service) Medicare program and Medicare health maintenance organizations (HMOs) in thirteen states with high rates of managed Medicare participation (Arizona, California, Colorado, Florida, Illinois, Massachusetts, Minnesota, New Mexico, New York, Oregon, Pennsylvania, Texas, and Washington State).

Except for physicians' knowledge of patients' medical histories, only about one-third of patients considered their physician's knowledge about them to be excellent or very good. The majority of patients considered their primary physician's knowledge about them and their life circumstances to be only good, fair, poor, or very poor. This constitutes poor performance on one of the defining features of primary care and one that in theory distinguishes primary care from other areas of medicine. The result is striking in the light of evidence for considerable continuity in U.S. primary care relationships. Three-quarters of adults in these samples report having been in their current primary physician's practice for three years or more.

The Performance of Primary Care Teams

The functioning of teams in primary care has important bearing on our ability to meet the objectives of whole-person care and sustained partnerships. As noted above, formal definitions of primary care have

Doctor's Knowledge of:	General Adult Population[a] (N = 6,083)		Adults Aged Sixty-Five and Older[b] (N = 8,433)	
	Excellent, Very Good	Good, Fair, Poor, Very Poor	Excellent, Very Good	Good, Fair, Poor, Very Poor
Your entire medical history	51%	49%	54%	46%
Your responsibilities at home or work	34	65	40	60
What worries you most about your health	36	64	40	60
You as a person (your values and beliefs)	29	71	39	61

Table 2.1. Patients' Views of How Well Their Primary Physicians Know Their Medical History and Life Circumstances.

[a]Based on a survey of insured adults in Massachusetts, all ages, 1996.

[b]Based on a survey of Medicare beneficiaries aged sixty-five and older in thirteen states nationwide, 1998.

posited that primary care can be provided by a team or by an individual clinician. Throughout the United States, medical practices rely substantially on teams to provide primary care. Yet available evidence from patients reveals a large gap between the reality of team care and the ideals of "sustained clinician-patient partnerships providing care in the context of family and the community." In fact, data from patients paint a picture that suggests that they experience the other clinicians on the team as a bewildering stream of providers who are "not my doctor," who know little about them, and whose role in their care is unclear to them.

Consider that there is a distinction between visible and invisible team care and that what most U.S. patients experience is care from invisible teams. *Visible team care* refers to situations in which the members of the primary care team and their respective roles in providing care are known to and understood by the patient. This is contrasted with care from the *invisible team,* wherein the roles and identities of the other clinicians involved in the patient's care are not clear or understood—where the patient perceives and relates to these others as "not my doctor" rather than as part of a team of clinicians with whom he or she has a sustained primary care partnership.

Among patients nationwide who report having a primary physician, most indicate that other clinicians in their primary physician's practice play an important role in their care. This tells us that there is team care, but not whether the team functions in a visible or invisible way from the patient's perspective. Roughly half of patients rate both the quality of care provided by these other clinicians and their coordination with the primary physician as excellent or very good, which is encouraging. However, the data reveal substantial failings in the interpersonal elements of team care. Table 2.2 illustrates this point, comparing patients' assessments of their primary physician with their assessments of the other clinicians on the team. Three-quarters of patients in practices that rely on teams rate the other clinicians' whole-person knowledge about them unfavorably, nearly two-thirds rate the clinicians' knowledge of their medical history unfavorably, and 55 percent rate their communication skills unfavorably. By comparison, patients' ratings of their primary physician's whole-person knowledge about them was slightly better, and their primary physician's knowledge of their medical history and communication skills were substantially better.

	Assessments of Other Clinicians in the Practice Whom Patients Consider to Play an Important Role in Their Care		Assessments of Primary Physician	
	Excellent, Very Good	Good, Fair, Poor, Very Poor	Excellent, Very Good	Good, Fair, Poor, Very Poor
Quality of care they provide	55%	45%	[a]	[a]
Coordination between them and your regular doctor	56	44	[a]	[a]
Their explanations of your health problems or treatments that you need	54	46	72	28
Their knowledge of your medical history[b]	37	63	56	44
Their knowledge of you as a person (your values and beliefs)	25	75	29	71

Table 2.2. Patients' Assessments of Care Provided by Their Primary Care Physician and Other Clinicians in the Practice.

[a]This item was not asked with reference to the primary physician.

[b]Data for this item are based on a survey of Medicare beneficiaries aged sixty-five and older in thirteen states nationwide, 1998 ($N = 8,433$). All other data are based on a survey of insured, employed adults in Massachusetts, 1996 ($N = 6,083$).

The data suggest that while many primary care practices embrace a team approach, we are a great distance from meeting the defining criteria of primary care through teams. Most particularly, it is clear that the criteria for sustained partnerships between patients and their primary care clinicians and a whole-person orientation to care are not currently being met by most team arrangements in primary care.

The weak performance of primary care teams may account for performance differences consistently observed in data from patients of open- and closed-model medical practices. *Closed-model practices* refer to those in which physicians work exclusively with one health plan on either a salaried or contractual basis (staff and group model HMOs). *Open-model practices* refer to those in which physicians have contractual relationships with multiple health plans. Closed-model practices have historically embraced the concept of primary care teams and generally structure their care processes accordingly. For example, the appointment-scheduling protocols of staff- and group-model HMOs that we have studied have almost uniformly prioritized patients' access to care over their continuity with particular clinicians. The underlying philosophy that gave rise to many of today's closed-model practices, and to the structures and processes through which they provide care, is that a clinician's technical expertise and clinical knowledge predominate in his or her ability to provide high-quality care, and therefore that care can appropriately be provided by whichever clinician from the team has the necessary level of expertise for the presenting problem (for example, physician, nurse practitioner, other clinician) regardless of that clinician's preexisting knowledge about the patient. Indeed, more patients in closed-model practices report that other clinicians play an important role in their care, yet their assessments of the care they provide are no better than those observed generally and reported in Table 2.2. Our data suggest that open-model practices also rely on teams, but to a lesser extent.

This use of teams, without the establishment of visible teams, may account for some of the differences in primary care experiences that are consistently reported by patients in closed- versus open-model practice settings. In studies conducted over the past twenty years and in varied populations and geographical areas, patients in closed-model practices consistently report less favorable communication quality and interpersonal treatment, feel that their primary physicians have less comprehensive knowledge about their medical history and life circumstances, and change primary physicians significantly more often than their counterparts in open-model practices (Safran, Tarlov, and

Rogers, 1994; Safran and others, 2000a, 2002; Rubin and others, 1993; Davies and others, 1986; Miller and Luft, 1994; Murray, 1988; Clement, Retchin, and Brown, 1994; Rossiter, Langwell, Wan, and Rivnyak, 1989).

There is considerable empirical evidence that underscores the high value that most patients place on the interpersonal aspects of care and that these have a significant relationship to outcomes, including patients' adherence to medical advice (Safran and others, 1998b, 2000b), health outcomes (Safran and others, 1998b; Greenfield, Kaplan, and Ware, 1985; Greenfield and others, 1988), and loyalty to their primary physician's practice (Safran and others, 2001). Indeed, available empirical evidence suggests that among adults who identify a primary physician, three-quarters place a high priority on seeing that physician when they require medical care. Within that group, most also want appointment times that meet their schedules. A small minority of patients with a primary physician say they prioritize access and appointment convenience over continuity (16 percent).

These patient priorities regarding the access-continuity trade-off may surprise many practice leaders and managers. In my experience, practices in the Northeast and other competitive health care markets presume that their patients prioritize access above all else, and they implement scheduling systems accordingly. In response to these data, one set of practices that we recently studied implemented a new appointment scheduling system that involved asking patients who called for an appointment to indicate their relative priorities with respect to seeing a particular clinician versus being seen at a particular time. Over the subsequent months, patients' evaluations of their primary care in these practices—and in particular, their continuity with their primary physician and the quality of their interactions with that physician—increased significantly. Although the practices implemented a number of other changes that may also have contributed to the shift in patients' experiences, the observed improvement occurred during a period when the overall trend in primary care relationship quality in that market was downward (Murphy and others, 2001).

The Declining Quality of Patients' Primary Care Experiences

This raises one final area for which empirical data from patients should inform our thinking about the future of primary care. Although there are no national tracking systems to monitor changes in the quality of primary care, data from our two longitudinal patient surveys raise concerns about the current trajectory of performance on several defining features of primary care. Murphy and others (2001) recently reported substantial declines in the quality of primary care relationships and in access to care among Massachusetts adults who retained the same primary physician over a three-year observation period (1996–1999). The observed decline in primary care relationship quality appears to generalize well beyond Massachusetts. Data from Medicare beneficiaries in thirteen states nationwide and collected between 1998 and 2000 reveal even larger declines than those seen in the three-year Massachusetts study. Over a twenty-four-month period, data from Medicare beneficiaries who retained the same primary physician showed substantial declines in communication quality, interpersonal treatment, thoroughness of physical examinations, visit-based continuity, and integration of care. Table 2.3 compares the results of these two longitudinal studies.

	Massachusetts Adults, 1996–1999		Medicare Enrollees, Thirteen States, 1998–2000	
	Observed Score Change (Mean)[a]	Effect Size[b]	Observed Score Change (Mean)[a]	Effect Size[b]
PHYSICIAN-PATIENT INTERACTIONS				
Communication	−1.51	0.10	−3.24	0.20
Interpersonal treatment	−2.06	0.12	−2.77	0.15
Physician's knowledge of patient	1.11	0.05	1.58	0.08
Thoroughness of physical exams	−2.97	0.17	−3.15	0.16
Patient trust	−0.68	0.05	0.86	0.06
STRUCTURAL AND ORGANIZATIONAL				
Financial access	0.46	0.02	−2.57	0.13
Organizational access	−2.72	0.17	0.74	0.04
Visit-based continuity	1.21	0.06	−4.10	0.24
Integration of care	0.38	0.02	−1.91	0.11

Table 2.3. Changes in Primary Care Performance Observed in Two Longitudinal Studies.

[a]For all respondents who retained the same primary care physician throughout the observation period, score changes were computed as the difference between the respondent's score at follow-up versus baseline ($time_2 - time_1$). Data in the table represent the mean score change observed for each scale.

[b]The effect size is computed as the absolute change in score divided by the standard deviation of the scale. This standardized metric allows comparison across scales and across studies regarding the magnitude of change observed.

Understanding how and why this erosion of primary care relationship quality is occurring is an urgent matter as we look to secure the future of primary care. In the context of the Massachusetts study, we generated eight hypotheses that might account for the observed decline in relationship quality. The study data afforded information to address seven of these hypotheses. Table 2.4 summarizes the hypotheses and what we found concerning each.

Of the seven hypotheses explored empirically, three appear to have played a significant role in the observed relationship quality decline: (1) changes in the amount of time that patients had with their primary physician during office visits, (2) changes in visit-based continuity, and (3) changes in patients' disease burden. The changes in visit-based continuity appear to have countered the effects of time and disease burden. That is, visit-based continuity increased, on average, for patients in this study, and the observed increases in visit-based continuity appear to have helped to forestall larger declines in relationship quality than would have been observed in the absence of these continuity increases. Both of the other two factors (time and disease burden) appear to have contributed to the observed decline in relationship quality between 1996 and 1999.

LOOKING TO THE FUTURE

As we consider the future of primary care, it seems clear that the challenges of creating sustained clinician-patient partnerships and providing care that is oriented to the whole person will increase rather than abate. The challenges are numerous and varied, and they come from all directions. They come from the Internet, with its around-the-clock availability and abundance of information, and from a population that hungers for that information. They come from a health insurance system set up such that established primary care relationships can be disrupted by a single business decision made by a medical practice, an employer, or a health plan. They come from the organization of medical practices, including primary care and specialty practices, and our failure to develop a means to truly integrate patient care within and across sites. And they come from a population that eagerly looks to "complementary therapies" as well as "conventional" ones (including pharmaceuticals learned about from television or print ads) to achieve the state of health that they long for. To meet the objectives of establishing sustained clinician-patient partnerships

Hypothesized Influence on Relationship Quality (RQ)	Hypothesized Direction of Effect on RQ	Analytic Approach	Findings	Magnitude of the Effect
1 Changes in the amount of time physician spends with the patient in visits	Negative	Patients' assessments of the adequacy of time physician spends and of changes in time spent 1996–1999 modeled as predictors of change in relationship quality scales.	There was compelling evidence that changes in the amount of time spent with patients (perceived and reported by patients) was a significant driver of the reduced RQ observed in 1999 versus 1996.	Changes in time accounted for approximately a 0.2 to 0.25 point decline in RQ scales (largest of all observed effects).
2 Turmoil at certain health plans	Negative	Comparison of changes in RQ reported by patients in plans that experienced extreme turmoil during the study period versus those that did not.	There was no evidence that plan turmoil had an effect on the observed changes in relationship quality. Patients in plans with and without turmoil showed equivalent change in all four elements of RQ.	None
3 Changes in patients' expectations	Negative	Analysis of report rating item pairs to see if patient expectations changed (for example, was there a lower rating of a given experience say, a ten-minute office wait, in 1999 versus 1996?).	There was minimal evidence that patients' expectations concerning their care changed during the study period.	Minimal to none
4 Changes in expectations of a subgroup of patients (higher socioeconomic status, SES)	Negative	Analysis of high-SES subgroup versus other patients to determine if that group is more demanding and if the pattern changed over the study period.	There is evidence that the high-SES group is more demanding regarding their care, but this effect appeared to remain constant over the study period and therefore does not explain the observed decline in RQ.	None

Table 2.4. Explaining the Observed Decline in Relationship Quality: A Summary of Analyses.

Hypothesized Influence on Relationship Quality (RQ)	Hypothesized Direction of Effect on RQ	Analytic Approach	Findings	Magnitude of the Effect
5 Decline in physician morale	Negative	Analysis of satisfaction data from the primary physicians whose patients participated in the study to see if a physician's satisfaction predicts his or her patients' assessment of care and/or predicts changes in the patient's assessments of care.	Physician satisfaction did not significantly predict patients' assessments of care. There was no effect cross-sectionally or longitudinally. While we observed substantial declines in physician satisfaction (Murphy and others, 2001), physicians appear to have buffered their patients from their increasing dissatisfaction with their professional life.	None
6 Increase in visit-based continuity	Positive	Analysis of changes in visit-based continuity as predictors of changes in RQ scales.	Changes in visit-based continuity significantly predicted changes in all four measures of RQ.	Changes in continuity corresponded with a 0.14 to 0.22 point increase in RQ scales (the increased continuity experienced in many settings offset the other factors that were driving RQ downward).
7 Occurrence of salient health event, acquisition of new medical conditions	Negative	Analysis of changes in the number and types of chronic medical conditions that patients reported over the study period as predictors of change in their assessments of their physicians' performance.	Acquisition of new health conditions was associated with significant declines in patients' assessments of their physician, particularly the relationship quality elements and integration of care.	Increased disease burden accounted for approximately a 0.1 point decline in RQ scales.
8 Patients' feeling "stuck," feeling a lack of options	Negative	No data to allow explicit study of this hypothesis.	Our population had increasing choice available to them over the study course, so if they felt stuck, it was due to concerns about "the devil you know vs. the devil you don't" rather than due to the imposition of constraints on their choice of physician.	Unknown

Table 2.4. Explaining the Observed Decline in Relationship Quality: A Summary of Analyses, Cont'd.

and whole-person care in the face of these challenges will require creative solutions and a commitment to the end goal. Consider the possible components.

Accepting and Embracing the Role of Teams

Primary care in the twenty-first century requires the involvement of a team of clinicians. Nationwide, primary care practices have evolved explicit and thoughtful systems to ensure that their patients have access to twenty-four-hour coverage all year. And while practices vary in the degree to which they prioritize continuity between patients and particular clinicians for appointments, the reliance on teams to ensure patients' access to information and care is virtually universal.

The problem (or at least part of it) is that no one told the patients. And thus, patients' expectations and preferences concerning the care that they receive when they go to their doctor's office have not shifted to make room for teams. Recall the baseball strike of 1994–1995. There were thirty-four weeks during which the players we knew did not play ball. Yet baseball got played—by teams that had names we recognized and players whom we had never heard of. It was disorienting to watch the Red Sox play with a cast of characters whose batting averages were unknown to us and whose abilities at first base, on the pitcher's mound, or behind home plate were mysteries to us. The data suggest that this is how patients experience teams in primary care practices today. It need not be this way.

To create the visible team will require two things. First, it will require communicating with patients about teams: making explicit from their initial visit and thereafter who the players are and what role each plays. That might be the easy part. Creating visible team care will also require that practices develop explicit strategies and systems to ensure that they too know the position played by each and that each clinician on the team be clear about his or her role in creating a sustained partnership with the patient. It is probably no accident that patients' experience of teams to date suggests a blur of clinicians who fill in for their "real" doctor but have no real vesting in them as a person or patient. The use of teams in primary care practices has primarily been about ensuring appointment access and after-hours coverage. But accessibility is only one of the defining criteria of primary care. And the data from patients make clear that several other essential elements of primary care have been missing in the team approach to primary care thus far.

Primary Care as a Contract

There is another aspect of primary care that we do not make explicit with patients: primary care requires a sustained clinician-patient partnership. The data reported here suggest that most patients enter into a primary care relationship with a presumption that it will continue over some substantial period of time—usually years. As noted, most Americans have a particular physician whom they consider to be their primary physician, and three-quarters of those who have a primary physician have been in that physician's practice for three years or more.

However, there is nothing to indicate whether patients consider their relationship with their primary physician to be a partnership. A partnership connotes something more than simply a relationship that endures over time. It connotes a particular type of relationship in which there are shared objectives and a shared understanding about the roles and individual accountabilities for accomplishing them. When a partnership is established, the objectives, roles, and accountabilities are typically made explicit in a written document—a verbal exchange of promises or some other formal means. We have nothing analogous to this as we establish primary care relationships. When a patient selects a primary care physician, perhaps it is clear (though probably rarely, if ever, made explicit) that the physician assumes a set of accountabilities to that patient. However, the patient's accountabilities to the physician and their shared objectives (presumably to the patient's health and well-being) are almost always left unspoken.

There seems the potential for a powerful shift in the nature of primary care relationships if the moment of a patient's selecting a primary physician (and the physician agreeing to assume that role) is marked by a purposeful process that includes outlining their shared objectives with regard to that patient's health and their individual roles and responsibilities for achieving them. This could include an explicit understanding about the role that the other clinicians (the "team") will play—and it should include this if we are to create visible team care in the ways posited above. Such a dialogue about the shared objectives for the patient's health would go beyond taking the patient's medical history and discussing his or her risk profile from a standardized list of behavioral characteristics. It would require a deliberate and guided discussion about the patient's principal health concerns and priorities and designing strategies to address them. The issues would undoubtedly extend to areas outside the realm that the physician's time and expertise enable him or her to address. But the process would identify the parameters in which they need to operate and would identify the other roles that need to be filled in order to meet that patient's objectives concerning their health. This brings us to the ever more critical role of integrating patients' care.

Integrating Care

Not so long ago, it was customary for a single physician, perhaps working in collaboration with a nurse, to provide most or all of a patient's medical care over a period of many years, or even a lifetime. Developments over the past half-century in our abilities to diagnose and treat patients' symptoms and diseases have changed that dramatically. Yet despite the profound shifts in medical practice and the fact that patient care invariably requires the involvement of multiple professionals within and outside the primary care setting, our ability to integrate the varied components of a patient's care to a coherent whole seems to have made little, if any, progress. Many of the structures and processes that we envisioned fifteen or more years ago as solutions to fragmented care are now in place. More than half of Americans are enrolled in a managed care plan that requires them to have a primary physician who is responsible for coordinating all care received from specialists and other health care professionals. There are integrated delivery systems. Acute care hospitals are now joined, under one corporate structure, with rehabilitation facilities, long-term care, and home care services. Yet most clinicians and patients would agree that care is no more integrated today than it was before these systems were in place. Why have these advances in our health care infrastructure and systems not made a noticeable difference in the integration of patient care?

Consider an analogy: we have built a new, architecturally spectacular theater and in this theater we produce plays with the same players who performed in the previous more rudimentary theater. The experience of going to the theater may now be substantially different, but the experience of the drama as it unfolds on the stage is unchanged because the ways that the actors comport themselves and address one another are unchanged. To continue this analogy, consider attending a performance of *Giselle* or *Swan Lake* or any other classical ballet. One thing that you will notice is that the experience of watching an American ballet company (*any* American ballet company) perform one of the classic ballets is entirely different from the experience of watching the Kirov, the Stuttgart, or any other European ballet company. Profound differences in the national cultures, and thus in the culture of the ballet companies, account for the different experience. When you watch an American ballet company, the soloists will leave you breathless with their technical expertise and their artistry. But if you turn your attention to the corps de ballet (the dozens of dancers who perform together in unison), your enchantment might be deflated. This is not because the dancers in the corps are not technically superb. Every one of them is. But they do not relish their role as a member of the corps de ballet; they do not dedicate their professional energies to becoming expert at being part of a team that dances in seamless unison. Every one of them wants to be a soloist, regrets that they are not yet, and bides their time in the corps hoping to be considered good enough for a solo. This is not surprising in the United States, whose culture glorifies and celebrates above all else the individual pioneer, athlete, dancer, business mogul, or doctor who stands head and shoulders above all others. Watching the corps de ballet in European companies is an entirely different experience. They dance in absolute breathtaking unison and create a visual effect unlike any other performance experience.

The processes of performing as an individual and that of performing in a group are different, and they require an entirely different type of focus and expertise. For a corps de ballet to create the magnificent effect of unison, each member must be keenly attentive to the group while simultaneously attending to her or his own dancing—making thousands of microadjustments to position, pace, and movement to ensure that the corps is performing as a single, graceful, powerful entity.

And so it is with medicine. We have collections of individuals who are highly trained to do a job that requires detailed knowledge, technical skill, and artistry. We train health care professionals, in the classroom and at the bedside, with an almost exclusive emphasis on honing their individual knowledge, skills, and techniques so that they can function at an extreme level of excellence as they go about their role in patient care. We do a superb job of teaching clinicians to be soloists in the ballet of medicine. But as illustrated above, excellence in the performance of groups (or team) requires more than just highly skilled individuals who are functioning individually. To function as a coherent team requires an additional set of skills and deliberate attention from each individual member to the performance of the whole. It is our failure to recognize this, and to attend to the sets of skills and behaviors required for effective team functioning, that has kept health care fragmented in the face of profound changes in our infrastructure that we thought would yield integrated care.

There is no question that integration of care remains a critical function and that it is one that the primary physician is uniquely positioned and uniquely qualified to fill. One of the physicians I interviewed in 1994, when exploring the definition of primary care, listed "first and last" as a distinguishing and essential feature of primary care. When asked to elaborate, she said, "You'll be the one to make the diagnosis, to decide if they need to see any specialists for further evaluation, and then, you'll be the person, if you're doing your job right, who will pull it all together; who will counsel the person around all the different opinions and help guide them through what has to be done. It's really first, middle and last" (Safran, 1994, p. 16).

It did not take the imposition of rules from managed care plans to motivate Americans to align themselves with a primary physician. As early as the 1970s and 1980s, when only a handful of Americans were enrolled in managed care plans, three-quarters of U.S. adults reported having a primary doctor. The onset of consumerism in American health care should not be taken to mean that patients now wish to single-handedly command their health care vessels or that they think they can. Americans have a seemingly insatiable appetite for information about how to get healthier, feel better, and live longer. And many are willing to combine conventional and nonconventional therapies to achieve the state of health that they long for. But they are also overwhelmed and bewildered by conflicting information and boundless choices with little to assure them of the safety or quality of the therapies or providers they choose. They need a skilled and knowledgeable partner to work with them in making choices that will help, not harm, them—and they know that. A large majority already see their primary physician as this cocaptain of their vessel, though many may wish to broaden the scope of the conversation to encompass aspects of health and health care that are not currently part of the agenda. In the context of formulating primary care partnerships with patients, the areas of the patient's health that are priorities to address, and the range of professionals whose involvement should be considered, will be apparent. The range of professionals will be broad, including those within and outside conventional medical disciplines. The primary physician will need resources and tools that are not currently available, including rich information systems that provide the data required to select individuals whose technical and interpersonal qualifications meet the patient's needs, and norms for interaction and teamwork that allow integration of care between the primary physician, the patient and those contributing to the patient's care in an episodic, consultative or ongoing way.

CONCLUSION: WHAT IS THE FUTURE OF PRIMARY CARE FROM THE PATIENT'S PERSPECTIVE?

More than three-quarters of American adults indicate that there is one doctor whom they consider to be their primary physician. This rate has remained remarkably stable over the past several decades, despite substantial changes in U.S. health care delivery systems. Moreover, it appears that the majority of primary care relationships endure for years. Thus, even in an era that has been dubbed consumerist with regard to health care, all available data suggest that Americans value having an established, long-term relationship with a primary physician.

However, data from patients summarized in this chapter highlight several areas where primary care performance appears poor, particularly with respect to providing care that is whole-person oriented, integrated, and based on clinician-patient partnerships. The data make clear that despite primary care relationships that have endured over several years, patients do not feel that their primary care physicians know much about them as human beings—about their values and preferences, about their life circumstances, and about their daily role responsibilities. Moreover, it is clear that despite the widespread use of teams in primary care practices, patients experience the other clinicians who work in their primary physician's practice as a bewildering array of individuals who are "not my doctor" and have no particular knowledge about them or investment in their care. Thus, we are a substantial distance from the ideal of primary care that is whole-person oriented. And we appear to be losing ground. Data from two large-scale longitudinal studies of patients who retained their primary physician over several years reveal substantial erosion in the quality of primary care relationships between 1986 and 2000.

Without our focused attention and effort, the task of ensuring that primary care is whole-person oriented, integrated, and founded on sustained clinician-patient relationships will grow more difficult in a health care system that is increasingly complex, in medical practices that are increasingly strained for time and resources (human, physical, and financial), and in a population that has ready access to a bewildering array of information and advice promising health outcomes that individuals long for. The discussion in this chapter has posited three elements as essential to securing the future of primary care in the face of these challenges: adapting the current functioning of primary care teams such that they become a visible, meaningful, and valued part of primary care from the patient's perspective; formalizing primary care as a partnership by making explicit the shared objectives and the roles and responsibilities that each party has for achieving them; and developing the norms, processes, and systems that will allow primary care physicians to integrate patient care in the face of the substantial barriers to integration that currently exist and that are likely to intensify.

From the patient's perspective, the future of primary care is a certainty. How it will be configured is not. But that it will be needed and desired by patients is. Americans are intensely interested in health and endlessly enamored with the idea of improving their health, feeling better, and living longer. There will remain, for the foreseeable future, a critical role for the group of professionals who will be their partner in achieving that.

References

Agency for Health Care Policy and Research, Center for Cost and Financing Studies. *1987 NMES Household Survey and Health Insurance Plans Survey Data.* Rockville, Md.: Agency for Health Care Policy and Research, 1998. CD-ROM.

Aiken, L. H., and others. "The Contribution of Specialists to the Delivery of Primary Care." *New England Journal of Medicine,* 1979, *300*(24), 1363–1370.

Alpert, J., and Charney, E. *The Education of Physicians for Primary Care.* Washington, D.C.: U.S. Department of Health, Education and Welfare, 1973.

American Association of Health Plans. *Health Plans and Employer-Sponsored Plans.* Washington, D.C.: American Association of Health Plans, 1999.

Clement, D. G., Retchin, S. M., and Brown, R. S. "Satisfaction with Access and Quality of Care in Medicare Risk Contract HMOs." In H. S. Luft (ed.), *HMOs and the Elderly.* Ann Arbor, Mich.: Health Administration Press, 1994.

Davies, A. R., and others. "Consumer Acceptance of Prepaid and Fee-for-Service Medical Care: Results from a Randomized Controlled Trial." *Health Services Research,* 1986, *21*(3), 429–452.

Donaldson, M. S., Yordy, K. D., Lohr, K. N., and Vanselow, N. A. (eds.). *Primary Care: America's Health in a New Era.* Washington, D.C.: National Academy Press, 1996.

Greenfield, S., Kaplan, S., and Ware, J. E. Jr. "Expanding Patient Involvement in Care: Effects on Patient Outcomes." *Annals of Internal Medicine,* 1985, *102*(4), 520–528.

Greenfield, S., and others. "Patients' Participation in Medical Care: Effects on Blood Sugar Control and Quality of Life in Diabetes." *Journal of General Internal Medicine,* 1988, *3*(5), 448–457.

Health Care Financing Administration. *Managed Care Trends.* [www.hcfa.gov/medicaid/trends00.pdf]. July 25, 2001a.

Health Care Financing Administration. *Medicare 2000: Thirty-Five Years of Improving Americans' Health and Security.* Rockville, Md.: Health Care Financing Administration, 2001b.

Health Care Financing Administration. *National Breakout of Managed Care Entities.* [www.hcfa.gov/medicaid/plansum0.pdf]. June 25, 2001c.

Institute of Medicine. *Report of a Study: A Manpower Policy for Primary Health Care.* Washington, D.C.: National Academy of Sciences, 1978.

Miller, R. H., and Luft, H. S. "Managed Care Plan Performance Since 1980: A Literature Analysis." *Journal of the American Medical Association,* 1994, *271*(19), 1512–1519.

Millis, J. S. *The Millis Commission Report.* Chicago: American Medical Association, 1966.

Murphy, J., and others. "The Quality of Physician-Patient Relationships: Patients' Experiences 1996–1999." *Journal of Family Practice,* 2001, *50,* 123–129.

Murray, J. P. "A Follow-Up Comparison of Patient Satisfaction Among Prepaid and Fee-for-Service Patients." *Journal of Family Practice,* 1988, *26*(5), 576–581.

Rosenblatt, R. A., and others. "The Generalist Role of Specialty Physicians: Is There a Hidden System of Primary Care?" *Journal of the American Medical Association,* 1998, *279*(17), 1364–1370.

Rossiter, L. F., Langwell, K., Wan, T. T., and Rivnyak, M. "Patient Satisfaction Among Elderly Enrollees and Disenrollees in Medicare Health

Maintenance Organizations: Results from the National Medicare Competition Evaluation." *Journal of the American Medical Association,* 1989, *262*(1), 57–63.

Rubin, H. R., and others. "Patients' Ratings of Outpatient Visits in Different Practice Settings: Results from the Medical Outcomes Study." *Journal of the American Medical Association,* 1993, *270,* 835–840.

Safran, D. G. "Defining Primary Care: A Background Paper for the Institute of Medicine Committee on the Future of Primary Care." Boston: New England Medical Center, 1994.

Safran, D. G., and Taira, D. A. *Health Care Delivery Systems and Primary Care Performance: Executive Summary.* Boston: Health Institute, 1999.

Safran, D. G., Tarlov, A. R., and Rogers, W. H. "Primary Care Performances in Fee-for-Service and Prepaid Health Care Systems: Results from the Medical Outcomes Study." *Journal of the American Medical Association,* 1994, *271*(20), 1579–1586.

Safran, D. G., and others. "The Primary Care Assessment Survey: Tests of Data Quality and Measurement Performance." *Medical Care,* 1998a, *36*(5), 728–739.

Safran, D. G., and others. "Linking Primary Care Performance to Outcomes of Care." *Journal of Family Practice,* 1998b, *47*(3), 213–220.

Safran, D. G., and others. "Organizational and Financial Characteristics of Health Plans: Are They Related to Primary Care Performance?" *Archives of Internal Medicine,* 2000a, *160,* 69–76.

Safran, D. G., and others. "Linking Doctor-Patient Relationship Quality to Outcomes." *Journal of General Internal Medicine,* 2000b, *15*(suppl.), 116.

Safran, D. G., and others. "Switching Doctors: Predictors of Voluntary Disenrollment from a Primary Physician's Practice." *Journal of Family Practice,* 2001, *50*(2), 130–136.

Safran, D. G., and others. "Primary Care Quality Performance in the Medicare Program: Comparing Primary Care of HMOs and Traditional Medicare." *Archives of Internal Medicine,* 2002, *162,* 757–765.

Smith, W. G., and Buesching, D. "Measures of Primary Medical Care and Patient Characteristics." *Journal of Ambulatory Care Management,* 1986, *9*(1), 49–57.

Starfield, B. *Primary Care: Concept, Evaluation and Policy.* New York: Oxford University Press, 1992.

Weinick, R. M., and Drilea, S. K. "Usual Source of Health Care and Barriers to Care, 1996." *Statistical Bulletin,* 1998, *79*(1), 11–17.

CHAPTER THREE

The Internet, Complementary and Alternative Medicine, and Self-Care

Bernard Lo

The explosion of medical information on the Internet, the growth of complementary and alternative medicine (CAM), and the development of self-care programs enable patients to be better informed and more active in their own care and obtain care outside the conventional medical system. They also challenge physician expertise and call into question the traditional doctor-patient relationship. Some physicians may feel rejected or threatened by these developments. However, the Internet, CAM, and self-care offer physicians an opportunity to consider how the usual doctor-patient relationship may fail to meet patient expectations and needs and suggest how it might be revitalized. This chapter analyzes how these developments have altered the doctor-patient relationship and suggest how physicians might reshape their role in response. The following three cases illustrate how these changes affect patient interactions with physicians:

- *Case 1: Request for intervention that the patient learned about on the Internet.* A fifty-four-year-old patient requests a heart scan that he learned about on the Internet as a way to detect asymptomatic heart disease. The medical literature discourages use of this magnetic resonance imaging (MRI) angiogram for screening because it frequently yields indeterminate results. The patient asked his primary physician whether the managed care plan refused to cover the scan because of costs. The ensuing discussion revealed that the patient had great anxiety over health and considerable stress at home and work. Rather than get the test, the patient agreed to see a cardiologist and a counselor.

- *Case 2: Use of CAM that may be causing medical complications.* A sixty-two-year-old woman had hypertension that was well controlled on hydrochlorthiazide. She started taking an herbal remedy that was recommended by the owner of a health food store for her weight gain and low energy level. Her blood pressure increased to 170/100. Her physician looked up the herbal remedy and found that it contained ephedra, a substance known to increase blood pressure. In the ensuing discussion, the physician learned that the patient was concerned about weight gain and low energy, desired more natural therapies, and worried about long-time use of medications.
- *Case 3: A self-care program for a patient who takes medications irregularly.* A nineteen-year-old man with asthma had frequent emergency department visits and hospitalizations, usually related to poor adherence to prescribed inhalers and delays in seeking care when his symptoms worsened. He did not take inhalers regularly because of his unpredictable work and school schedule. He also did not believe that taking medications regularly would significantly improve his asthma. The insurance plan suggested that the patient enter a self-care program, which provided asthma education, daily self-monitoring of peak flow rates, and guidelines for adjusting medications in response to changes in peak flows without a physician visit or telephone call. The patient's need for hospitalizations and emergency visits decreased. However, the next year, the insurance company dropped the program for financial reasons.

TRADITIONAL VIEW OF THE DOCTOR-PATIENT RELATIONSHIP

The traditional view of the doctor-patient relationship rests on several assumptions. Patients are viewed as dependent on physicians, who have medical knowledge, experience, and clinical judgment (Pellegrino and Thomasma, 1988; Lo, 2000). Patients cannot get information or recommendations about health care providers or medical care other than by consulting physicians. Illness often compromises the patient's ability to gather information or make decisions about personal medical care. Furthermore, because physicians need to order medical tests and provide prescriptions, patients depend on them for access to services. Decisions about health care are regarded as different from decisions about consumer purchases. Because consumers often have prior experience with purchases, they can readily compare brands and manufacturers and usually have time to gather information. Physicians are bound by both professional ethics and the law to act in the best interests of patients. This obligation promotes patient trust in physicians.

Under managed care, the traditional role of the physician has been challenged. As in case 2, patients may be suspicious that primary care physicians are serving as gatekeepers for tests, referrals, and therapies (Bodenheimer, Lo, and Casalino, 1999). They may fear that primary care physicians are not acting in their best interests but instead responding to financial incentives to save money for managed care organizations or to increase their own incomes. Furthermore, patients may fear that physicians are no longer professionals making independent decisions based on their best judgment but merely following authorization decisions, practice guidelines, and formulary restrictions established by bureaucrats in managed care organizations.

MEDICAL INFORMATION ON THE INTERNET

Patients are increasingly turning to the Internet for health and medical information. Over half of Americans with Internet access use it to obtain health information, a higher percentage than use the Internet to look up sports scores or stock prices, or to purchase merchandise (Pew Internet and American Life Project, 2000).

The Internet offers a broad array of health information and services. Patients can access peer-reviewed journal articles, other medical information, referrals to providers, medical advice, support groups, and chatrooms. There is information on a wide range of conditions, from weight loss to rare, serious diseases. In addition, patients can obtain prescription drugs, CAM, and other products, often without consulting a physician. A variety of entities post information and offer products, including established health care institutions like the National Cancer Institute and academic health centers, patient advocacy groups, laypeople with little or no medical training, and businesses trying to sell a product. Information and services on the Internet are convenient to access because patients can log on at any time and from their homes.

Information on the Internet can help patients be better informed about their condition and their options for care. It is particularly useful for patients with serious conditions for which several treatment options have similar effectiveness but quite different side effects or time courses. For example, patients with early-stage breast cancer can choose between mastectomy or a lesser breast operation combined with a longer course of radiation therapy. Similarly, patients with early-stage prostate cancer need to choose among different treatment options. Furthermore, patients may benefit from learning how other patients with the condition made these difficult choices.

The weakness of the Internet is that information is not regulated. Studies on a variety of medical conditions have found that much medical information on the Internet is scientifically inaccurate, and clinical advice offered on the Internet often is not consistent with evidence-based guidelines (Biermann, Golladay, Greenfield, and Baker, 1999; Impicciatore, Pandolfini, Casella, and Bonati, 1997; Jadad and Gagliardi, 1998; Soot, Moneta, and Edwards, 1999; Wyatt, 1997; Berland and others, 2001). In case 1, the Web site of a radiology group that owned an MRI scanner presented testimonials from customers but did not refer to scientific studies that evaluated the sensitivity and specificity of the test. Moreover, it is difficult for patients who do not understand the design of clinical trials to evaluate the quality of health information on the Internet. Testimonials from other patients may seem more compelling than rigorous scientific studies. Efforts to rate the quality of information on health Web sites may be unsuccessful because patients who start at one site frequently move to another Web site using hyperlinks. As in case 1, patients may learn about interventions on the Internet and request them. Some Web sites may encourage patients to request specific interventions, particularly prescription drugs. Physicians may feel frustrated at spending precious time clearing up misconceptions, explaining why the test is not appropriate in the patient's situation, and responding to patient concerns that physicians withhold beneficial care in order to save money. In the Internet era, physicians no longer control access to medical information or even access to medical services. Prescription drugs may be available on Internet with little or no clinical evaluation to exclude those with contraindications (Armstrong, Schwartz, and Asch, 1999).

Patients may also use the Internet to communicate with their physicians (Spielberg, 1998). They may be able to ask their physician questions, alert the physician to changes in their condition, and provide follow-up. Thus, the Internet may be a convenient substitute for an office visit.

Case 1 suggests that physicians might react in different ways when patients bring in information from the Internet. The physician may concentrate on the specific question the patient asked: whether he should get the heart scan. Such a conversation might focus on technical issues, such as the limitations of the test and the evaluation of diagnostic tests. Or the physician may try to understand the underlying concerns that led the patient to search the Internet and bring in the information. In case 1, the physician learned about the patient's concerns regarding serious undiagnosed illness and also discussed the role of stress in his life. Rather than focus solely on the MRI scan, the physician paid attention to the patient as a person and developed a comprehensive plan of care that addressed the underlying concerns and problems.

COMPLEMENTARY AND ALTERNATIVE MEDICINE

Over 42 percent of Americans have used CAM, and its popularity is increasing (Eisenberg and others, 1998). Patients often are willing to spend significant amounts of money out of pocket on CAM—often as much as they spend for prescription drugs (Eisenberg and others, 1998). Many forms of CAM, such as herbal remedies, can be used without a physician's approval, although certain types of CAM, such as acupuncture or chiropractic, are obtained through CAM providers.

There are many reasons for the popularity of CAM (Astin, 1998). As in case 2, CAM may address unmet patient needs and expectations regarding health care. Patients may seek CAM because they have concerns that health care is overly medicalized or desire therapies that they believe may have fewer side effects or are more "natural." Also, patients may want more attention paid to prevention and health maintenance. CAM may be more consistent with their spiritual or philosophical beliefs. Finally, CAM may attract patients who believe that doctors do not spend time with them, listen to them, or are interested in them as persons. In contrast, practitioners of CAM may be considered more likely to meet these expectations.

Physicians may find it hard to evaluate the safety and effectiveness of herbal remedies. It is difficult to determine the ingredients and dosage of CAM preparations because herbal preparations are often not standardized. Furthermore, there may be no rigorous scientific studies regarding the safety, side effects, and effectiveness of specific herbal therapies. Even when such studies have been carried out, it is often impractical for busy physicians to find such information in a timely manner when patients ask about herbal remedies at an office visit.

Although patients often regard herbal remedies as "natural," such products may cause serious adverse events (Angell and Kassirer, 1998). It may be hard for physicians to persuade patients that CAM can have serious adverse effects. Patients may give little weight to the lack of Food and Drug Administration (FDA) review of herbal therapies or may even mistrust the federal government. They may not understand that herbal therapies, like prescription drugs, may have adverse as well as beneficial effects. As in case 2, herbal remedies have been reported to contain ephedra, which may raise blood pressure, cause palpitations, or worsen coronary artery disease (Mashour, Lin, and Frishman, 1998). Herbal remedies may also interact with other drugs the patient is taking.

In case 2, physicians might react on several different levels to the patient's use of herbal remedies and the increase in blood pressure. The physician may concentrate on the question of whether the patient should stop taking the herbal remedy. In such discussions, physicians might explain case reports on the adverse effects of ephedra or the standards by which new drugs are evaluated in the peer-reviewed literature and by the FDA. This approach focuses on the biomedical aspects of disease: the patient's blood pressure and the clinical effects of the herbal preparation. Alternatively, the physician may address the underlying concerns that led the patient to be interested in CAM. This approach requires the physician to inquire about what the patient was hoping the herbal remedy would accomplish and to acknowledge her concerns about weight gain, low energy, and the long-term effects of medications. A comprehensive plan for care would address these issues, as well as her blood pressure. This latter approach focuses more on the patient and her concerns about her health and the impact of illness and treatment on her life instead of concentrating on her medical condition.

SELF-CARE

The term *self-care* includes a variety of actions that patients take to improve their health. Disease management programs have been developed for several chronic conditions, such as asthma, diabetes, and congestive heart failure (Ansell, 1999; Bailey and others, 1999; Cote and others, 1997; Gallefoss, Bakke, and Rsgaard, 1999; Turner, Taylor, Bennett, and Fitzgerald, 1998). These disease management programs are intended to correct three problems. First, patients with these conditions often are not prescribed effective therapies as recommended in consensus, evidence-based guidelines, such as steroid inhalers for moderate or severe asthma. Disease management programs may identify patients who are not receiving effective therapies. Second, as in case 3, patients often do not take medications as recommended, even if they are prescribed appropriately. In these conditions, health outcomes are compromised when patients do not take medications regularly or act promptly if an exacerbation occurs. Thus, disease management programs may fill a gap in standard care: once physicians prescribe a therapy, they often pay little attention to whether the patient takes the medication as prescribed. Third, when exacerbations occur, patients often do not take timely steps to prevent subsequent clinical deterioration and the need for an emergency department visit or hospitalization. Thus, disease management programs teach patients to recognize significant changes in their condition and alter medications based on these clinical changes without consulting a physician (Von Korff and others, 1997). The goal is not just to increase patient knowledge but to increase their health-promoting behaviors and self-efficacy (Holman and Lorig, 1997). *Self-efficacy* refers to a person's sense of personal ability to affect the consequences of his or her disease. This third type of program may not be integrated with care by the principal physician. Although the physician may have input into the guidelines that the patient learns, typically the patient changes therapy without consulting the physician. The reason for having patients modify their regimen without contacting their primary physician is that doctors may not respond in timely manner. Sometimes there is a nurse available by telephone or by e-mail for patients to contact with specific questions regarding their management (Piette, Weinberger, Kraemer, and McPhee, 2001; Piette and others, 2000). Some disease management plans use interactive Internet-based programs to allow patients to send the results of their monitoring to a central office, which can check that appropriate changes in therapy were made.

In other chronic conditions, such as arthritis, self-care programs have different goals (Holman and Lorig, 1997; Lorig, 1999; Mazzuca and others, 1997, 1999; Scholten and others, 1999). In most types of arthritis, standard therapies generally do not alter the long-term course of illness and may provide only partial relief of symptoms. The same is true of conditions such as neuropathy and chronic obstructive lung disease. Rather than helping patients change their medications in response to clinical changes, self-care programs in this condition help patients optimize their function and quality of life using such techniques as distraction, visualization, deep breathing, and positive self-talk (Lorig, 1994). These programs commonly include group meetings, which also serve as support groups.

Self-care programs for self-limited problems, such as upper respiratory infections and musculoskeletal strains, have still different objectives. These programs discourage patients from unnecessary tests and physician visits. However, these programs may be based on a thin understanding of concerns that lead patients to seek medical care. Often there is no test or therapy that physicians would order routinely in a self-limited illness. However, patients may seek care because they fear that their condition is more serious than usual, because they have conditions such as anxiety or depression, or because they expect a prescription. Unless these concerns are addressed, patients may not accept that a physician visit is unnecessary.

Cost savings may be the principal reason that health care organizations support self-care programs. Many disease management programs have been shown to reduce costs while often improving patient outcomes (Bodenheimer, 2000). Similarly, self-care programs for arthritis and for self-limited problems have been shown to reduce health care costs. However, after insurers achieve the most dramatic savings, through reducing hospitalizations or emergency department visits, the savings diminish. Furthermore, the savings may not be gained by the organization paying for the disease management program (Bodenheimer, 2000). As health care organizations face increasing financial pressures from increasing costs, they may cut back on self-care programs in order to save money or require patients to pay out of pocket for them.

THE IMPACT OF THESE DEVELOPMENTS ON THE DOCTOR-PATIENT RELATIONSHIP

The popularity of the Internet, CAM, and self-care may indicate shortcomings in standard medical care. Health information on the Internet allows patients to have more information on their condition and to check that their physicians are up to date. These developments also suggest that physicians pay insufficient attention to illness as contrasted with disease. Although patients want their doctors to be competent in the technical aspects of medicine, they also want their doctors to be skilled at the human aspects of illness. Patients may turn to CAM or the Internet because they feel that doctors do not listen to them or are not interested in them. They may want doctors to be interested in how the illness affects them as people in addition to being skilled at making the right diagnosis and ordering appropriate tests and therapies. Patients may want doctors to spend more time explaining their condition and the options for care. They may believe that doctors are insensitive to the impact of chronic illness on the quality of their lives. In addition, patients may believe that doctors give more attention to disease than to health and prevention. The traditional doctor-patient relationship may also give insufficient attention to the psychosocial aspects of health care. As case 2 illustrates, patients may have serious concerns about standard medical care. They may worry about side effects of prescription drugs or desire more "natural" therapies. Furthermore, they may not accept the importance of taking medications regularly for the rest of their lives. Often patients find it difficult to fit medications into their daily routines. Physicians commonly fail to address the practical obstacles to implementing plans of care based on evidence-based guidelines.

The growth of health information on the Internet, CAM, and self-care has helped make patients more informed and more active in their care. The assumptions underlying the traditional view of patients as dependent and passive may no longer hold. First, patients no longer depend on physicians for medical information or recommendations. Indeed, inequalities in information may be reversed. Patients with chronic illness or rare conditions who spend considerable time on the Internet may have more information than physicians, particularly nonspecialists. Even patients with serious illness need not depend on physicians for information, because family members commonly use the Internet to obtain medical information for them. Second, physicians no longer control access to testing and therapies. Patients intent on obtaining a test or therapy can probably find a provider on the Internet who is willing to provide it. Third, the self-perception of patients has changed. Patients feel more informed about their condition and options for referral and care. In addition, they are more confident in their ability to choose providers, make suggestions about care, and choose among feasible options for care. Furthermore, they may feel more capable of implementing a plan of care, monitoring their health, and responding to significant changes in their conditions. Fourth, their expectations of the physician role have changed. Patients may defer to physicians less often and be more likely to ask questions, make suggestions, and take control over decisions. In addition, CAM and self-care programs show that physicians are not essential for health care.

The growth of the Internet, CAM, and self-care may cause tension in the doctor-patient relationship. Some physicians may see their role and expertise denigrated. Others may feel frustrated at spending time correcting misinformation that patients find on the Internet or explaining why a test or therapy they have heard about is not right for them. CAM may present emotional challenges to physicians, since they may feel that they have failed or that patients are rejecting them or their recommendations.

These developments may have more impact on primary care physicians who care for patients with a variety of illnesses and whose patients commonly have several chronic conditions. A specialist needs to keep up with information on a restricted set of conditions, including new medical developments, popular forms of CAM, and disease management programs. A primary care physician needs to be familiar with such information for a broader range of problems. Also, primary care doctors may feel more constrained than specialists by time limits on patient visits. They may feel they have less time to discuss information from the Internet or the patient's use of CAM, particularly since they are now urged to give more attention to a range of issues, such as domestic violence, cancer screening, and depression. Finally, primary care physicians who discourage patients from seeking interventions described on the Internet may be mistrusted because patients fear that primary physicians are serving as gatekeepers motivated by self-interest or by bureaucratic regulations rather than patients' best interests.

NEW ROLES FOR PRIMARY CARE PHYSICIANS

How should the role of primary care physicians change in the light of these developments? Physicians need to take advantage of the unique skills they bring to the doctor-patient relationship and recognize that some traditional physician tasks may now be better done by other persons or by new technologies.

Physicians can no longer expect to be the primary source of medical information for patients. Retrieving information electronically on the Internet is more accessible and reliable than searching the physician's memory or filing cabinets. Patients can gather medical information about their condition, practice guidelines, and therapies from the Internet.

If physicians are no longer experts in health information, what expertise do they bring to the doctor-patient relationship? I believe that there are two types of physician expertise that the Internet, CAM, and self-care highlight: clinical judgment and the psychosocial aspects of illness and health care.

Physicians can still be experts in clinical judgment, even though they may no longer be experts in health information. After obtaining information from the Internet, patients often want to have a physician put the information in context and check whether it is reliable and applicable to their situation. Medical judgment has several components. First, physicians can evaluate the reliability of information from the Internet or about CAM using the standards developed for evidence-based medicine. Thus, they can help patients put into perspective information they obtain from other sources. Second, physicians can apply general knowledge to an individual patient's specific situation. Pertinent clinical considerations may be the stage of illness, coexisting medical conditions, and other subtle factors that are difficult to capture in explicit algorithms. Third, physicians can help patients deliberate about decisions and take into account their preferences and values regarding risk, uncertainty, and side effects. Often patients develop their preferences only when confronted by an important medical decision with several possible approaches, as in the treatment of localized breast cancer or prostate cancer. Physicians can help patients clarify and articulate their preferences. Fourth, physicians can tailor the decision-making process to the individual patient. Some patients want to play a more active role in decisions. Others may prefer to review the evidence and reasoning underlying the physician's recommendations but defer to the physician's views.

The growth of the Internet, CAM, and self-care has accelerated and amplified changes in the doctor-patient relationship that have already occurred. Over the past generation, the guiding principle of the doctor-patient relationship has shifted from a paternalism to informed consent. These developments allow patients to be even more informed and active in their own care.

Physicians can also be experts in the psychosocial aspects of illness and health care. They can make patients feel listened to, understood, and cared for. Much of what physicians do is technical in nature: making a diagnosis, ordering tests, and prescribing therapies for the biological disease. As we have seen, physician expertise in these biotechnical areas is being reduced because of computers, the development of evidence-based practice guidelines, information on the Internet, and self-care. However, the patient's experience of illness encompasses a great deal more than diagnosis, testing, and therapy. Illness, particularly chronic illness, may have an impact on the patient's ability to function, cause psychological suffering, and alter relationships with family, friends, and coworkers. As healers, doctors need to address these psychosocial aspects of illness. One reason for the popularity of support groups on the Internet, CAM providers, and self-care programs is that they give patients a sense that someone has heard them and understands what they are experiencing (Jonas, 1999). Commonly patients complain that their doctors are too busy, do not listen to them, or do not really understand them. Yet part of the physician's expertise is to give patients the sense that they are understood and cared for. To elicit and understand the patient's concern and needs, physicians need interpersonal skills, such as using open-ended questions, making empathic comments, listening carefully, and following the patient's lead. Through their interactions with patients, physicians can provide appropriate comfort, reassurance, and hope.

Physicians also can develop their expertise in the psychosocial aspects of health care. The popularity of CAM and self-help illustrates that a plan for care must fit the patient's values, preferences, and practical constraints. After making the correct diagnosis and prescribing effective treatments as recommended in evidence-based practice guidelines, physicians need to address whether the patient is willing and able to follow the recommendations. Does the patient agree with the plan of care shown in the literature as being the most effective?

Does the patient have concerns about long-term effects of medications? What are the practical barriers to the patient's taking medications regularly, and how might they be overcome? Traditionally, this issue is termed *adherence* or *compliance*, terms that imply that there is a best treatment plan and the problem is that patients fail to carry it out consistently (Funnell and Anderson, 2000). An alternative perspective leaves open the question of whether evidence-based guidelines are appropriate for a particular patient. For individuals with great concerns about the long-term risks of medications, the optimal decision might differ from the decision for most other patients. Furthermore, the concept of compliance stigmatizes patients who do not follow treatment plans scrupulously, even though it is difficult and uncommon for anyone to take many pills a day regularly. Physicians can learn from the experience of self-care programs that help patients identify and overcome barriers to following treatment regimens.

The idea that physicians should attend to the psychosocial aspects of illness as well as the biotechnical aspects of disease is not new. Almost seventy-five years ago, Peabody (1927) declared, "The treatment of a disease may be entirely impersonal; the care of a patient must be completely personal" (p. 878). Noting the "amazing progress of science" and the "enormous mass of scientific material which must be made available to the modern physician" (p. 877) Peabody also warned that physicians must pay attention to the impact of the patient's life on his symptoms and how illness affects the patient's emotions and relationships at home and at work. In treating a disease, physicians need to "compromise" (p. 881) with the practical barriers to following a prescribed regimen. Furthermore, Peabody warned that if the physician does not form a "personal bond" with patients, they may turn to alternative sources of care, "chiropractice, or perhaps it is Christian Science" (p. 879).

What is new is that the Internet, CAM, and self-care provide contemporary evidence that patients expect more than a correct diagnosis, the right test, or appropriate prescriptions. Furthermore, the Internet, CAM, and self-care suggest how physicians might learn these psychosocial skills. Physicians might learn from Internet support groups and self-help groups. What are the concerns that patients believe are not addressed adequately in usual health care? What statements or actions do patients find helpful? How might these insights be incorporated into the physician's role? Similarly, physicians might learn from CAM providers how to help patients feel that their concerns have been understood and addressed (Jonas, 1999). Do CAM providers simply spend more time with patients, or do they also interact in different ways? Finally, at successful self-care programs, physicians can learn how to assess barriers to implementing care plans and suggest strategies for helping patients achieve their health goals.

CHALLENGES AND BARRIERS

Information Needs

To fulfill the new roles that we have suggested, physicians need improved information technologies, including Internet access to pertinent information, in their offices. With the explosion of medical knowledge and the proliferation of critical reviews of the evidence pertaining to clinical questions, it becomes increasingly difficult for primary care physicians to keep in their minds practice guidelines that are soundly based on rigorous evidence. Having such information readily accessible gives physicians confidence that their recommendations are technically competent and frees them to attend to the psychosocial aspects of illness and the practical issues of forming a feasible plan of care with the patient. Furthermore, timely access to medical information helps doctors respond to patient questions about information they found on the Internet. Similarly, physicians who want to discuss with patients how to integrate CAM with prescription drugs will need the latest information about the safety and effectiveness of specific CAM modalities. Doctors who want to integrate self-care with their office care will need on-line access to algorithms used in these programs, as well as a flow sheet of the patient's measured parameters.

Lack of Physician Skills

Physicians need to develop or strengthen their skills in several areas. First, they need to understand evidence-based medicine and how to interpret the medical literature in order to answer patient questions about information from the Internet, about CAM, or about self-care. Second, they need to learn how to help patients develop their ability to manage their care. Doctors need to identify the barriers to implementing a care plan, help patients devise strategies to overcome them and maintain behavioral changes, and provide positive reinforcement for self-care. Third, physicians need to strengthen their communication skills in order to elicit patient concerns, values, and preferences;

explain evidence-based medicine; and help patients develop self-care skills. Although physicians need not become experts in these areas, they need to know enough to raise the issues, start the discussion, and provide positive feedback and encouragement.

Health Care Organizations

Physicians need appropriate incentives to embrace the new role that is suggested in this chapter. In our market-driven health care system, activities and programs may be dropped if they are not cost-saving or cost-effective from the perspective of the party paying for the program. In the region where I practice, which has high managed care penetration, a number of insurers have dropped self-care programs when they face increasing costs and budget deficits.

Indirect incentives also need to be reexamined. Individual providers and health care organizations are often rated using quality measures such as ordering mammograms, referring diabetic patients to ophthalmology, and prescribing beta blockers after myocardial infarction. These outcomes can be readily determined using administrative and billing data. Physicians naturally focus their attention on tests and therapies that are measured and compared. It is unrealistic to expect physicians to give equal attention to other activities that are not directly measured and rewarded, even if they are beneficial to patients (Casalino, 1999). However, the new roles defined here are much harder to measure and benchmark. It is possible that physicians filling the roles suggested may have lower ratings on common quality measures: a patient may decide against a screening test because the benefits seem small, because he or she wants to focus on prevention rather than early detection, or because he or she wants to spend more time talking to the physician about managing an active chronic illness rather than problems that might develop in the future.

Concerns About Inequity

The reconfigured doctor-patient relationship described here may develop predominantly among wealthier and better-educated patients. Such persons may have Internet access, disposable income to spend on CAM, and a greater sense of self-efficacy and willingness to accept the responsibility of managing their own care. In contrast, persons who are poor or poorly educated may lack computer skills, access to the Internet, self-care skills, and a sense of self-efficacy. Hence, the benefits of more personalized health care, which is more consistent with the patient's values and concerns, may also be more widespread among well-educated groups, who are better able to articulate their concerns and preferences and are used to making choices in their lives. Thus, the benefits of the Internet, CAM, and self-care may accrue primarily to higher socioeconomic groups. The new physician role thus may serve to widen discrepancies in health care and in health outcomes, even though the overall or average level of health outcomes may improve.

Targeted programs using the Internet and self-care can improve health outcomes for the least well off. Medicaid patients who receive Internet access and training have improved health outcomes and quality of life (Science Panel on Interactive Communication and Health, 1999). Patients from disadvantaged backgrounds with chronic illness, who often are high users of emergency departments and hospitalizations, benefit from disease management programs (Mazzuca and others, 1999). These interventions can have a multiplier effect because in addition to improving care for a specific medical condition, they can increase self-efficacy, teach skills, and help people form social networks. The technologies of the Internet and self-care are neutral with regard to the distribution of benefits across society; it is a moral and political decision as to whether the benefits will fall primarily on those already at the top of the socioeconomic ladder or will be distributed more equitably across society to help those most in need.

CONCLUSION

Over the past generation, the guiding principle of the doctor-patient relationship has shifted from paternalism to informed consent. The Internet, CAM, and self-care have amplified these changes. These developments make patients less dependent on physicians and better able to play an active role in their care. Physicians need to reconsider the nature of their expertise and their appropriate role. Although they certainly need to be highly competent at the technical aspects of care, their most important expertise may be to provide clinical judgment, individualize decisions for patients, and attend to the psychosocial aspects of illness and health care.

References

Angell, M., and Kassirer, J. P. "Alternative Medicine: The Risks of Untested and Unregulated Remedies." *New England Journal of Medicine,* 1998, *339,* 839–841.

Ansell, J. E. "Empowering Patients to Monitor and Manage Oral Anticoagulation Therapy." *Journal of the American Medical Association,* 1999, *281,* 182–183.

Armstrong, K., Schwartz, J. S., and Asch, D. A. "Direct Sale of Sildenafil (Viagra) to Consumers over the Internet." *New England Journal of Medicine,* 1999, *341,* 1389–1392.

Astin, J. A. "Why Patients Use Alternative Medicine: Results of a National Study." *Journal of the American Medical Association,* 1998, *279,* 1548–1553.

Bailey, W. C., and others. "Asthma Self-Management: Do Patient Education Programs Always Have an Impact?" *Archives of Internal Medicine,* 1999, *159,* 2422–2428.

Berland, G. K., and others. "Health Information on the Internet: Accessibility, Quality, and Readability in English and Spanish." *Journal of the American Medical Association,* 2001, *285,* 2612–2621.

Biermann, J. S., Golladay, G. J., Greenfield, M.V.V.H., and Baker, L. H. "Evaluation of Cancer Information on the Internet." *Cancer,* 1999, *86,* 381–390.

Bodenheimer, T. "Disease Management in the American Market." *British Medical Journal,* 2000, *320,* 563–566.

Bodenheimer, T., Lo, B., and Casalino, L. "Primary Care Physicians Should Be Coordinators, Not Gatekeepers." *Journal of the American Medical Association,* June 2, 1999, *281,* 2045–2049.

Casalino, L. P. "The Unintended Consequences of Measuring Quality on the Quality of Health Care." *New England Journal of Medicine,* 1999, *341,* 1147–1150.

Cote, J., and others. "Influence on Asthma Morbidity of Asthma Education Programs Based on Self-Management Plans Following Treatment Optimization." *American Journal of Respiratory and Critical Care Medicine,* 1997, *155,* 1509–1514.

Eisenberg, D. M., and others. "Trends in Alternative Medicine Use in the United States, 1990–1997: Results of a Follow-Up National Survey." *Journal of the American Medical Association,* 1998, *280,* 1569–1575.

Funnell, M. M., and Anderson, R. M. "The Problem with Compliance in Diabetes." *Journal of the American Medical Association,* 2000, *284,* 1709.

Gallefoss, F., Bakke, P. S., and Rsgaard, P. K. "Quality of Life Assessment After Patient Education in a Randomized Controlled Study on Asthma and Chronic Obstructive Pulmonary Disease." *American Journal of Respiratory and Critical Care Medicine,* 1999, *159,* 812–817.

Holman, H. R., and Lorig, K. R. "Patient Education: Essential to Good Health Care for Patients with Chronic Arthritis." *Arthritis and Rheumatism,* 1997, *40,* 1371–1373.

Impicciatore, P., Pandolfini, C., Casella, N., and Bonati, M. "Reliability of Health Information for the Public on the World Wide Web: Systematic Survey of Advice on Managing Fever in Children at Home." *British Medical Journal,* 1997, *314,* 1875–1879.

Jadad, A. R., and Gagliardi, A. "Rating Health Information on the Internet." *Journal of the American Medical Association,* 1998, *279,* 611–614.

Jonas, W. "Alternative Medicine—Learning from the Past, Examining the Present, Advancing to the Future." *Journal of the American Medical Association,* 1999, *280,* 1616–1617.

Lo, B. *Resolving Ethical Dilemmas: A Guide for Clinicians.* (2nd ed.) Philadelphia: Lippincott Williams and Wilkins, 2000.

Lorig, K. *Living a Healthy Life with Chronic Conditions.* Palo Alto, Calif.: Bell Publishing, 1994.

Lorig, K. "Evidence Suggesting That a Chronic Disease Self-Management Program Can Improve Health Status While Reducing Hospitalization." *Medical Care,* 1999, *37,* 5–14.

Mashour, N. H., Lin, G. I., and Frishman, W. H. "Herbal Medicine for the Treatment of Cardiovascular Disease: Clinical Considerations." *Archives of Internal Medicine,* 1998, *158,* 2225–2234.

Mazzuca, S. A., and others. "Effects of Self-Care Education on the Health Status of Inner-City Patients with Osteoarthritis of the Knee." *Arthritis and Rheumatism,* 1997, *40,* 1466–1474.

Mazzuca, S. A., and others. "Reduced Utilization and Cost of Primary Care Clinic Visits Resulting from Self-Care Education for Patients with Osteoarthritis of the Knee." *Arthritis and Rheumatism,* 1999, *42,* 1267–1273.

Peabody, F. W. "The Care of the Patient." *Journal of the American Medical Association,* 1927, *88,* 877–882.

Pellegrino, E. D., and Thomasma, D. G. *For the Patient's Good: The Restoration of Beneficence in Health Care.* New York: Oxford University Press, 1988.

Pew Internet and American Life Project. *The Online Health Care Revolution: How the Web Helps Americans Take Better Care of Themselves.* Washington, D.C.: Pew Internet and American Life Project, 2000.

Piette, J. D., Weinberger, M., Kraemer, F. B., and McPhee, S. J. "Impact of Automated Calls with Nurse Follow-Up on Diabetes Treatment Outcomes in a Department of Veterans Affairs Health Care System: A Randomized Controlled Trial." *Diabetes Care,* 2001, *24,* 202–208.

Piette, J. D., and others. "Do Automated Calls with Nurse Follow-Up Improve Self-Care and Glycemic Control Among Vulnerable Patients with Diabetes?" *American Journal of Medicine,* 2000, *108,* 20–27.

Scholten, C., and others. "Persistent Functional and Social Benefit Five Years After a Multidisciplinary Arthritis Training Program." *Archives of Physical Medicine and Rehabilitation,* 1999, *80,* 1282–1287.

Science Panel on Interactive Communication and Health. *Wired for Health and Well-Being: The Emergence of Interactive Health Communication.* Washington, D.C.: U.S. Government Printing Office, 1999.

Soot, L. C., Moneta, G. L., and Edwards, J. M. "Vascular Surgery and the Internet: A Poor Source of Patient-Oriented Information." *Journal of Vascular Surgery,* 1999, *30,* 84–91.

Spielberg, A. R. "On Call and Online: Sociohistorical, Legal, and Ethical Implications of E-Mail for the Patient-Physician Relationship." *Journal of the American Medical Association,* 1998, *280,* 1353–1359.

Turner, M. O., Taylor, D., Bennett, R., and Fitzgerald, J. M. "A Randomized Trial Comparing Peak Expiratory Flow and Symptom Self-Management Plans for Patients with Asthma Attending a Primary Care Clinic." *American Journal of Respiratory and Critical Care Medicine,* 1998, *157,* 540–546.

Von Korff, M., and others. "Collaborative Management of Chronic Illness." *Annals of Internal Medicine,* 1997, *127,* 1097–1102.

Wyatt, J. C. "Measuring Quality and Impact of the World Wide Web." *British Medical Journal,* 1997, *314,* 1879–1881.

PART TWO

The Components of Primary Care

Processes and Providers

Part Two provides a basis for the deconstruction of primary care. Assessing the individual elements of primary care may be useful to determine the relative value of each element to the future of primary care. In Chapter Four, Barbara Starfield describes the characteristics of primary care and the significant evidence of primary care's contribution to the overall health of our population. In Chapter Five, Helen Burstin and Carolyn Clancy describe and assess alternative sites and circumstances where primary care may be provided. In Chapter Six, Harry Kimball provides a specialist perspective and argues that, in some circumstances, it is appropriate for specialists to assume the primary care of a patient. In Chapter Seven, Mary Mundinger offers a nursing perspective and argues that advanced practice nurses are the preferred primary care provider based on their abilities and training.

CHAPTER FOUR

Deconstructing Primary Care

Barbara Starfield

The seminal documents that define primary care do so in terms of combinations of characteristics, including those such as first contact; longitudinal responsibility for patients or "sustained partnership"; integration of physical, psychological, and social aspects of health or "majority of personal health care needs"; accessibility; coordination; accountability; and "context of family and community" (Starfield, 1998; Institute of Medicine Committee on the Future of Primary Care, 1996). Despite the widespread consensus that primary care consists of these several elements in combination, not everyone understands primary care in this way. In much of the developing world, primary care is considered basic care, often limited to a set of specific interventions such as immunizations and oral rehydration for diarrhea, and widely regarded as the care provided to disadvantaged segments of the population rather than to everyone. In some industrialized countries, most notably the United States, primary care is widely believed to be essentially a gatekeeper, functioning largely as care for conditions not requiring a specialist.

Studies over the past decade in a variety of countries have provided much information about the nature of primary care. In fact, there is now more knowledge about the characteristics and importance of primary care than there is about specialty care, an ironic thought for countries (such as the United States) that are so invested in specialty care.

This chapter documents what is known about the characteristics of primary care and its importance to health, and, in contrast, indicates what little is known about specialty care. It then suggests that a more concerted focus on achieving primary care will, concomitantly, result in higher quality of care in the specialties as well as in primary care.

COMPONENTS OF PRIMARY CARE: THEIR MEASUREMENT AND THEIR UTILITY

Primary care is that level of health care systems that provides person-focused care over time, taking responsibility for dealing with all health problems that occur with reasonable frequency, that is sufficiently accessible to provide needed first contact care, and that coordinates care provided at others levels of services. It is distinguished from emergency care, consultative care, and referral care by these four characteristics, when present together. By virtue of these functions, it provides the infrastructure of most well-organized health systems and the basis for achieving better outcomes, as well as better distribution of health services across the population.

The functions of primary care can be defined in such a way as to make them measurable, and hence amenable to accountability within a health services system. Measurement can take place at various units of analysis: populations, subpopulations, clinical populations, facilities, or the health system as a whole. The basis for measurement of the four functions involves consideration of both the capacity of a health system and the achievement of the functions at the point of delivery of health services to patients and populations.

Measurement of Primary Care

Figure 4.1 provides the framework for choosing those aspects of structure (capacity) and those aspects of performance that uniquely characterize each of the functions. This diagram splits the health services system into three parts—structure, process, and outcome—which cor-

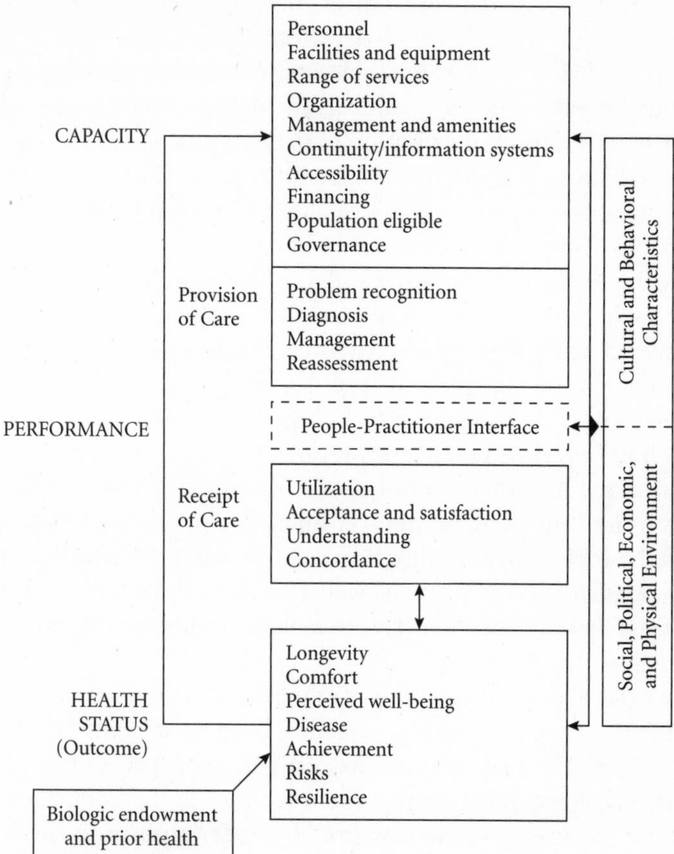

Figure 4.1. The Health Services System

Source: From *Primary Care: Concept, Evaluation, and Policy,* 2e by Barbara Starfield © 1999 by Oxford University Press, Inc. Used by permission of Oxford University Press, Inc.

respond to the more current terms of *capacity, performance,* and *health status.* The diagram contains the individual characteristics of each.

Evaluation of each of the special features of primary care involves determining if there is a capacity to accomplish each one and whether they are actually accomplished. Each of the four features of primary care is measured by measuring the structural feature that reflects the capacity to accomplish the function and the relevant performance feature.

First contact care requires services to be accessible (the structural feature) and be received (utilization) from the primary care source (rather than elsewhere) for each new need.

Longitudinality (person-focused care over time) requires a mutual affiliation between a primary care facility or practitioner and patients (the structural feature of definition of the eligible population), and its translation into good interpersonal relationships that last over time (generally at least two years) as well as for all nonreferred visits (utilization) to be made there.

If services are to be comprehensive, they must be designed to meet people's needs (range of services available), and they also must be delivered when they are needed; thus, people's needs must be recognized when they are present (problem/needs recognition). Comprehensiveness does not imply that the same package of services be available everywhere. It does require that all problems, except those that are too uncommonly encountered in the population to permit practitioners to maintain competence in dealing with them, need to be included. Coordination requires a mechanism of information transfer (continuity) as well as recognition of information from visits that patients may have to make elsewhere (problem/needs recognition).

Thus, there are eight characteristics that need to be assessed in evaluating the adequacy of primary care: four of them structural and four performance. The Primary Care Assessment Tools (PCAT) family of tools makes it possible to assess them from both the perspective of consumer experiences as well as from provider reports on the characteristics of their services. (See Starfield, 1998.)

Family-centered care, culturally competent care, and community orientation are often included in the definition of primary care, and, indeed, the PCAT tools assess them in addition to the four seminal characteristics. However, it is apparent that these three characteristics are derivative in the sense that optimal achievement of the four cardinal features necessarily achieves these additional "domains" by virtue of the requirement for adequate needs recognition and adequate interpersonal relationships that are integral to comprehensiveness and to longitudinality. (In our empirical analyses and psychometric testing of the PCAT, we found that these three derivative features do not factor out separately but rather become part of the four dimensions of primary care; Shi, Starfield, and Xu, 2001.)

EVIDENCE FOR THE BENEFITS OF THE FOUR COMPONENTS OF PRIMARY CARE

The benefits of each of the four features of primary care have been amply documented and need only be summarized here briefly. (They are catalogued in Starfield, 1998, and buttressed by additional research literature in the time since it was written.)

With Regard to First Contact

Evidence shows that the better the achievement of first contact care, the lower the costs, the more efficient the use of specialists, and the better the outcomes of care for primary care problems (Starfield, 1998). Forrest and Starfield (1996) categorized ambulatory care episodes, that is, each episode of care reported by people in the Medical Expenditure Panel Survey (MEPS) survey into those that involved preventive care and those that involved sick care. They demonstrated that episodes that start with a visit to the primary care physician have much lower costs, whether for sick visits or for preventive care, for all but two of the twenty-three clinically different episode types. The lower cost is especially notable in the case of sick episodes of care, and more so than for preventive episodes.

With Regard to Longitudinality

The benefits of longitudinality are well demonstrated by a large number of studies (Table 4.1). In studies that explore the benefits of a relationship with a particular practitioner, there is better recognition of patients' problems and needs, more accurate diagnosis, better concordance with appointment keeping and with treatment advice, fewer hospitalizations, fewer emergency visits, lower costs, better prevention of some types, better prescribing, fewer reported unmet needs, and more satisfaction if there is a long-term relationship between patient and an individual practitioner. If the individual identifies a place (rather than no place) as the regular source of care, appointment keeping is better and there are fewer hospitalizations, but the effect on the latter is minimal. There is also better prevention of most types, especially those that are not associated with specific organ systems; that is, if

	Identification with a Person	Identification with a Place
Better problem and needs recognition	XX	
More accurate and earlier diagnosis	XX	
Better concordance		
Appointment keeping	XX	XX
Treatment advice	XX	
Less emergency room use	XX	
Fewer hospitalizations	XX	X
Lower costs	XX	X
Better prevention (some types)	XX	XX
Better monitoring	X	
Fewer drug prescriptions	X	
Fewer unmet needs	XX	XX
Increased satisfaction	X	

Table 4.1. Benefits of Longitudinality, Based on Evidence from the Literature.

Note: XX: Good evidence. X: Moderate evidence.

patients identify with a place rather than no place, there are benefits but not nearly as many as when the identification is with a person.

Many studies conducted in diverse countries show the importance to patient satisfaction and outcomes of several facets of the doctor-patient relationship: communication involving the patients' ideas about their problems, finding common ground on their management, discussions of how to stay healthy and feeling understood, and how their illness affects their lives (Little and others, 2001; Stewart, 2001).

With Regard to Coordination

Empirical studies of coordination also show benefits. There is a difference in recognition (incorporation into practice) of information about patients according to what type of practitioner is generating and receiving the information. If a physician is following up after himself or herself, information is best recognized. If a physician is following up information generated by another physician, the recognition of the information is less. If a nurse is following up on information generated by a physician, information recognition is even less, and if a physician is following up on information generated by the nurse, there is almost no recognition of the information. Moreover, recognition of information from visits to other facilities, such as emergency department visits, is generally very poor, especially if the patient makes these visits without a specific referral from the primary care practitioner (Starfield, Simborg, Horn, and Yourtee, 1976).

THE ROLE AND BENEFIT OF PRIMARY CARE WITHIN HEALTH SERVICES SYSTEMS

Primary care has an important influence on a population's health. In a major cross-national comparison done in the late 1980s and again five years later, strength of primary care was assessed by scoring components of health systems that are conducive to primary care. Systems or policy characteristics include such things as professional earnings of primary care physicians relative to specialists. Six characteristics address the achievement of the functions of primary care: first contact care, person-focused care over time, comprehensive care, coordinated care, family-centered care, and community orientation. Countries with strong primary care systems had lower health care costs than did countries with weaker primary care infrastructures. Although there is not a linear relationship between the strength of primary care and health outcomes (many other types of factors influence both overall levels of health as well as equity in distribution of health), there is a relationship such that populations of countries with poor primary care services generally have worse health (see the top group of countries in Tables 4.2 to 4.4), although there are important caveats depending on other characteristics of the countries (Starfield and Shi, 2002).

The optimum balance of those features (eleven in the earlier study and fifteen in the later study) that predispose to good outcomes is unknown, but the data provide important clues. The countries with poor primary care and generally poorer outcomes lack policies that attempt to distribute resources according to needs, lack government-provided universal financial coverage for health services, have higher cost sharing for primary care services, have worse comprehensiveness of primary care services, and have services that are not family centered (Starfield and Shi, 2002).

Even within countries, the impact of primary care remains strong on various manifestations of health. For example, states in the United States that have more primary care resources have better health outcomes for just those indicators that would be expected to respond to primary care alone, without also involving specialty care (Shi,

Primary Care Orientation	Low Birth Weight (1993)	Neonatal Mortality (1993)	Postneonatal Mortality (1993)	Infant Mortality (1996)
LOWEST (Belgium, France, Germany, United States)	9.5	7.8	11.5	8.8
MIDDLE (Australia, Canada, Japan, Sweden)	7.3	5.3	5.5	6.0
HIGHEST (Denmark, Finland, Netherlands, Spain, United Kingdom[a])	4.8	7.8	4.6	6.4

Table 4.2. Average Rankings for Health Indicators in Infancy for Thirteen Countries, Grouped by Primary Care Orientation.

Note: The best level of health indicator is ranked 1; worst is ranked 13; thus, lower average ranks indicate better performance.

[a]England and Wales only.

Source: Organization for Economic Cooperation and Development (1998).

	All Except Suicide		Suicide		All Except External	
Primary Care Orientation	Female	Male	Female	Male	Female	Male
LOWEST (Belgium, France, Germany, United States)	9.5	10.8	7.3	8.3	8.8	10.8
MIDDLE (Australia, Canada, Japan, Sweden)	3.8	2.8	7.0	7.3	3.8	3.5
HIGHEST (Denmark, Finland, Netherlands, Spain, United Kingdom[a])	7.6	7.4	6.8	5.8	8.2	7.0

Table 4.3. Average Rankings for Health Indicators, Years of Potential Life Lost (Total and Suicide) in Thirteen Countries, Grouped by Primary Care Orientation.

Note: The best level of health indicator is ranked 1; worst is ranked 13; thus, lower average ranks indicate better performance.

[a]England and Wales only.

Source: Organization for Economic Cooperation and Development (1998).

<table>
<tr><th>Primary Care Orientation</th><th>DALEs[a]</th><th></th><th>Child Survival Equity[b]</th><th></th><th>Overall Health[c]</th><th></th></tr>
<tr><td>LOWEST (Belgium, France, Germany, United States)</td><td>16.3</td><td></td><td>22.5</td><td></td><td>36.3</td><td></td></tr>
<tr><td>MIDDLE (Australia, Canada, Japan, Sweden)</td><td>4.8</td><td rowspan="2">11.0</td><td>16.5</td><td rowspan="2">15.08</td><td>26.0</td><td rowspan="2">29.1</td></tr>
<tr><td>HIGHEST (Denmark, Finland, Netherlands, Spain, United Kingdom)</td><td>16.0</td><td>15.2</td><td>31.6</td></tr>
</table>

Table 4.4. Average Rankings for Health Indicators for Countries Grouped by Primary Care Orientation: World Health Report, 2000.

Note: 1 = highest-ranking country (higher numbers mean poorer ranking). The bracketed figures are the mental health indicator for the middle and highest groups.

[a]DALE = disability-adjusted life expectancy (life lived in good health).

[b]Child survival: survival to age five, adjusted for socioeconomic factors.

[c]Overall health: $\frac{\text{DALE minus DALE in absence of a health system}}{\text{Maximum DALE for health expenditures minus same in absence of a health system}}$

Source: Starfield (1998).

Starfield, Kennedy, and Kawachi, 1999), even when income inequalities within the states are taken into account. (The opposite is the case when the supply of specialists is concerned: health levels are worse with a greater ratio of specialists to population.) While income inequality is significantly related to higher total mortality, higher infant mortality, lower life expectancy, and higher low birth weight ratios, primary care physician availability is independently associated with lower total mortality, lower infant mortality (which is primarily due to its very significant effect on postneonatal mortality), stroke mortality, and higher life expectancy (see Figure 4.2). The effect of primary care is quite strong: each additional primary care physician per 10,000 population reduces total mortality by .34 per 100,000 population in state-level analyses. These conclusions have been confirmed by analyses from the 283 metropolitan areas in the United States, although the effect is much greater for white populations in these areas

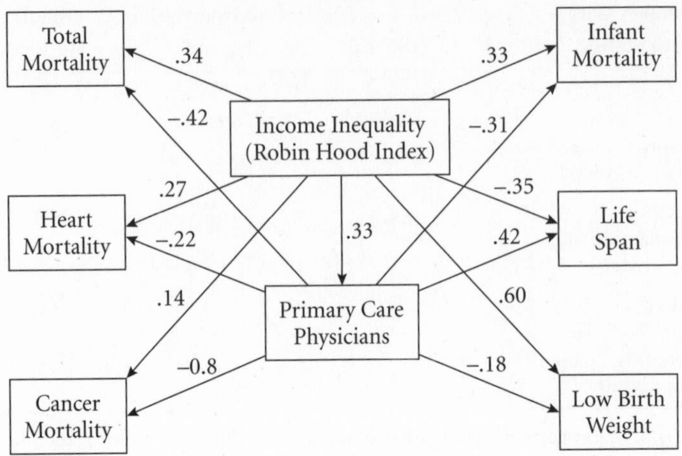

Figure 4.2. Path Coefficients for the Effects of Income Inequality and Primary Care on Mortality, United States, 1990

Note: Coefficients above .03 are significant.

Source: Based on data in Shi, Starfield, Kennedy, and Kawachi (1999).

than for the black populations, for which income inequality is the overwhelmingly more important determinant of mortality (Shi and Starfield, 2001). The findings have also been confirmed in sixty communities in the United States for which there are data on self-reported health, which is better in communities with higher ratios of primary care physician to population (Shi and Starfield, 2000). Clearly, primary care cannot solve all of the adverse effects of an inequitable society, but it can do a lot to reduce their ill effects.

A study conducted in Spain showed the effect of primary care reform on mortality rates for several major causes of death (Villalbi and others, 1999). The researchers divided Barcelona into zones based on how early primary reform was implemented. Theory about the impact of primary care would suggest that deaths associated with hypertension and stroke would be responsive to primary care alone, whereas death from perinatal causes, cervical cancer, and cirrhosis would also require improvements in specialty care for mortality to be reduced. Ten years after the reform was implemented, death rates associated with hypertension and stroke in those zones in which reform was implemented first fell the most. For perinatal causes, death rates fell, but not more in the zones with earlier primary care reform. The same was the case for deaths associated with cervical cancer and cirrhosis. For tuberculosis, rates in all three zones decreased concomitantly with a citywide public health campaign to address the problem.

A recent report from the United Kingdom demonstrated the high salience of the primary care physician to population ratio in the case of in-hospital standardized mortality rates. This factor was more important than the percentage of patients admitted as emergencies, the number of hospital doctors per one hundred hospital beds, and the admission ratio (Jarman and others, 1999). Thus, where it has been examined, primary care makes a major contribution to reductions in mortality in populations.

Primary-care-to-population ratios have been shown to reduce the rate of hospitalizations for at least six ambulatory-care-sensitive conditions among adults in the United States (Parchman and Culler, 1994). There is no relationship between the internists-to-population ratio and the rates of hospitalization for these conditions, which are thought to be preventable by good primary care, but there is a strong and very significant negative relationship between the family physician-to-population ratios and hospitalization rates for these conditions, such that the higher the ratio, the lower the hospitalization rate. The same is the case for children. That is, there is no relationship between the pediatrician-to-population ratio and the rates of hospitalization for the two ambulatory-care-sensitive conditions that were studied, but there is a strong and significant negative relationship between the family-physician-to-population ratio and rates of hospitalization for these conditions.

Another recent national study of the impact of primary care on health showed that adults in the United States with a primary care physician rather than a specialist as their personal physician had one-third lower costs of care and were one-fifth less likely to die, after controlling for the effects of age, gender, income, insurance, smoking, perceived initial health, and eleven major conditions (Franks and Fiscella, 1998).

A summary of the evidence regarding the value of a primary care–led health system indicates substantial benefits. Countries with strong primary care have lower costs and generally healthier populations. Within countries, areas with higher primary care physician-to-population ratios have healthier populations by a variety of measures.

QUALITY OF CARE FROM THE VANTAGE OF PRIMARY CARE

Health is determined by a spectrum of antecedents, including the social and political context in which people find themselves (see Figure 4.1). Although we may continue to think of health as mainly determined by genetic and biological predispositions, these predispositions are heavily conditioned by the context in which they exist. A parsimonious depiction of the variety of types of "causes" of ill health divides them into the political context, the social context, personal exposures and characteristics, as well as the pathophysiological mechanisms through which they operate to increase or decrease risks to illness and the genetic and biological characteristics. Any such simple categorization fails to show the innumerable interactions that undoubtedly exist between and among these types of influences on health. Also unrecognized in such a two-dimensional framework is the influence of time and trajectories over the life course. The influence on adult health of events in very early life and continuing through childhood is now undeniable, although the mechanisms of the trajectories are still unclear. Does early damage always increase risk of subsequent pathology, and under what conditions might it not? Might the effects of early insults be occult, only to be manifested later? Are they mostly gradually accumulating, with each increment leading to progressively greater risks to health later? Or are there vulnerable "incubation" periods during which individuals are particularly susceptible to incurring risks that will be manifested later (Hertzman, Frank, and Evans, 1994)? It is also certain that the pathway of determinants does not act in the same way in all countries, all cultures, and all population subgroups.

The increasing recognition of the multiple causes of illness poses new challenges for both primary care and specialist practice. Although appropriate clinical care for specific conditions is better than inappropriate care, the vision of high-quality primary and specialty care needs better focus.

Because of its centrality within health care systems and its responsibility for coordination of care, quality of health services depends critically on primary care. In the past, and even into the present, the focus of quality assessment and assurance has been mainly on adherence to professional standards (whether based on expert opinion or on evidence from research) for performance of a myriad of diagnostic and therapeutic interventions for specific conditions. However, future challenges for quality of care will increasingly be based on achievement of better health at least cost and with fewest adverse effects. Not all guidelines or standards will lead to better outcomes even when adherence to them is high, largely because the evidence on which they are based is not generalizable to the populations for which they are intended. Low volunteer rates, exclusion of populations with comorbidity, and lack of attention to population representation among the participants in controlled clinical trials make it hazardous to apply the findings to the general population of patients and, especially, of subpopulations. Aging of the population as well as better survival resulting from medical interventions is resulting in greater prevalence of comorbidity within the population. The extent of adverse effects of interventions, whether from frank error or from physiological or psychological responses that could not be anticipated, is increasingly recognized as an important facet of quality of care. Similarly, the influence of the way in which services are delivered has not received the attention it deserves, given its major impact on health outcomes apart from the specific technical interventions that are administered. Last, the new imperative to reduce mortality and improve health-related quality of life for socially disadvantaged populations received special emphasis in the U.S. Health Objectives for the Nation for the year 2010. These national goals make it clear that elimination, not merely reduction, of disparities in health across population subgroups characterized by socioeconomic status, race, ethnicity, disability status, gender, and age is a national priority, along with improving average levels of mortality, morbidity, and health-related quality of life.

Thus, to the conventional focus on technical aspects of diagnosis and treatment, concern for quality of care needs broadening to include four specific and measurable aspects of the provision of health services to populations and subpopulations.

Person-Focused Care and the Importance of Comorbidity

The increasing importance of person-focused assessments, rather than disease-focused assessments, derives largely from the recognition that comorbidity is the rule rather than the exception and that discomfort, dysfunction, and disability result not only from specific medical conditions but from combinations of conditions, as well as the social conditions under which they co-occur. Ten examples show the high salience of comorbidity as a challenge to health services:

- Roos, Carriere, and Friesen (1998) showed that in an entire population of Canadian adult patients with hypertension, only one-third of visits made by these patients in any one year are for that diagnosis. The next most common reason for their visits was diabetes, which accounted for 3 percent of visits. Thus, 63 percent of visits made by patients with hypertension are for a large number of reasons, no one of them accounting for more than 1 percent of visits. It clearly does not make sense to limit considerations of quality of care for patients with hypertension to care of their hypertension, or even to care of their hypertension and their diabetes.
- Clouse and Osterhaus (1994) demonstrated that adults with a diagnosis of migraine have 33 percent greater costs for conditions unrelated to migraine than other patients matched for age, gender, and length of enrollment in a managed care plan.
- One-eighth of the costs of asthma and chronic otitis media and eustachian tube disorders are attributable to diagnosis and treatment of just one comorbidity, sinusitis, rather than the indicator condition (Ray and others, 1999).
- In children with chronic illness, the observed coprevalence for the most common pairs of childhood chronic conditions is one and one-half to four times greater than predicted on the basis of random distribution of these conditions (Newacheck and Stoddard, 1994).
- Insights about the demonstrated relationships of low-grade and largely asymptomatic systemic infections or even low birth weight (Barker and others, 1989) and subsequent coronary heart disease provide powerful evidence of the interrelationships among apparently unrelated types of morbidities and extend these observations even further to considering the impact of clustering of morbidity over the life span from fetal health to old age (Mendall, 1998). That is, diseases cluster in a whole variety of different ways in different individuals (Kunitz, 2002).
- The average number of diagnosed conditions in adults over the age of sixty is two. Over 80 percent of females of between the ages of sixty-five and eighty-five have at least one chronic condition; 50 percent have more than one, and 25 percent have three or more.
- For the U.S. population as a whole, 41 percent have one type of morbidity, 33 percent have two to three types, 6 percent have four to five types, and 1 percent have six to nine types—and these data are

based on diagnoses made in medical visits and thus underrepresent the extent of comorbidity as it exists in populations (unpublished data).

- U.S. national data show that considering only the co-occurrence of obesity, hypertension, diabetes, and hypercholesterolemia, 75 percent of U.S. adults are sick (Schwartz and Woloshin, 1999). Almost one-third of the U.S. adult population have two of these conditions, one-seventh have three, and 3 percent have all four—and this just considers these four conditions.
- Over three in five (63 percent) of those over age sixty-five have more than one type of chronic condition. Per capita Medicare expenditures increase more than linearly with increasing number of types of chronic conditions, from $1,049 for those with one type, $2,374 for two types, $4,269 for three types, and $13,923 for four or more types. Rates of hospitalizations overall and for ambulatory-care-sensitive conditions separately also increase more than linearly, as does the occurrence of preventable complications of hospitalization (Wolff, Starfield, and Anderson, 2002).
- Although the occurrence of comorbidity rises with age, the excess of comorbidity (as compared with what would be expected from chance co-occurrence) is much greater among the young (van den Akker and others, 1998).

A disease-by-disease focus, which has characterized approaches to health services, is becoming increasingly dysfunctional. Existing clinical guidelines apply to individual diagnoses, and even the best ones derive from clinical trials that exclude people with coexisting illnesses. For example, a recent study (Duggan, Elliott, and Logan, 1999) showed that the sensitivity and specificity of a test for *Helicobacter pylori* was much lower when tested in primary care practices than the published values, which came from studies in specialty care. Other recent studies have confirmed the inappropriateness (in primary care) of guidelines developed by specialists in tertiary medical centers. Research by primary care physicians shows how inappropriate such guidelines can be for common conditions such as otitis media, headaches, or hypertension. For example, adherence to guidelines for management of febrile infants leads to no better outcomes (Culpepper and Gilbert, 1999; Green, Hames, and Nutting, 1994; Hetlevik, Holmen, and Kruger, 1999; Kendrick, 2000; Pantell and others, 2000). Evidence-based medicine is surely a desirable approach to ensuring the quality of practice, but existing evidence is not, for the most part, appropriate for primary care. The criteria by which the quality of evidence is based rely heavily on elegance of research methods and internal validity, particularly as manifested by the randomized controlled clinical trial. Unfortunately, the requirements for external validity, or generalizability of the findings to populations other than the ones studied, have not been a major criterion for judging the adequacy of guidelines. Individuals with comorbidity are usually excluded from participation in clinical trials, and the average rate of participation in these trials, even among eligible individuals, is about 15 percent. Minorities participate less in such trials. Trial reports usually report average responses and not the range of responses within the trial group (Guyatt and others, 2000; Naylor, 1995; Maynard, 1997; Mant, 1999). Thus, there is now little evidence for most diagnostic and management interventions in primary care, where the populations, the nature of the problems, and the extent of comorbidity make questionable the application of many, if not most, clinical guidelines.

Minimization of Adverse Effects of Medical Interventions

Health services harm as well as benefit people. It stands to reason that the more the interference with human physiology, which has been adapting to its micro- and macroenvironments for many millennia, the greater the likelihood of unanticipated adverse effects. This is equally the case for people with major health problems as for those without them. The imperative, then, is to do more good than harm. Unfortunately, our ability to detect harm, short of death or major pathology, is now poorer than our ability to detect benefit. Benefit is detected by assessing selected changes in biophysiological characteristics, as well as by assessing increases in life expectancy or improved functional status associated with disease progression. Adverse effects are often not associated with the disease itself but rather relate more generally to derangements in systems that may not be involved in the disease under treatment. Thus, their ascertainment requires a much broader examination of effects than those associated with the disease.

The possibilities for occurrence of adverse effects are of staggering magnitude. The variability in use of technology among Western industrialized nations is extraordinary. In Japan, there are 69.7 CAT scanners per 1 million population; in the United Kingdom, there are 6.3. In Japan, there are 18.8 magnetic resonance imagers per 1 million people; in Canada, there are 1.3. The cascade effect of diagnostic technology is well documented but poorly recognized. For each diagnostic intervention, there is a finite possibility of an adverse effect, even death. The burgeoning use of technology can only increase the number of adverse effects, even if the rate of each decreases due to safer individual ones. It has been determined, for example, that if each prospective jogger is subjected to a diagnostic workup to assess the likelihood of occult cardiac diseases, more people will be killed by the cascade effect of tests than would die simply from unexpected death during jogging (Graboys, 1979).

Per capita expenditures on pharmaceuticals range from $352 per person per year in France to $207 in New Zealand. Since 1990, the rate of introduction of new medications has skyrocketed, with most of the new medications adding little to improve health but much to increased costs of health care systems. The U.S. Institute of Medicine estimated that somewhere between forty-four thousand and ninety-eight thousand deaths per year in the United States result from errors in hospitals (Kohn, Corrigan, and Donaldson, 1999). Deaths due to medication errors are skyrocketing (Phillips, Christenfeld, and Glynn, 1998). Adverse effects of medications due not to medical error but to unanticipated ill effects are calculated to be somewhere between the fourth and sixth leading cause of death in the United States today. When iatrogenic causes of death associated with unnecessary surgery, errors in medication administration, other errors in hospital care, and nosocomial infections (infections acquired in the hospital) are added to the toll of death, then iatrogenic causes amount to the third leading cause of death—225,000 deaths annually—in the United States, after heart disease deaths and cancer deaths and more than cerebrovascular diseases (Starfield, 2000). These figures are underestimates because they derive primarily from studies in hospitals and exclude adverse effects that lead to discomfort and disability rather than death. One analysis of adverse effects in outpatient care determined that 4 to 18 percent (depending on the study) of consecutive patients suffered adverse effects, at a total cost of $77 billion and including 116 million extra doctor visits, 77 million extra prescriptions, 17 million emergency department visits, 8 million hospital admissions, 3 million long-term care admissions, and 199 million additional deaths (Weingart, Wilson, Gibberd, and Harrison, 2000). Moreover, the dangers of iatrogenic illness are not well recognized. The routes by which harm may occur are many (Fisher and Welch, 1999). No current quality assessment program is designed to systematically monitor ill effects from medications, although much anecdotal evidence, particularly in the elderly, indicates that symptomatic side effects are frequently worse than the symptoms from the underlying condition for which the medication is prescribed. Primary care practitioners face the greatest challenge for detecting adverse effects because of their focus on people instead of diseases and because of their coordinating function.

Primary Care as an Influence on Outcomes

The evidence cited above regarding the importance of primary care suggests that the adequacy of primary care should be an intervening variable in clinical trials. If a good relationship with a particular provider leads to better outcomes, shouldn't all clinical trials include it as a modifying or mediating factor?

The Imperative for Equity

Equity is the absence of systematic and potentially remediable differences in one or more aspects of health across populations or population groups defined socially, economically, demographically, or geographically (Starfield, 2001a, 2001b; International Society for Equity in Health, 2003). The imperative to eliminate differences in health and health services across population groups distinguished by race/ethnicity, gender, age, educational attainment, income level, and disability status is made clear in the most recent goals and objectives for the nation (U.S. Department of Health and Human Services, 2000). The imperative to achieve equity is thus clear, at least in the United States.

Although there are few studies of the impact of health services in reducing inequities, some show that achievement of equity is at least partly facilitated by better primary care services. That is, primary care has an equity-producing effect that is most pronounced for measures of health that are especially responsive to primary care, such as postneonatal mortality, stroke mortality, and self-perceived health (Shi and Starfield, 2000).

There are new techniques that make it possible to characterize comorbidity, detect adverse effects, measure the effect of different ways of organizing and delivering services (especially primary care), and visualize how primary care contributes to equity in health. The necessary tools are available.

Comorbidity can be represented by techniques such as the Adjusted Clinical Group (formerly Ambulatory Care Groups) system developed at the Johns Hopkins University (Starfield, Weiner, Mumford, and Steinwachs, 1991; Johns Hopkins University, 2003). This system takes all diagnoses made on each individual in a year and combines them in such a way as to provide a "burden of morbidity" pattern unique to each individual or aggregated to describe a population of people.

The International Classification of Primary Care (Lamberts, Wood, and Hofmans-Okkes, 1993) is a well-developed and well-tested system of coding and classifying symptoms and signs, which could be put to good use in documenting and monitoring the occurrence of adverse effects of interventions, including medications.

Every evaluation of effectiveness of an intervention should include among its study variables important characteristics of the health delivery system, including the level of care at which the intervention is provided (specialty care or primary care), the type of practitioner prescribing the intervention, and the duration and nature of the relationship between the practitioner and the patient, as these have been amply demonstrated to influence the outcome of care. All evaluations of the quality of care should include consideration of the adequacy of primary care characteristics as well as clinical characteristics. Validated instruments such as the Primary Care Assessment Tools (PCAT; Shi, Starfield, and Xu, 2001), which is available in comparable form for adults, children, and the providers, make it possible to do this in a standard way.

All consideration of the determinants of disease, whether in patients or in populations and including both conventional epidemiological and clinical investigations, should include variables that reflect the ecological context in which people live. At the very least, information should be obtained to make it possible to link individual or population characteristics with area characteristics from census and other data, with due regard for the assurance of confidentiality and security of the data. Only in this way can the imperative to understand and eliminate inequity be accomplished.

LESSONS FOR SPECIALTY CARE FROM PRIMARY CARE

Concerted research over the past ten years has contributed extensive knowledge about the special contributions of primary care and of its centrality within health services systems. It has been constructed, deconstructed, and reconstructed, so that the knowledge gained provides a sound basis for policy and decision making.

The same cannot be said for specialty care, about which little is known. It is commonly assumed that specialists should carry the burden of disease management in the area of their specialty. Clinical classification systems for diseases often take on the name of the specialist rather than the disease type (for example, *cardiology* rather than *heart disease* and *dermatology* rather than *skin disease*) despite the fact that the vast majority of diseases are seen more commonly in primary care than in specialty care (Starfield and others, 2003). The following account demonstrates how little is known about the responsibilities of specialty care. In the course of a research project to ascertain the primary care experiences of individual children being seen in specialty clinics, the specialists seeing the patients in the specialty clinic were asked to indicate about how long they expected to be caring for the individual patient before returning the patient to primary care. None of the specialists was able to answer the question for any of the patients. The specialists had never considered their care in the context of the overall care of the patient.

The challenge now is to take what has been learned about primary care and make it useful for learning about specialty care and about the relationship between primary care and specialty care. The challenge is particularly acute in the United States, where specialists practice in the community alongside primary care physicians. In many other countries, specialty care is clearly distinguished from primary care because specialists customarily are limited to practice in hospitals, with clearer roles and expectations.

Developing a Framework for Conceptualizing Specialty Care Is Needed

The elements of such a framework might start with descriptions of the types of problems dealt with by specialists. The National Ambulatory Care Surveys provide data on the problems appearing in the practices of different specialists as well as the diagnoses made. However, there has been no attempt to determine the variability of these problems and diagnoses within specialty practice or the reasons that patients self-refer or are referred to specialists. A recent study documented the variability among primary care physicians in decisions about which specialty to target referrals (Forrest, Nutting, Starfield, and von Schrader, 2002). At least two different specialties were reported as the target for referrals for patients with the same specific diagnosis. The reasons for this variability are unclear. Is it a result of different perceptions of primary care physicians as to the domain of different specialties, or is it associated with differences in the problems prompting referral? For example, referred patients with low back pain are sent to physical therapists 28 percent of the time and to orthopedists 23 percent of the time; the other half of referred patients with back pain are sent to a variety of other specialists (Starfield, Forrest, Nutting, and von Schrader, 2002). Is this the case because there are differences according to whether the primary care physician just needs advice on management or whether the need is for a definitive intervention that is provided only by one of the possible types of specialists? To what extent do different types of specialists provide different services, even when the patient's problem is the same?

A second consideration for conceptualizing the province of specialty care concerns the nature of the care provided. To what extent does specialty care address the various functions of referral? What is the balance among the three main purposes of referral: need for advice and guidance on diagnosis and management (consultative care), short-term care consisting primarily of technically challenging diagnostic tests or procedures that cannot be provided in primary care, or long-term transferral of patients for management of technically complex or very unusual disease challenges? Although studies of reasons for referral and coordination of care are sparse, studies in the United States indicate that about half of referrals are for one-time advice and guidance on diagnosis or management (Forrest, Nutting, Starfield, and von Schrader, 2002; Forrest and others, 1999).

Explicitly Recognizing That Prevention Is in the Province of Both Specialists as Well as Primary Care Physicians

Although primary care physicians generally provide better preventive care for those aspects of prevention that are person focused rather than disease focused and primary prevention rather than secondary prevention, specialists often do better for preventive activities and secondary prevention (screening) in the specific area of their specialty. Prevention is not a defining feature of primary care any more than curative care is a defining feature of specialty care. The challenge is to determine what types of prevention are more effectively and efficiently done by which types of health professionals.

Developing Mechanisms of Communication Between Primary Care and Specialty Care to Enhance Coordination

Specialist care consists of specific functions, although the nature and extent of the balance between these functions are unknown.

The consultative function, wherein there is need for only one-time advice and guidance to the primary care function, is a short-term reason for referral. Customarily, patients are referred to the specialist, who often conveys the advice to the patients rather than back to the referring physician. Could the bulk of these referrals be replaced with systems wherein specialists provide the advice directly to the primary care physician rather than requiring a visit of the patient to the specialist? Videoconferencing is making it possible to do this when primary care physicians and their patients are located at great distance from the specialists. Could it not be done routinely when the need is solely for advice to the primary care physician?

Need for surgery constitutes about one-fifth of all reasons for referral, and either surgery or a nonsurgical technical procedure is a reason for referral in about three of eight referrals. The extent to which specialists retain patients longer than expected by either the patient or the primary care physician is unknown (Forrest, Nutting, Starfield, and von Schrader, 2002) but has major implications for costs and organization of services.

Shared care is an increasingly recognized aspect of primary care–specialist interrelationships and a potentially useful way to improve coordination of care. The extent to which primary care physicians receive and follow up on the care provided by specialists to whom they refer patients is unknown, as is the variability in this aspect of coordination. It is almost certainly unusual for a primary care physician to receive information about the care provided to patients who have self-referred to specialists, although there is undoubtedly great variability in this aspect of coordination of care. Experiments with shared care seem to be more common in the United Kingdom than in the United States, possibly because most specialist care is provided by hospital-based specialists and there is greater flexibility in developing new ways of organizing services because lines of responsibility for primary care and specialty care are clearer than in the United States. In these experiments, shared care arrangements are highly diverse, including specialist consultations directly in the primary care physicians' offices; e-mail with a common database with multiple access ports; computer-assisted shared care with an agreed-on database to be collected; shared patient cards either held by the patient or mailed back and forth between primary care physician and specialist; liaison meetings; or even sharing of resources in which consultants do not see patients but provide education, support, and strategic planning to the primary care physician (Greenhalgh, 1994). A preliminary descriptive study in U.S. pediatrician offices found that the pediatricians scheduled the referred patient to see the specialist and sent patient information to the specialist in about half the referrals. The odds of a referral completion were increased threefold when the primary care physician scheduled the appointment and communicated with the specialist about the patient (Forrest and others, 2000). The primary care physician expressed interest in subsequent shared care with the specialist in three-fourths of all referrals (Forrest and others, 1999). Knowledge about these types of practices and attempts at coordination, even in organized health services delivery settings, is extremely sparse but appears important in helping to specify appropriate educational and continuing education experiences of primary care physicians as well as of specialists.

CONCLUSION

The construction, deconstruction, reconstruction, and revisualization of the roles of primary care suggest that broad policy changes will have to occur before primary care can assume its place in the U.S. health care system. No one change is likely to be effective in making the transition from specialty orientation to primary care orientation with strong and appropriate specialty support.

In 1993, Starfield and Simpson posed a dozen changes to U.S. policy that would be required to elevate primary care to its proper place within the health care system. Ten years later, few, if any, of the changes have occurred. Costs continue to rise, and outcomes, relative to those of other industrialized countries, have not improved. The World Health Organization, in its evaluation of 191 countries (2000), including the poorest developing nations as well as the richer industrialized ones, ranked the United States twenty-fourth in disability-adjusted life expectancy, thirty-second in child survival equity, and fifty-fourth to fifty-fifth on fairness of financial contributions to health systems. It is time to take stock of what primary care can achieve if it is properly organized and financed. Recent "reforms," although often undertaken in the name of primary care, have been in the wrong direction because the reformers have not understood the spirit of primary care: person-focused care over time, comprehensive, coordinating, and first contact. Only major changes in national health policy can change the course.

References

Barker, L. R., and others. "Recognition of Information and Coordination of Ambulatory Care by Medical Residents." *Medical Care,* 1989, *27,* 558–562.

Clouse, J. C., and Osterhaus, J. T. "Healthcare Resource Use and Costs Associated with Migraine in a Managed Healthcare Setting." *Annals of Pharmacotherapy,* 1994, *28,* 659–664.

Culpepper, L., and Gilbert, T. T. "Evidence and Ethics." *Lancet,* 1999, *353,* 829–831.

Duggan, A. E., Elliott, C., and Logan, R. F. "Testing for *Helicobacter pylori* Infection: Validation and Diagnostic Yield of a Near Patient Test in Primary Care." *British Medical Journal,* 1999, *319,* 1236–1239.

Fisher, E. S., and Welch, H. G. "Avoiding the Unintended Consequences of Growth in Medical Care: How Might More Be Worse?" *Journal of the American Medical Association,* 1999, *281,* 446–453.

Forrest, C. B., Nutting, P. A., Starfield, B., and von Schrader, S. "Family Physicians' Referral Decisions: Results from the ASPN Referral Study." *Journal of Family Practice,* 2002, *51,* 215–222.

Forrest, C. B., and Starfield, B. "The Effect of First-Contact Care with Primary Care Clinicians on Ambulatory Health Care Expenditures." *Journal of Family Practice,* 1996, *43,* 40–48.

Forrest, C. B., and others. "The Pediatric Primary-Specialty Care Interface: How Pediatricians Refer Children and Adolescents to Specialty Care." *Archives of Pediatric and Adolescent Medicine,* 1999, *153,* 705–714.

Forrest, C. B., and others. "Coordination of Specialty Referrals and Physician Satisfaction with Referral Care." *Archives of Pediatric and Adolescent Medicine,* 2000, *154,* 499–506.

Franks, P., and Fiscella, K. "Primary Care Physicians and Specialists as Personal Physicians: Health Care Expenditures and Mortality Experience." *Journal of Family Practice,* 1998, *47,* 105–109.

Graboys, T. B. "The Economics of Screening Joggers." *New England Journal of Medicine,* 1979, *301,* 1067.

Green, L. A., Hames, C.G.S., and Nutting, P. A. "Potential of Practice-Based Research Networks: Experiences from ASPN. Ambulatory Sentinel Practice Network." *Journal of Family Practice,* 1994, *38,* 400–406.

Greenhalgh, P. M. *Shared Care for Diabetes: A Systematic Review.* London: Royal College of General Practitioners, 1994.

Guyatt, G. H., and others. "Users' Guides to the Medical Literature: XXV. Evidence-Based Medicine: Principles for Applying the Users' Guides to Patient Care. Evidence-Based Medicine Working Group." *Journal of the American Medical Association,* 2000, *284,* 1290–1296.

Hertzman, C., Frank, J., and Evans, R. G. "Heterogeneities in Health Status and the Determinants of Population Health." In R. G. Evans, M. Barer, and T. Marmor (eds.), *Why Are Some People Healthy and Others Not?* New York: Aldine de Gruyer, 1994.

Hetlevik, I., Holmen, J., and Kruger, O. "Implementing Clinical Guidelines in the Treatment of Hypertension in General Practice: Evaluation of Patient Outcome Related to Implementation of a Computer-Based Clinical Decision Support System." *Scandinavian Journal of Primary Health Care,* 1999, *17,* 35–40.

Institute of Medicine Committee on the Future of Primary Care. *Primary Care: America's Health in a New Era.* Washington, D.C.: National Academy Press, 1996.

International Society for Equity in Health. Sept. 2003. [www.iseqh.org].

Jarman, B., and others. "Explaining Differences in English Hospital Death Rates Using Routinely Collected Data." *British Medical Journal,* 1999, *318,* 1515–1520.

Johns Hopkins University. ACG Case-Mix System. [http://acg.jhsph.edu]. Sept. 2003.

Kendrick, T. "Why Can't GPs Follow Guidelines on Depression? We Must Question the Basis of the Guidelines Themselves." *British Medical Journal,* 2000, *320,* 200–201.

Kohn, L., Corrigan, J., and Donaldson, M. *To Err Is Human: Building a Safer Health System.* Washington, D.C.: National Academy Press, 1999.

Kunitz, S. J. "Holism and the Idea of General Susceptibility to Disease." *International Journal of Epidemiology,* 2002, *31,* 722–729.

Lamberts, H., Wood, M., and Hofmans-Okkes, I. *The International Classification of Primary Care in the European Community.* New York: Oxford University Press, 1993.

Little, P., and others. "Preferences of Patients for Patient Centred Approach to Consultation in Primary Care: Observational Study." *British Medical Journal,* 2001, *322,* 468–472.

Mant, D. "Can Randomised Trials Inform Clinical Decisions About Individual Patients?" *Lancet,* 1999, *353,* 743–746.

Maynard, A. "Evidence-Based Medicine: An Incomplete Method for Informing Treatment Choices." *Lancet,* 1997, *349,* 126–128.

Mendall, M. A. "Inflammatory Responses and Coronary Heart Disease." *British Medical Journal,* 1998, *316,* 953–954.

Naylor, C. D. "Grey Zones of Clinical Practice: Some Limits to Evidence-Based Medicine." *Lancet,* 1995, *345,* 840–842.

Newacheck, P. W., and Stoddard, J. J. "Prevalence and Impact of Multiple Childhood Chronic Illnesses." *Journal of Pediatrics,* 1994, *124,* 40–48.

Organization for Economic Cooperation and Development. *OECD Health Data 1998.* Paris: OECD, 1998.

Pantell, R., and others. "Detecting Serious Bacterial Illness in Febrile Infants: Do Guidelines Help?" Paper presented at the 2000 Pediatric Academic Societies meeting, 2000. [http://www.aap.org/research/pros/biblio.htm].

Parchman, M. L., and Culler, S. "Primary Care Physicians and Avoidable Hospitalizations." *Journal of Family Practice,* 1994, *39,* 123–128.

Phillips, D. P., Christenfeld, N., and Glynn, L. M. "Increase in U.S. Medication-Error Deaths Between 1983 and 1993." *Lancet,* 1998, *351,* 643–644.

Ray, N. F., and others. "Healthcare Expenditures for Sinusitis in 1996: Contributions of Asthma, Rhinitis, and Other Airway Disorders." *Journal of Allergy and Clinical Immunology,* 1999, *103,* 408–414.

Roos, N. P., Carriere, K. C., and Friesen, D. "Factors Influencing the Frequency of Visits by Hypertensive Patients to Primary Care Physicians in Winnipeg." *Canadian Medical Association Journal,* 1998, *159,* 777–783.

Schwartz, L. M., and Woloshin, S. "Changing Disease Definitions: Implications for Disease Prevalence. Analysis of the Third National Health and Nutrition Examination Survey, 1988–1994." *Effective Clinical Practice,* 1999, *2,* 76–85.

Shi, L., and Starfield, B. "Primary Care, Income Inequality, and Self-Rated

Health in the United States: A Mixed-Level Analysis." *International Journal of Health Services,* 2000, *30,* 541–555.

Shi, L., and Starfield, B. "The Effect of Primary Care Physician Supply and Income Inequality on Mortality Among Blacks and Whites in US Metropolitan Areas." *American Journal of Public Health,* 2001, *91,* 1246–1250.

Shi, L., Starfield, B., Kennedy, B. P., and Kawachi, I. "Income Inequality, Primary Care, and Health Indicators." *Journal of Family Practice,* 1999, *48,* 275–284.

Shi, L., Starfield, B., and Xu, J. "Validating the Adult Primary Care Assessment Tool." *Journal of Family Practice,* 2001, *50,* 161W–175W. [http://jfponline.com/content/2001/02/jfp_0201_01610.asp].

Starfield, B. *Primary Care: Balancing Health Needs, Services, and Technology.* New York: Oxford University Press, 1998.

Starfield, B. *Primary Care: Concept, Evaluation, and Policy. (2nd ed.)* New York: Oxford University Press, 1999.

Starfield, B. "Is U.S. Health Really the Best in the World?" *Journal of the American Medical Association,* 2000, *284,* 483–485.

Starfield B. "Basic Concepts in Population Health and Health Care." *Journal of Epidemiology and Community Health,* 2001a, *55,* 452–454.

Starfield B. "Improving Equity in Health: A Research Agenda." *International Journal of Health Services,* 2001b, *31,* 545–566.

Starfield, B., Forrest, C. B., Nutting, P. A., and von Schrader, S. "Variability in Physician Referral Decisions." *Journal of the American Board of Family Practice,* 2002, *15,* 473–480.

Starfield, B., and Shi, L. "Policy Relevant Determinants of Health: An International Perspective." *Health Policy,* 2002, *60,* 201–218.

Starfield, B., Simborg, D. W., Horn, S. D., and Yourtee, S. A. "Continuity and Coordination in Primary Care: Their Achievement and Utility." *Medical Care,* 1976, *14,* 625–636.

Starfield, B., and Simpson, L. "Primary Care as Part of U.S. Health Services Reform." *Journal of the American Medical Association,* 1993, *269,* 3136–3139.

Starfield, B., Weiner, J., Mumford, L., and Steinwachs, D. "Ambulatory Care Groups: A Categorization of Diagnoses for Research and Management." *Health Services Research,* 1991, *26,* 53–74.

Starfield, B., and others. "Co-Morbidity: Implications for the Importance of Primary Care in 'Case' Management." *Annals of Family Medicine,* 2003, *1,* 8–14.

Stewart, M. "Towards a Global Definition of Patient Centred Care." *British Medical Journal,* 2001, *322,* 444–445.

U.S. Department of Health and Human Services. *Healthy People 2010: Understanding and Improving Health and Objectives for Improving Health.* (2nd ed.) Washington, D.C.: U.S. Government Printing Office, 2000.

van den Akker, M., and others. "Multimorbidity in General Practice: Prevalence, Incidence, and Determinants of Co-Occurring Chronic and Recurrent Diseases." *Journal of Clinical Epidemiology,* 1998, *51,* 367–375.

Villalbi, J. R., and others. "An Evaluation of the Impact of Primary Care Reform on Health." *Atencion Primaria,* 1999, *24,* 468–474.

Weingart, S. N., Wilson, R. M., Gibberd, R. W., and Harrison, B. "Epidemiology of Medical Error." *British Medical Journal,* 2000, *320,* 774–777.

Wolff, J. L., Starfield, B., and Anderson, G. "Prevalence, Expenditures, and Complications of Multiple Chronic Conditions in the Elderly." *Archives of Internal Medicine,* 2002, *162,* 2269–2276.

World Health Organization. *The World Health Report 2000. Health Systems: Improving Performance.* Geneva: World Health Organization, 2000.

CHAPTER FIVE

Nontraditional Approaches to Primary Care Delivery

Helen Burstin
Carolyn Clancy

> *Patients, too, must recognize these trends and adapt to them. Greater knowledge and the resulting rise in specialization, the increasing institutionalization of medical practice and its greater concentration in urban areas, greater reliance upon diagnostic tests and equipment and upon skilled aides all permit higher quality of medical service to a larger number of patients. Patients must recognize that the benefits of these changes far outweigh the loss of the greater amount of personal attention, the more frequent house calls, and the more leisurely pace of medical practice a generation ago.*
>
> —*Citizens Commission on Graduate Medical Education, 1966*

The opinions expressed in this chapter are those of the authors and do not necessarily reflect those of the Agency for Healthcare Research and Quality or the U.S. Department of Health and Human Services.

Although this passage was written as part of the Millis Commission Report in 1966, it provides an appropriate assessment of what has happened to primary care through 2001. The perspective that "patients will adapt" has clearly driven many of the changes in modern health care. Although patients may recognize the advantages that modern medicine has brought in terms of improved diagnosis and treatment, something has been steadily lost from primary care practice for many years. The idealized version of primary care would include an ongoing, continuous, comprehensive relationship with a provider who can provide primary access to the health care system and help navigate the increasingly complex maze of modern health care. With the continued proliferation of interventions and information sources, navigation has never been more critical. The primary care provider would be compassionate, considerate, and able to assist with a patient's total health and illness needs, and he or she would consider the patient in the context of family and community. The patient would receive the "great amount of personal attention" that was apparently lost in the modern medical era.

In this chapter, we review what has happened to many of the core constructs of primary care, particularly focusing on the forces within medicine and society that have shaped the changes in primary care that we have witnessed. We then examine nontraditional approaches to primary care delivery, such as e-health, urgent care services, self-care, complementary medicine, and specialty care for chronic illness, which may provide valuable insights for primary care. This reconstruction of primary care will depend on a thorough assessment of the forces that led to the deconstruction, as well as how and why patients have moved to these nontraditional approaches for care once thought to be the domain of the primary care physician. As we review what has been lost from the core constructs of primary care, we can begin to see the elements from these nontraditional approaches that can be reconstructed into a more patient-centered and patient-responsive primary care system.

CORE CONSTRUCTS OF PRIMARY CARE

Primary care is defined as care "which provides integrated, accessible health care services by clinicians who are accountable for addressing a large majority of personal health care needs, developing a sustained partnership with patients, and practicing in the context of family and community" (Donaldson, Yordy, Lohr, and Vanselow, 1996, p. 1). Starfield's criteria (1992) for primary care emphasize seven important features: continuous, first contact, comprehensive, coordinated, community oriented, family centered, and culturally competent. A review of the forces that have influenced these core constructs may help us better understand primary care in the current context of health care in the twenty-first century.

The concept of a continuous, "sustained partnership with patients" has been an enduring hallmark of the definition of primary care (Leopold, Cooper, and Clancy, 1996). In a recent comparison of primary care providers, American patients were more likely to value continuity with their doctor than were their British counterparts. This higher value assigned to continuity of care was associated with a higher level of trust with the provider (Mainous and others, 2001). An individual's trust in his or her primary care physician has been demonstrated by Safran to be predictive of willingness to attempt difficult lifestyle changes (Safran and others, 1998), and negative perceptions of the physician-patient relationship are associated with voluntary disenrollment (Safran and others, 2001). Patients unable to choose their own physician may also be less satisfied with care received (Schmittdiel, Selby, Grumbach, and Quesenberry, 1997). Greater continuity has been associated with improved outcomes, such as less emergency department utilization (Christakis and others, 2001). As managed care has forced some patients to discontinue care with their usual provider for the sake of staying within a health plan, patients' access to care has worsened (Burstin and others, 1998). For example, patients who changed providers in a given year were more likely to report that they delayed getting care when they needed it. However, in some circumstances, patients are willing to make trade-offs in continuity for easier access. For example, with an acute illness, some patients would prefer to see another provider rather than wait for their own provider (Love and Mainous, 1999).

Another key feature of primary care is first contact use. There are reasonable data to suggest that first contact with a primary care provider can reduce use of specialists and emergency departments. In a study from the 1987 National Medical Expenditure Survey, Forrest and Starfield (1998) found that several features of practice resulted in fewer first contact visits with a primary care provider, including absence of extended office hours and longer travel times. Overall, generalists provided more first contact care than specialists due to more accessible office practices. As specialty-trained physicians increasingly provide primary care services, it will be important to examine the persistence of access barriers to first contact care (Rosenblatt and others, 1995). Rosenblatt's study (Rosenblatt and others, 1998) assessing the contribution made by specialists to primary care for Medicare beneficiaries demonstrated that older patients whose principal physician is a specialist are less likely to receive recommended preventive services than those seen by a generalist physician.

Although a distinguishing characteristic in the definition of primary care explicitly articulates "addressing a large majority of personal health care needs," this may be an area in which primary care has fallen short. In a study by Levinson, Gorawara-Bhat, and Lamb (2000), patients frequently offered clues to their emotional or social feelings that went undetected by providers. Overall, primary care providers missed opportunities to respond to patients' clues in 79 percent of cases. Given that most clues were emotional in nature, this reticence to respond to clues may reflect underlying physician discomfort in dealing with these issues. Perhaps most disturbing from the primary care perspective, the surgeons in the study performed slightly better than primary care physicians in responding to patient clues.

The role of the primary care provider has shifted with the changing dynamics of the rapidly evolving health care system. As health care has grown more complex and technical, there has been a systemic shift that favors expensive, high-tech, and specialized care. With the rise of managed care, the role of the primary care provider has changed in many ways that may not be desirable to patients and providers alike. In some ways, primary care can be a lens through which one can witness some of the least welcomed and anticipated changes in the health care system. In its latest iteration, it could be argued that primary care has evolved from a conceptual model to a structural model defined by health insurance companies, encompassed by the phrase, "Primary care is everything you can get without a referral." In this more structural model, primary care is defined as much by what it is not—procedurally oriented specialty care—rather than the essence of what it is. The primary care provider may be increasingly viewed as the way station on the way to the "real" care that the patient desires.

Although managed care has been perceived as a strong, often negative, force in primary care, many physician decisions are more strongly influenced by personal characteristics, such as age, gender and training, and practice setting (Landon, Reschovsky, Reed, and Blumenthal, 2001). The practice setting, such as group or individual practice, can also play an important role. In the Community Tracking Survey of the Center for Studying Health System Change, primary care providers did not demonstrate significant influence in decision making by managed care or financial arrangements.

Although the primary care provider is supposed to provide accessible health care services, this provider is often viewed as the bottleneck to needed health care services. The gatekeeping role assigned to primary care often places primary care physicians in an adversarial role with other providers, as well as patients. As outlined by Eisenberg in 1985, the gatekeeper role "goes beyond the concept of the primary care physician as manager of the patient's medical care who ensures quality and coordination" to the "fulcrum for containing costs" (p. 537). One potential role of gatekeeping was to avoid specialty services for care that would be best addressed by primary care (Franks, Clancy, and Nutting, 1992). These gatekeeping models were clearly intended to reduce costs, though they have not made a significant impact on specialty use, as compared to point-of-service health maintenance organization (HMO) plans (Joyce, Kapur, Van Vorst, and Escarce, 2000). In a study by Grumbach and others (1999), patients who had difficulty obtaining referrals were much more likely to report low trust and low satisfaction with their primary provider.

While the gatekeeper role offered primary care a prominent role in the managed care system, the gatekeeper who denied access to services likely left a negative impression on patients and providers alike. The primary care providers' perception of the gatekeeper role may also be leading providers to care for patients beyond their own comfort level. In a disturbing study, St. Peter, Reed, Kemper, and Blumenthal (1999) found that one in four primary care physicians reported that the scope of care that they were expected to provide exceeded their own perception of what would be an appropriate scope for their practice. The concern over excessive scope was more common among pediatricians and general internists, compared to family or general practitioners. Perhaps most disturbing, physicians who derived part of the revenue from capitation were more likely to report concern about excessive scope of practice.

NONTRADITIONAL APPROACHES TO PRIMARY CARE DELIVERY

The growth in the delivery of primary care–type services by nontraditional sources and providers of primary care services likely reflects dissatisfaction with the devolution of the primary care model. If viewed as a set of modular services, including physical examinations, first-line treatment for common ailments, preventive services, and psychosocial needs, it is easy to see how other providers could deliver these services. Some of these nontraditional approaches, such as utilization of the emergency department, complementary and alternative medicine, and self-care, address selected elements of primary care, though the care is often provided outside the traditional realm of the primary care provider.

Emergency Services

Particularly for uninsured and low-income populations, the emergency department often serves as the path into the health care system. This reliance on emergency department services for nonurgent conditions has been well documented. Many patients use emergency department services as a substitute for primary care. Although it is also known that patients who rely on emergency departments use costlier services and often receive unnecessary treatment that could have been avoided, there are clearly lessons for primary care in the reasons that patients seek emergency department care, especially for nonurgent conditions.

Although a core construct of primary care is accessibility, the lack of universal access in the United States creates formidable barriers for poor and uninsured patients to office-based primary care services. For uninsured and low-income patients, the emergency department may provide more accessible services than primary care providers. The 1986 Emergency Medical Treatment and Active Labor Act requires that all patients who arrive in the emergency department be seen by a provider and stabilized or treated, regardless of their ability to pay. This ability to access emergency services without fear of being turned away may draw in patients with limited access to the health care system. As required payment at the time of service has grown more prevalent in health care systems, the emergency department often remains a site of care that will bill for services rendered.

While only approximately 6.3 percent of the population used nonurgent emergency department visits (Cunningham, Clancy, Cohen, and Wilets, 1995), this usage has been associated with important access barriers to primary care. For example, Medicaid patients are more likely to use emergency departments in part due to difficulties accessing office-based physicians willing to accept Medicaid fee schedules. In addition, Cunningham, Clancy, Cohen, and Wilets (1995) found that very young children were more likely to access the emergency department for nonurgent care, possibly related to parents' inability to reach their usual provider after hours. Patients who use emergency departments for ambulatory care were more likely to report nonfinancial barriers to care, such as inability to access evening services or get off work, no timely clinic appointments, and failed attempts to get care elsewhere (Young and others, 1996). In a cross-sectional survey of patients presenting to fifty-six emergency departments over a twenty-four-hour period, patients who used emergency departments for ambulatory care were more likely to report nonfinancial barriers rather than financial barriers to care. These nonfinancial barriers included an inability to access evening services or get off work, inaccessible clinic services at the time they were needed, and failed attempts to get care elsewhere (Young and others, 1996).

In a New York City study, 34 percent reported convenience as the primary reason for using emergency room services, and only 21 percent reported any contact with a physician or other health care provider prior to their visit to the emergency department. While emergency departments may not offer continuous care and a sustained partnership with a provider over time, the use of emergency care may reflect the higher relative value that patients put on accessibility over the other core constructs of primary care.

While emergency department use for nonurgent conditions may offer important insights into the failings of the primary care system, an ongoing relationship with a primary care provider has been found to be an important mitigating factor for nonurgent emergency department use, regardless of insurance status or health status (Petersen and others, 1998). In addition, access to a primary care provider can help to reduce perceived delays in needed emergency care (Rucker, Brennan, and Burstin, 2001). While a relationship with a primary care provider can reduce the perceived need for emergency department visits, it does not appear to eliminate nonurgent use (Baker and others, 1994).

An attempt to codify the level of emergency department use by primary care accessibility was recently developed by Billings (Billings, Parikh, and Mihanovich, 2000). This classification system has four categories: nonemergent (immediate medical care was not required within twelve hours); emergent or primary care treatable (treatment was required within twelve hours but could have been provided in a primary care setting); emergent or emergency department care required but potentially preventable or avoidable if timely and effective primary care were available; and emergent or emergency department care required and not preventable or avoidable. Excluding emergency department patients who were admitted to the hospital, Billings (Billings, Parikh, and Mihanovich, 2000) found that only one of five emergency department visits in New York City was provided for emergency conditions that were not preventable. These data would suggest that patients are using emergency department services because of identified failings of the primary care system.

Another perspective on nonurgent emergency department use was offered by a Canadian study that found that among a largely insured cohort, patients reported that their primary care physicians did not educate them about when to see emergency care or the kinds of services that were available in the office (Boushy and Dubinsky, 1999). In addition, the authors found that 55 percent of patients used the emergency department because it was more convenient for them. This and multiple other studies suggest that the more traditional office hours of primary care physicians are leading patients to seek care when it is convenient for them. The apparent overuse of emergency services is quite complex, related to access, payment, knowledge, and convenience. Primary care needs to be more responsive to the stated needs and preferences of patients that are driving nonurgent emergency department use.

Primary Care On-Line

Although health and disease education for patients has been viewed as a critical role for primary care providers, patients are increasingly accessing needed health care information on their own. The new e-health consumers are searching for three elements: convenience, control, and choice (Ball and Lillis, 2001). The Internet and health care Web sites have opened a portal of information on health care previously unavailable to the lay public and provided mainly in health care encounters. With these health interactive technologies, patients can become more active partners in their own care. If patients are more knowledgeable about their own health care needs, a more seamless connection could be forged between patients and providers. Alternatively, the use of on-line services could reflect public sentiment that primary care is falling short on the core construct of "addressing the majority of personal health needs." This perceived need for patients to address their own personal health needs likely reflects an inability or unwillingness of primary care providers to share information in a way that patients can understand it. While only 8 percent of U.S. households had a computer in 1984, it was estimated that 51 percent had computers in 2000. At least half of U.S. users of the Internet reported spending time looking for health information or support (Eng and others, 1998). With limited face-to-face time with physicians, patients are taking a more active role in their care and turning to the Internet for health information (Kolata, 2000). The Internet allows patients to access health care information in a timely and flexible manner, not constrained by the office hours of their primary care provider. In August 2000, a Harris Interactive poll found that 98 million adults used the Internet to find health information. This represented an 81 percent increase in use in two years.

Informed health care consumers are advocating an open portal of electronic communication with providers. Interactive technology, such as e-mail with providers, encourages continuous, seamless primary care with patients and their families. E-mail has been identified as an important tool for timely communication between patients and providers. An e-mail relationship with providers can allow patients to become more active partners in their own care, assist with chronic disease management, and enhance joint decision making. Nearly all online patients report that they would like to exchange e-mail with their doctors. However, the use of e-mail by providers is limited by fear of the additional burden of patient e-mail, lack of payment for electronic communication, and uneasiness about more informed patients (Ferguson, 2000). Additional barriers include concerns about the privacy and security of e-mail and potential liability concerns. According to the Pew Internet and American Life Project, 55 percent of patients used the Internet to access health information, while only 9 percent used e-mail to communicate with a doctor. Although the number of physicians willing to use e-mail with patients has increased, it is still lagging behind patient expectations.

The unheralded increase in health and medical information sites offers significant opportunities for self-help and peer support. Some have advocated the idea of a "patient helper" who can guide patients through their search of the myriad of available on-line services for the highest-quality materials (Davidoff and Florance, 2000). If on-line resources are less accessible to certain populations due to cost, low literacy, or access to computers, then increased use of the Internet could result in a growing digital divide that may exacerbate existing health care disparities (Burstin, 2000).

There are also concerns about the uneven quality of health information for patients on the Internet and the questionable use of patient information by Internet vendors. Much of the health care information that can be found on-line is of poor quality and misleading to patients (Berland and others, 2001). The American Medical Association published standards on the appropriate disclosure of the use of personal information and financial support for health care Web sites (Winker and others, 2000). However, most providers are not helping patients find high-quality information on the Internet. Although some physicians may be challenged by the concept of the informed health care consumer, patients have indicated that they would like their primary care physician to serve as their navigator to the Internet. Primary care providers have been slow to fully engage in this new world of Internet connectivity and on-line health care. To promote the idea of patient informatics, it has been recommended that it be incorporated into clinical skills education (Bader and Braude, 1998).

Self-Care and Shared Decision Making

From the perspective of many health insurers, self-care has now been defined as the beginning of primary care (Bischoff and Kelley, 1999). Although many view education about chronic illness management as a core element of primary care, the data would suggest that it is not being done effectively. For example, while comprehensive diabetes education is strongly recommended, fewer than half of those with insulin-treated diabetes reported that they had received formal training (Harris, Eastman, and Siebert, 1994). These data would suggest that the core primary care construct of a sustained partnership has been compromised. Novel self-care approaches have demonstrated increasing success. For example, patients with knee osteoarthritis who were randomized to self-care education demonstrated fewer primary care visits in the subsequent year (Mazzuca and others, 1999). In a randomized trial, patients who participated in a chronic disease self-management education program were able to maintain or improve health status, while decreasing the likelihood of hospitalization (Lorig, Sobel, and Stewart, 1999). The value of peer-to-peer teaching in primary care practice has only recently been tapped through examples such as "drop-in group medical visits" (Noffsinger and Scott, 2000). In these visits, a patient is seen by his or her physician in a supportive group setting that may include other patients, family members, and members of the health care team.

Several studies have also demonstrated the effectiveness of Internet-based information and support groups (Gustafson and others, 1999a). In a study of patients with HIV, Gustafson and others (1999b) demonstrated decreased costs, length of stay, and improved quality of life among users of an on-line information and support program. In an Internet-based intervention for diabetes, researchers were able to demonstrate that even older, less computer-literate adults could effectively participate in on-line self-management programs (Feil, Glasgow, Boles, and McKay, 2000). In many novel Internet-based disease management programs, the most frequently used feature was the social support groups with other patients. In addition, patients with chronic illness who seek information about their illness on-line reported better adherence to their medications following a visit to a disease-specific Web site (Zrebiec and Jacobson, 2001). While primary care providers have not been consistent and effective advocates of shared decision making and patient self-education, these alternate paths have begun to reap benefits. If collaborative care models of shared decision making and strategies for enhanced patient self-care could develop between primary care providers, health educators, and patients, the benefits to health status and outcomes could be substantial.

Other Health Professionals

The role of health professionals outside the typical primary care provider offers important insights into the state of primary care practice. Although medication management has always been viewed as a critical element of primary care practice, the role of the pharmacist in primary care has recently received more attention ("ASHP Statement on the Pharmacist's Role in Primary Care," 1999). There has always been an assumption that pharmacists would play a role in patient education in the community, and that role has increasingly been more formalized to include a collaborative drug management model. In this model, pharmacists directly provide "a limited range of primary care functions in addition to those encompassed by pharmaceutical care, either independently or in collaboration with other members of a primary care team" ("ASHP Statement on the Pharmacist's Role in Primary Care," 1999, p. 1665). In some localities, pharmacists have begun to bill for provision of services to patients with common illnesses, such as diabetes mellitus or hyperlipidemia.

Patients tend to seek complementary therapy for common primary care conditions that Western medicine cannot effectively eradicate, such as chronic low back pain (Elder, Gillcrist, and Minz, 1997). Their use of complementary services may relate somewhat to the kind of care that they experience outside the traditional medical setting. In a survey of British patients who were using complementary therapies, patients reported feeling cared for and that they were "getting somewhere" with a chronic problem or symptom (Luff and Thomas, 2000). Patients often seek complementary therapies at the urging of their primary care provider. In a study from a California HMO, nearly 90 percent of providers reported that they recommended at least one alternative therapy, most commonly for pain management (Gordon, Sobel, and Tarazona, 1998). However, most of the patients in the HMO needed to go outside their health plan to access these complementary therapies, and only half of the patients disclosed their use of alternative therapies to their physicians. A recent British study by White (2000) identified a set of key issues that describe why patients choose complementary therapies: dissatisfaction with conventional medicine, lack of holism in conventional medicine, a greater sense of self-control, and support in chronic illness. Complementary providers have been identified as better communicators with better bedside manners. Patients who used complementary therapies also reported a better sense of control over their health and illness.

Providers focused on certain patient populations offer different delivery models of primary care. For example, in the case of women's health, midwives are perceived to address more personal health care needs for women, including greater attention to preventive services across the life cycle (DeSandre, 2000). Although many primary care providers view the care of midwives during pregnancy as a specialized form of care, midwives' attention to an inclusive, woman-centered approach have led some women to select them as their regular source of primary care services. In a study that examined the relationships between nurse practitioners, physician assistants, and obstetrician-gynecologists, well-woman care, preventive services, and psychosocial care were provided to women by the midlevel providers due in part to the lack of interest by physicians in offering this care (Coulter, Jacobson, and Parker, 2000). The specialized site of care for women, such as women's health centers, often staffed by a variety of generalist physicians, obstetrician-gynecologists, and midlevel providers, has been shown to improve the delivery of gender-specific services, such as mammography and Pap smear screening (Harpole and others, 2000). By integrating multidisciplinary primary and specialty services for women, it could be argued that quality of care would increase through greater access to needed consultations with specialists (Carlson, 2000).

A shift in role of the primary care provider to coordinator of specialty services, rather than the gatekeeper to these services, has been proposed as an alternative model for primary care (Bodenheimer, Lo, and Casalino, 1999). These efforts would likely lead to greater coordination and integration with primary care services—returning to core constructs of primary care that attenuated during the heyday of managed care. Recent efforts supported by the Robert Wood Johnson Foundation to improve chronic illness care suggest that patient advocacy groups identify coordination of services as a critical unmet need (G. Anderson, personal communication, June 2001). Improved collaborative and multidisciplinary relationships between primary care providers and other health professionals needs to be enhanced for the benefit of patients' need and outcomes.

Nontraditional Sites of Primary Care

Primary care services provided at sites maximally accessible to patients, such as work site– and school-based clinics, offer important insights about access barriers to traditional primary care services. Several innovative studies have demonstrated the role of providers in the work site to promote health promotion and disease management for chronic illness. There is a growing literature of the benefits of providing health promotion activities at the work site. In a recent randomized controlled trial, Allen, Stoddard, Mays, and Sorensen (2001) found that a peer-delivered intervention to improve breast and cervical screening at the workplace significantly improved the use of Pap smears. In an example of work site disease management, a targeted diabetes management program with a work site diabetic health educator significantly improved diabetes lab parameters (Burton and Connerty, 1998).

Similarly, the ability for children, especially adolescents and chronically ill children, to access care services at school has the potential to improve access to care significantly. In a recent example, a school-based health clinic reduced costs, through fewer emergency department services, while improving the use of preventive services for children at risk (Adams and Johnson, 2000). There has been a high degree of acceptance of these school-based services among children and adolescents, especially among students at high risk for health and social problems. However, few studies have been able to document a significant effect on health behaviors, though one interesting study demonstrated that teaching children about management of asthma could be linked with broader education goals (Lurie, Straub, Goodman, and Bauer, 1998). School-based clinics meet many of the attributes of primary care, but the lack of coordination and collaboration with other community-based providers has been identified as problem areas (Ryan, Jones, and Weitzman, 1996).

CONCLUSION

Although the current state of primary care offers many opportunities for improvement, the basic constructs of primary care remain an important and necessary part of our health care system. While negative forces have adversely affected the practice of primary care, patients still need the positive force of a relationship with a primary care provider who can serve as teacher, advocate, and coordinator. Certainly, the nontraditional approaches to primary care delivery cannot incorporate all of the desired features of primary care, yet it is important to consider the features that have led patients to vote with their feet. Based on this review of nontraditional approaches to primary care delivery, a reconstructed model of primary care would need to be more patient centered and responsive to patients' needs, provide information to patients in ways that they can understand, and coordinate all needed patient services.

Several important themes should drive the reconstructed vision of primary care. One is the sense of a true partnership with patients, which includes elements of patient-centered care, self-efficacy, and supportive care for chronic illness. As we recall that the Latin root for *doctor* means "teacher," we should weave patient education back into primary care, while respecting the critical role that patients play in their own health care. A new model of primary care services would also incorporate shared decision making, requiring primary care providers to establish new relationships with patients, families, and other members of the health care team. In this context, the role of the primary care clinician as teacher focuses greater attention on patient skill development rather than simply providing content. As primary care providers evolve from gatekeepers to more robust coordinators of comprehensive health care services, enhanced working relationships with specialists and other members of the health care team will be critical success factors. Primary care needs to effectively incorporate the Internet and electronic communication into practice, or patients will embark on the information revolution and leave their primary care providers behind. In this age of accountability, if we are serious about the transformation of primary care, we need a serious and concerted focus on developing valid measures for assessing these constructs.

References

Adams, E. K., and Johnson, V. "An Elementary School-Based Health Clinic: Can It Reduce Medicaid Costs?" *Pediatrics,* 2000, *105,* 780–788.

Allen, J. D., Stoddard, A. M., Mays, J., and Sorensen, G. "Promoting Breast and Cervical Cancer Screening at the Workplace: Results from the Woman to Woman Study." *American Journal of Public Health,* 2001, *91*(4), 584–590.

"ASHP Statement on the Pharmacist's Role in Primary Care." *American Journal of Health System Pharmacy,* Aug. 15, 1999, pp. 1665–1667.

Bader, S. A., and Braude, R. M. "Patient Informatics: Creating New Partnerships in Medical Decision Making." *Academic Medicine,* 1998, *73,* 408–411.

Baker, D. W., and others. "Regular Source of Ambulatory Care and Medical Care Utilization by Patients Presenting to a Public Hospital Emergency Department." *Journal of the American Medical Association,* 1994, *271,* 1909–1912.

Ball, M. J., and Lillis, J. "E-Health: Transforming the Physician/Patient Relationship." *International Journal of Medical Informatics,* 2001, *61*(1), 1–10.

Berland, G. K., and others. "Health Information on the Internet: Accessibility, Quality, and Readability in English and Spanish." *Journal of the American Medical Association,* 2001, *285,* 2612–2621.

Billings, J., Parikh, N., and Mihanovich, T. *Emergency Department Use in New York City: A Substitute for Primary Care?* New York: Commonwealth Fund, Nov. 2000.

Bischoff, W. R., and Kelley, S. J. "Twenty-First Century House Call: The Internet and the World Wide Web." *Holistic Nursing Practice,* 1999, *13*(4), 42–50.

Bodenheimer, T., Lo, B., and Casalino, L. "Primary Care Physicians Should Be Coordinators, Not Gatekeepers." *Journal of the American Medical Association,* June 2, 1999, *281,* 2045–2049.

Boushy, D., and Dubinsky, I. "Primary Care Physician and Patient Factors That Result in Patients Seeking Emergency Care in a Hospital Setting: The Patient's Perspective." *Journal of Emergency Medicine,* 1999, *17*(3), 405–412.

Burstin, H. "Traversing the Digital Divide." *Health Affairs,* 2000, *19,* 245–249.

Burstin, H. R., and others. "The Effect of Change of Health Insurance on Access to Care." *Inquiry,* 1998, *35,* 389–397.

Burton, W. N., and Connerty, C. M. "Evaluation of a Worksite-Based Patient Education Intervention Targeted at Employees with Diabetes Mellitus." *Journal of Occupational and Environmental Medicine,* 1998, *40*(8), 702–706.

Carlson, K. J. "Multidisciplinary Women's Health Care and Quality of Care." *Women's Health Issues,* 2000, *10*(5), 219–225.

Christakis, D. A., and others. "Association of Lower Continuity of Care with Greater Risk of Emergency Department Use and Hospitalization in Children." *Pediatrics,* 2001, *107*(3), 524–529.

Citizens Commission on Graduate Medical Education. *The Graduate Education of Physicians: Report of the Citizens Commission on Graduate Medical Education Commissioned by John S. Millis, Chairman.* Chicago: Council on Medical Education, American Medical Association, 1966.

Coulter, I., Jacobson, P., and Parker, L. E. "Sharing the Mantle of Primary Female Care: Physicians, Nurse Practitioners, and Physician Assistants." *Journal of American Medical Women's Association,* 2000, *55*(2), 100–103.

Cunningham, P. J., Clancy, C. M., Cohen, J. W., and Wilets, M. "The Use of Hospital Emergency Departments for Nonurgent Health Problems:

A National Perspective." *Medical Care Research and Review,* 1995, *52*(4), 453–474.

Davidoff, F., and Florance, V. "The Informationist: A New Health Profession?" *Annals of Internal Medicine,* 2000, *132,* 996–998.

DeSandre, C. A. "Midwives as Primary Care Providers." *Journal of Midwifery and Women's Health,* 2000, *45*(1), 81–83.

Donaldson, M. S., Yordy, K. D., Lohr, K. N., and Vanselow, N. A. (eds.). *Primary Care: America's Health in a New Era.* Washington, D.C.: National Academy Press, 1996.

Eisenberg, J. M. "The Internist as Gatekeeper: Preparing the General Internist for a New Role." *Annals of Internal Medicine,* 1985, *102*(4), 537–543.

Elder, N. C., Gillcrist, A., and Minz, R. "Use of Alternative Health Care by Family Practice Patients." *Archives of Family Medicine,* 1997, *6*(2), 181–184.

Eng, T. R., and others. "Access to Health Information and Support: A Public Highway or a Private Road." *Journal of the American Medical Association,* 1998, *280,* 1371–1375.

Feil, E. G., Glasgow, R. E., Boles, S., and McKay, H. G. "Who Participates in Internet-Based Self-Management Programs? A Study Among Novice Computer Users in a Primary Care Setting." *Diabetes Education,* 2000, *26*(5), 806–811.

Ferguson, T. "Online Patient-Helpers and Physicians Working Together: A New Partnership for High Quality Health Care." *British Medical Journal,* Nov. 4, 2000, pp. 1129–1132.

Forrest, C. B., and Starfield, B. "Entry into Primary Care and Continuity: The Effects of Access." *American Journal of Public Health,* 1998, *88*(9), 1330–1336

Franks, P., Clancy, C. M., and Nutting, P. A. "Gatekeeping Revisited—Protecting Patients from Overtreatment." *New England Journal of Medicine,* 1992, *327,* 424–429.

Gordon, N. P., Sobel, D. S., and Tarazona, E. Z. "Use of and Interest in Alternative Therapies Among Adult Primary Care Clinicians and Adult Members in a Large Health Maintenance Organization." *Western Journal of Medicine,* 1998, *169*(3), 153–161.

Grumbach, K., and others. "Resolving the Gatekeeper Conundrum: What Patients Value in Primary Care and Referrals to Specialists." *Journal of the American Medical Association, 282*(3), 1999, 261–266.

Gustafson, D. H., and others. "Empowering Patients Using Computer Based Health Support Systems." *Quality in Health Care,* 1999a, *8,* 49–56.

Gustafson, D. H., and others. "Impact of a Patient-Centered, Computer-Based Health Information/Support System." *American Journal of Preventive Medicine,* 1999b, *16,* 1–19.

Harpole, L. H., and others. "A Comparison of the Preventive Health Care Provided by Women's Health Centers and General Internal Medicine Practices." *Journal of General Internal Medicine,* 2000, *15,* 1–7.

Harris, M. I., Eastman, R. C., and Siebert, C. "The DCCT and Medical Care for Diabetes in the U.S." *Diabetes Care,* 1994, *17,* 761–764.

Institute of Medicine, Committee on Quality Health Care in America. *Crossing the Quality Chasm: A New Health System for the Twenty-First Century.* Washington, D.C.: National Academy Press, 2001.

Joyce, G. F., Kapur, K., Van Vorst, K. A., and Escarce, J. J. "Visits to Primary Care Physicians and to Specialists Under Gatekeeper and Point-of-Service Arrangements." *American Journal of Managed Care,* Nov. 6, 2000, pp. 1189–1196.

Kolata, G. "Web Research Transforms Visit to the Doctor." *New York Times,* Mar. 6, 2000, p. A1.

Landon, B. E., Reschovsky, J., Reed, M., and Blumenthal, D. "Personal, Organizational, and Market Level Influences on Physicians' Practice Patterns Results of a National Survey of Primary Care Physicians." *Medical Care,* 2001, *39*(8), 889–905.

Leopold, N., Cooper, J., and Clancy, C. "Sustained Partnership in Primary Care." *Journal of Family Practice,* 1996, *42*(2), 129–137.

Levinson, W., Gorawara-Bhat, R., and Lamb, J. "A Study of Patient Clues and Physician Responses in Primary Care and Surgical Settings." *Journal of the American Medical Association, 284*(8), 2000, 1021–1027.

Lorig, K. R., Sobel, D. S., and Stewart, A. L. "Evidence Suggesting That a Chronic Disease Self-Management Program Can Improve Health Status While Reducing Hospitalization." *Medical Care,* 1999, *37*(1), 5–14.

Love, M. M., and Mainous, A. G. "Commitment to a Regular Physician: How Long Will Patients Wait to See Their Own Physician for Acute Illness?" *Journal of Family Practice,* 1999, *48,* 202–207.

Luff, D., and Thomas, K. J. "'Getting Somewhere,' Feeling Cared For: Patients' Perspectives on Complementary Therapies in the NHS." *Complementary Therapies in Medicine,* 2000, *8*(4), 253–259.

Lurie, N., Straub, M. J., Goodman, N., and Bauer, E. J. "Incorporating Asthma Education into a Traditional School Curriculum." *American Journal of Public Health,* 1998, *88,* 822–823.

Mainous, A. G. III, and others. "Continuity of Care and Trust in One's Physician: Evidence from Primary Care in the United States and the United Kingdom." *Family Medicine,* 2001, *33*(1), 22–27.

Mazzuca, S. A., and others. "Reduced Utilization and Cost of Primary Care Clinic Visits Resulting from Self-Care Education for Patients with Osteoarthritis of the Knee." *Arthritis and Rheumatism,* 1999, *42*(6), 1267–1273.

Noffsinger, E. B., and Scott, J. C. "Understanding Today's Group Visit Models." *Group Practice Journal,* 2000, *49*(2), 46–58.

Petersen, L. A., and others. "Non-Urgent Emergency Department Visits: The Effect of Having a Regular Doctor." *Medical Care,* 1998, *36*(8), 1249–1255.

Rosenblatt, R. A., and others. "Identifying Primary Care Disciplines by Analyzing the Diagnostic Content of Ambulatory Care." *Journal of the American Board of Family Practice,* 1995, *8*(1), 34–45.

Rosenblatt, R. A., and others. "The Generalist Role of Specialty Physicians: Is There a Hidden System of Primary Care?" *Journal of the American Medical Association,* 1998, *279,* 1364–1370.

Rucker, D., Brennan, T., and Burstin, H. "Delay in Seeking Emergency Care." *Academic Emergency Medicine,* 2001, *8*(2), 163–169.

Ryan, S., Jones, M., and Weitzman, M. "School-Based Health Services." *Current Opinion in Pediatrics,* 1996, *8*(5), 453–458.

Safran, D. G., and others. "Linking Primary Care Performance to Outcomes of Care." *Journal of Family Practice,* 1998, *47,* 213–220.

Safran, D. G., and others. "Switching Doctors: Predictors of Voluntary Disenrollment from a Primary Physician's Practice." *Journal of Family Practice,* 2001, *50,* 130–136.

Schmittdiel, J., Selby, J. V., Grumbach, K., and Quesenberry, C. P. "Choice of a Personal Physician and Patient Satisfaction in a Health Maintenance Organization." *Journal of the American Medical Association,* 1997, *278,* 1596–1599.

St. Peter, R. F., Reed, M. C., Kemper, P., and Blumenthal, D. "Changes in the Scope of Care Provided by Primary Care Physicians." *New England Journal of Medicine,* 1999, *341*(26), 1980–1985.

Starfield, B. *Primary Care: Concept Evaluation and Policy.* New York: Oxford University Press, 1992.

White, P. "What Can General Practice Learn from Complementary Medicine?" *British Journal of General Practice,* 2000, *50*(459), 821–823.

Winker, M. A., and others. "Guidelines for Medical and Health Information Sites on the Internet: Principles Governing AMA

Web Sites." *Journal of the American Medical Association,* 2000, *283,* 1600–1606.

Young, G. P., and others. "Ambulatory Visits to Hospital Emergency Departments. Patterns and Reasons for Use. Twenty-Four Hours in the ED Study Group." *Journal of the American Medical Association, 276*(6), 1996, 460–465.

Zrebiec, J. F., and Jacobson, A. M. "What Attracts Patients with Diabetes to an Internet Support Group? A Twenty-One-Month Longitudinal Website Study." *Diabetic Medicine,* 2001, *18*(2), 154–158.

CHAPTER SIX

The Specialist as Primary Care Provider

Harry R. Kimball

One of the unresolved issues in the debate about primary care in the United States is whether and how much of these services are, or should be, provided by physicians trained as surgical and medical specialists or subspecialists. The question is vexing because of the limited data about the scope of practice within specialty medicine, the variability in physician activities within a single specialty, confusion about what services constitute primary care, and the overlapping training in both primary and specialty care in internal medicine and pediatrics. Although everyone agrees that surgical or medical specialists and subspecialists provide some primary care, estimates about the frequency, quality, and cost of such services often rests on soft data and anecdotal evidence.

PRIMARY CARE, GENERALISM, AND SPECIALISM

The definition of primary care continues to evolve. In 1978, the Institute of Medicine defined primary care as the "3 C's and 2 A's": "accessible, comprehensive, coordinated, and continual care delivered by accountable providers of personal health care services" (Donaldson, Yordy, Lohr, and Vanselow, 1996, p. 29). In 1996, this definition was expanded to "the provision of integrated, accessible health care services by clinicians who are accountable for addressing a large majority of personal health care needs, developing a sustained partnership with patients, and practicing in the context of family and community." (Donaldson, Yordy, Lohr, and Vanselow, 1996, p. 31). While legitimate quibbles are possible, the general framework of these definitions of primary care is reasonable and has been widely accepted.

The term *generalist* regained favor during the national debate on health care reform in the 1990s. In common usage, generalists were physicians who provided "continuous, comprehensive, and coordinated care to a population undifferentiated by gender, sex, or organ system" (Young and Kimball, 1994, p. 315). In practice, the generalist designation was usually reserved for general internists, general pediatricians, and family physicians who also assumed the care of patients with chronic, complex illness. Internists and pediatricians were especially fond of the "generalist" label because the term *primary care provider* had been widely used by managed care organizations to describe clinicians who provided a bundle of medical services such as various screening procedures, immunizations, gatekeeping, and other relatively uncomplicated medical services. *Generalists* had more cachet in part because they were perceived as capable of managing more serious and complicated conditions in both outpatient and hospital settings.

Specialists or *subspecialists* have advanced training in a single organ system (such as cardiology), disease category (such as infectious diseases), or a technology or procedure (such as radiology or plastic surgery). Almost every specialist has some clinical experience in medicine, surgery, or pediatrics, although the extent of such training may be quite variable. Some, such as internal medicine and pediatric subspecialists, must be fully trained and certified in their primary discipline before they can enter, train, and be certified as a subspecialist. Other specialists have much less experience and training. This variability is an important point to keep in mind when the appropriateness of specialist-delivered primary care is at issue. More confusing, advanced training and certification in aspects of generalism exist even within primary care disciplines. Geriatric medicine and adolescent medicine are good examples of this situation. These physicians regard themselves as specialists, yet many others continue to think of them as bona fide primary care clinicians despite their specialty label and focused scope of practice.

As a consequence, primary care physicians in the United States do not fit neatly into a single mold as elsewhere around the world. In Europe, for example, health care is often sharply segmented by clinicians (general practitioners and specialty consultants) and by site of practice (outpatient offices and inpatient hospitals). In the United Kingdom, only general practitioners provide primary care services to the community; consultants treat patients in the hospital or related clinics. These divisions can be very rigid. In the United Kingdom, patients covered by the National Health Service (virtually everyone) can be referred to a consultant only by their general practitioner. In France, it is illegal for consultants to have private outpatient practices.

The pluralistic nature of primary care (family practice, internal medicine, and pediatrics) in the United States is often confusing to physicians and health care planners from abroad, yet it is well accepted (if not completely understood) by the American public and medical community. In fact, physicians are increasingly organized across specialty lines to form primary care groups consisting of family physicians, general internists, pediatricians, and even the occasional obstetrics-gynecology (OB/GYN) specialist. These newly configured groups offer greater efficiency and the convenience of all-inclusive care. As a result, these groups are often better positioned to negotiate more effectively with health plans to provide full-service care to increasingly diverse populations.

THE EDUCATIONAL PROCESS FOR PRIMARY CARE

Like all other specialties, the training curricula for the three major primary care specialties (internal medicine, family practice, and pediatrics) are governed by the Accreditation Council for Graduate Medical Education (ACGME) and the Residency Review Committee (RRC) for each discipline (American Medical Association, 2001). Each RRC reviews and accredits all training programs (up to six years) based on their compliance with the program training requirements. These requirements are developed by each RRC with broad input by the specialty discipline. In 2001, family practice had the most training programs (498), followed by internal medicine (397) and pediatrics (208). These programs recruit approximately seven thousand (internal medicine), thirty-five hundred (family practice), and twenty-five hundred (pediatrics) new residents each year from medical school graduates in the United States and abroad. The total (thirteen thousand) represents a slim majority of all entering residents, estimated at twenty-four thousand. At the present time, the proportion of international medical graduates (IMGs) to U.S. graduates (one-to-two) entering primary care training programs is higher than for nonprimary care training disciplines.

Although the training curriculum varies in each primary care specialty, all have extended periods of training in ambulatory settings (one to two years), and each has specific requirements for continuity clinics in which a panel of patients is followed throughout the three years of residency training.

The continuity experience accounts for a minimum 20 percent of all training for family physicians and 10 percent for internists and pediatricians. In addition, each primary care specialty requires specific experiences in emergency medicine and adolescent medicine, although they vary with respect to exposure to adults, children, and gender-specific illnesses and prevention (women's health). Family physicians especially (but not always) have significant training in obstetrics and surgery.

During the past decade, OB/GYN has sought to be officially recognized as primary care physicians for women, including women in the geriatric age group. To acquire necessary added knowledge and skills, OB/GYN residents are now required to provide continuous care to a panel of patients one-half day per week for three years and to rotate through month-long rotations in internal medicine or family practice, emergency medicine, and geriatric medicine. The total time required for training in these primary care experiences must be the equivalent of six months during the four-year training program.

Residents in surgical and related specialties have less formal training in primary care, although general surgeons often assume the regular care of patients with undifferentiated abdominal pain or colon cancer. Some specialties, such as radiology, require one year of training in a general medical, pediatric, or surgical residency to acquire the clinical experience necessary to perform invasive radiology procedures with greater safety.

In addition to allopathic residents, about fifteen hundred graduates of osteopathic medical schools enter primary care training programs accredited by the American Osteopathic Association (J. B. Crosby, personal communication, Sept. 2001). During the past decade, osteopathic medical schools have restructured their educational programs to emphasize primary care education, with the goal of becoming a greater factor in the health care delivery system.

Except for the military, a valid state medical license is required to practice medicine in the United States. Licensure is generally awarded following graduation from medical school, satisfactory completion of the U.S. Medical Licensing Examination (USMLE), and at least one year of postgraduate training. Some states, such as California and Florida, require additional licensing examinations. The USMLE and other licensing examinations test general medical knowledge and are not specialty specific. IMGs are required to be certified by the Educational Commission for Foreign Medical Graduates (ECFMG) to be licensed to practice medicine and to be eligible to enter ACGME-accredited training programs in the United States. ECFMG certification requires passage of the USMLE, a hands-on clinical skills examination, and documentation of English-language proficiency.

Following satisfactory completion of residency training, virtually all residents sit for certification examinations offered by one of the twenty-four member boards that comprise the American Board of Medical Specialties. These examinations are lengthy and cover the scope of each discipline. Pass rates in the primary care disciplines are approximately 83 percent (pediatrics), 84 percent (internal medicine), and 95 percent (family practice) for first-time-taker graduates of U.S. training programs. Pass rates for graduates of non-U.S. and Canadian schools are lower but have steadily improved during the past decade. The validity of certification is time limited (seven years for family practice and pediatrics, ten years for internal medicine). Certification is renewed (maintained) by completing a structured recertification program that includes passing a written examination of medical knowledge. All ABMS Member Board recertification programs are evolving to evaluate other components of clinical competence, among them clinical skills, professionalism, and clinical performance, including medical outcomes.

FREQUENCY AND QUALITY OF PRIMARY CARE SERVICES BY SPECIALISTS

Several studies have addressed the issue of primary care delivered by specialty physicians. The now-classic Mendenhall studies of the late 1970s stand alone in their scope (they sampled over fifty thousand internists and subspecialists) but cannot provide a completely accurate picture of contemporary primary care activities (Mendenhall and others, 1979). In the Mendenhall studies, the term *primary care* was avoided because of its varied meanings. Instead, patient interactions were categorized as first encounter, episodic care, consultative care, principal care, and specialized care. Continuity of care was a characteristic of only the last two patient interactions. Principal care was defined as encounters in which physicians provided a "majority of care" to a cadre of "regular patients." Comprehensiveness and continuity were felt to be satisfied by the "regular" and "majority of care" criteria. Specialized care was defined as "the provision of limited services" (that is, not majority care) to a regular patient (neither a consultation nor a first visit).

Using these definitional criteria, the practice activities of physicians in eight of the eleven subspecialties of internal medicine provided more than 50 percent principal care encounters in office-based practice arrangements. Not unexpectedly, principal care was more common in ambulatory encounters than in hospital or other settings. Surprisingly, oncologists and nephrologists were found to provide more principal care than did general internists. Mendenhall and others (1979) concluded that internal medicine subspecialists are assuming ongoing and comprehensive responsibility for the management of very substantial numbers of patients and have an appreciable commitment to entry level care. The data were believed to refute the notion that subspecialization by necessity alters patterns of physician-patient encounters. A second study (Aiken and others, 1979) confirmed that one of five Americans received continuing care from specialist physicians but also documented that general practitioners (80 percent) and family practitioners (77 percent) headed the list of principal care providers, followed by pediatricians (72 percent), OB/GYN (65 percent), and internists (62 percent).

More recently, Rosenblatt and others (1998) examined the ambulatory practices for Medicare-age patients in Washington State during 1994 and 1995. He documented that in this age group, family practitioners and general internists provided the most "majority of care" to outpatients (50 percent) compared with 21 percent for medical subspecialists and 11 percent for surgical specialists. Not surprising, the range of medical problems treated by family practitioners and general internists was much broader than occurred in medical or surgical subspecialty practices. Specialists providing the greatest amount of out-of-specialty care were pulmonologists, general surgeons, and gynecologists. The care provided by these specialists met the criteria of being continuous ("majority of care"), was reasonably comprehensive, and included common preventive measures. Coordination, cost, and quality were not addressed. Rosenblatt concluded that "most specialists do not assume principal care responsibility for elderly patients" (p. 1364). Nonetheless, a substantial number of patients, 15 percent of the total, received care only from physician specialists during the two-year period of study. This finding is not too dissimilar to the one-in-five frequency reported in the Mendenhall and the Aiken studies.

For this chapter, data were obtained from a 1999 American College of Physicians–American Society of Internal Medicine survey of 1,767 internists about the scope of their practice activities (J. Tooker, personal communication, Sept. 2001). The resulting practice profile is set out in Table 6.1

Although self-reported and not explicit about principal and primary care definitions (four practice scenarios were offered), the data confirm that internal medicine subspecialists currently devote an appreciable amount of time (26 percent) to "primary care" activities.

Data about the quality of primary care provided by specialists are mixed. As Franks, Nutting, and Clancy (1993) summarized, most comparisons have shown few or no differences; others have favored either primary care physicians or specialists. More recently, a study of primary care and specialty physicians at Kaiser Permanente (Northern California) found only minor differences in patient satisfaction ratings among general internists, family physicians, and medical specialists (Grumbach, Selby, Schmittdiel, and Quesenberry, 1999). These surveys asked patients about coordination, comprehensiveness, accessibility, prevention, lifestyle, and social issues. It is important to keep in mind that generalizations to the larger health care system may be limited because of the practice setting and the strong institutional

	Percentage of Clinical Time	
	Generalists (1,150)	Subspecialists (405)
Principal care[a]	23	18
Primary care[b]	64	8
Specialty care[c]	9	42
Consultative care[d]	4	32

Table 6.1. Practice Profile of Sample of Internists, 1999.

[a]Providing primary care to general or subspecialty patients.

[b]Providing primary care to nonsubspecialty patients.

[c]Providing only subspecialty care to subspecialty patients.

[d]Referred by another physician.

culture of this closed-panel HMO. Data from the ongoing Medical Outcomes Studies indicate that health care services provided by primary care physicians are generally less intense and less costly, but precise comparisons with specialty physicians are difficult because severity-of-illness adjustments are complex, and variations in regional cost patterns can be marked (S. Greenfield, personal communication, Aug. 2001).

CONTEMPORARY ISSUES FOR PRIMARY CARE PROVIDED BY SPECIALISTS

Is There a Role for the Specialist in Primary Care?

There appear to be sufficient data to conclude that medical specialists provide a substantial amount of primary care to the public. Although it is hard to pin down a precise estimate, it is probably in the range of 15 to 25 percent for internal medicine and 10 to 15 percent for pediatric subspecialists (J. Stockman, personal communication, Sept. 2001). Available data suggest that the provision of primary care is much less common in the surgical subspecialties with the exception of OB/GYN and perhaps general surgery. Data are lacking to confirm the suspicion that the quality of such care is inferior, although it may be more costly. The reason that quality differences are difficult to document may relate to both formal and informal communications between generalists and specialists (S. Greenfield, personal communication, Aug. 2001). While it is standard procedure for primary care physicians to consult with specialists about the management of patients with complicated diseases, the reverse is also common: specialists consult with generalists, often informally, when managing out-of-specialty conditions in patients being treated on a regular basis for a specialty disorder. The appropriate management of hypertension or of acute urinary tract infections are common examples of such reverse consultation. When necessary, preventive services are arranged with primary care providers (including nurse practitioners) without the actual transfer of ongoing care. Unfortunately, there is little hard information about when and under what circumstances these interactions take place, but they are more commonplace than is appreciated.

Which specialists are qualified to provide primary care is a sensitive issue. A relatively good case can be made for internal medicine and pediatric subspecialists because all have been fully trained and certified in the primary discipline, at least at one point in their medical career. If they have recently completed formal training, their primary care skills are likely satisfactory. Even if distant from training, these specialists may require relatively little assistance to acquire proficiency in primary care and prevention. The case may be less firm for OB/GYN specialists because of their relatively brief (six months) training in primary care and much less firm for surgical and other specialties with little knowledge of or experience with primary care issues. But even if trained, a specialist should not be automatically assumed to have adequate primary care skills. Such determinations can be made only on the basis of credible assessments of clinical performance.

What Do Patients Want?

Regardless of how physicians think primary care should be provided, it is important to understand and respond to the needs of patients. It is clear that Americans want to choose their own doctors, and they resent being denied access to specialty physicians or being shuttled from physician to physician to get their problems resolved. In the case of serious chronic disease, patients usually do not want referrals to other physicians for routine out-of-specialty problems. "Can't you take care of it?" is a common response. Referrals to other physicians are inconvenient, expensive, and anxiety producing. Patients also know that multiprovider care can lead to other problems (such as drug interactions or unnecessary testing) when miscommunication occurs.

Effects of an Aging Population, Diversity, and Scientific Advances on Primary Care Provided by Specialists

The increasing number of older patients inevitably translates to a greater need for chronic disease care, pain management, and end-of-life care. A similar outcome will result from future scientific advances that will keep patients functioning to advanced ages (the over-eighty-five age group is the fastest-growing segment of the population). Because of the complexity of chronic disease such as cancer, heart disease, and arthritis, it seems likely that medical subspecialists will become the principal care providers for many of these patients. In this role, they will be called on to provide primary care services because patients will demand it and because many of these physicians will be reasonably confident about their ability to provide out-of-specialty care.

With respect to cultural diversity, patients can be expected to gravitate toward physicians who understand or, better yet, are part of their culture. This understandable preference will limit their choice of doctors. In the Chinese community, for example, cultural factors can outweigh considerations about which kind of physician will manage their health care. Multiculturalism has introduced an entirely new metric into the generalist-specialist debate.

Workforce Considerations for the Specialist as Primary Care Provider

It is generally fruitless to speculate about the future of the medical workforce. Nonetheless, it is reasonable for such analyses to consider the contributions of specialists in meeting future primary care needs. Doing so will cause a downward adjustment in the number of primary care and generalist physicians called for.

CONCLUSION

Generalizations about the specialist as primary care provider come with many caveats. Nonetheless, it is undeniable that specialists, and particularly medical specialists, currently provide a substantial amount of primary care. Moreover, there is no convincing evidence available to document that this care is of inferior quality (although it may be somewhat more costly). With this in mind, the following observations are offered:

- When it comes to their doctors, America is prochoice. Regardless of health status or personal bias, it would be unwise to force patients to receive all primary care services from primary care clinicians.
- Medical politics and turf considerations should not determine whether specialists can or should have a role in delivering primary care services. The focus must be kept on outcomes of care, including efficient use of resources. Policy decisions should be guided by such results and by common sense.
- In some circumstances, it is appropriate for specialty physicians to assume the primary care of a patient. With adequate training and experience, such physicians can assume responsibility for providing accessible care, coordinating other medical services, and communicating with patients and their families. A special obligation exists to

avoid fragmentation of medical care for older patients with serious chronic disease and patients at the end of life.

- Not all specialty physicians can or should assume the role of a primary care physician. Physicians must be confident of their primary care knowledge and skills, a confidence that can come only with formal training or lengthy experience in managing medical problems outside their primary specialty. Developing guidelines for such situations would be difficult but very helpful to both patients and the medical profession.

References

Aiken, L., and others. "The Contribution of Specialists to the Delivery of Primary Care." *New England Journal of Medicine,* 1979, *300,* 1363–1370.

American Medical Association. "Program Requirements for Residency Education in Obstetrics and Gynecology." In *Graduate Medical Education Directory, 2001–2002.* Chicago: American Medical Association, 2001.

Donaldson, M. S., Yordy, K. D., Lohr, K. N., and Vanselow, N. A. (eds.). *Primary Care: America's Health in a New Era.* Washington, D.C.: National Academy Press, 1996.

Franks, P., Nutting, P., and Clancy, C. "Health Care Reform, Primary Care, and the Need for Research." *Journal of the American Medical Association,* 1993, *270,* 1449–1453.

Grumbach, K., Selby, J. V., Schmittdiel, J. A., and Quesenberry, C. P. Jr. "Outcomes and Physician Specialty: Quality of Primary Care Practice in a Large HMO According to Physician Specialty." *Health Services Research,* 1999, *34*(2), 485–502.

Mendenhall, R., and others. "A National Study of Internal Medicine and Its Specialties: II. Primary Care in Internal Medicine." *Annals of Internal Medicine,* 1979, *91,* 275–287.

Rosenblatt, R., and others. "The Generalist Role of Specialty Physicians: Is There a Hidden System of Primary Care?" *Journal of the American Medical Association,* 1998, *279,* 1364–1370.

Young, P., and Kimball, H. "A Statement on the Generalist Physician from the American Boards of Family Practice and Internal Medicine." *Journal of the American Medical Association,* 1994, *271,* 315–316.

CHAPTER SEVEN

Advanced Practice Nurses

The Preferred Primary Care Providers for the Twenty-First Century

Mary O'Neil Mundinger

In the 1970s, primary care gained great public interest, but the ambitious definitions outdistanced actual practice. Widely promoted as the five "C's" of first *c*ontact, *c*omprehensive, *c*oordinated, *c*ontinuous, *c*ommunity-based care, rarely did conventional primary care meet these criteria. Primary care, was in fact, the practice of internal medicine for those who sought regular medical assessments or symptomatic treatment. Essentially this is still the paradigm today, with the additional but now eroding role of gatekeeper for specialist care or interventions. Primary care, as envisioned by policymakers, has always been more a promise than a reality.

Today, the goal of fully establishing the multidimensional nature of primary care is far more likely, due to the rising interest in cost reductions through disease prevention, health promotion, and better coordination of care, especially for those with multiple medical conditions, and the growing public attention to error reduction. Primary care that provides this multiplicity of approaches has rarely been available. It is costly in time commitment, and physicians are not trained in the broad spectrum of skills. Advanced practice nurses, however, do have this full armamentarium of education, training, and experience to provide the new style of primary care, and the time-intensive approaches that primary care, in its most valuable form, requires. Advanced practice nurses, with the increased regulatory authority being granted, now hold the potential position in the health care system of being recognized as the preferred primary care providers.

The definition of primary care published in the Institute of Medicine study, *Primary Care: America's Health in a New Era* (Donaldson, Yordy, Lohr, and Vanselow, 1996), makes very clear that primary care is not about disease, physicians, or medicine. In fact, a close reading suggests that primary care is all about protecting and returning patients to good health, and that nurses are the clinicians being described: "Primary care is the provision of integrated, accessible health care services by clinicians who are accountable for addressing a large majority of personal health care needs, developing a sustained partnership with patients, and practicing in the context of family and community" (p. 31).

DIFFERENTIATED PRACTICE OF NURSES

Several measurable factors make primary care by advanced practice nurses different from primary care by physicians (or physician assistants). First, those who choose nursing with the goal of achieving independent practice in primary care have a different worldview from those who choose medicine. At Columbia University, all students entering nursing are already college graduates; three-quarters have been out of college for one to five years and have been engaged in careers perhaps only peripherally related to health care. Most choose nursing because of a personal or volunteer experience with illness, where they were involved in the care or decision making of someone struggling with disability or disease, and they felt a great sense of worthiness in achieving competence as a comprehensive and authoritative caregiver.

Most of our nursing students would qualify for acceptance into medical school. They do not take the Medical College Admission Test, but their grade point averages from competitive universities and their science backgrounds are similar (although rarely is organic chemistry listed on their transcripts), and their articulate commitment to helping sick people is very evident. Many have considered medicine, but very rarely is there an applicant who has tried and failed to be admitted to medical school. Instead, the students at Columbia Nursing have identified the caring role as central to their career plans, and they have also identified advanced practice nursing as a parallel role to primary care medicine, and one that may take less educational time to complete.

This educational time commitment is a second reason that many college graduates choose nursing over medicine: a college graduate entering medical school contemplates four years of studies plus three years of training for primary care, whereas traditional nursing education is four years of studies plus two years of training for primary care. Although the value of the current four-year medical school curriculum is under discussion for its appropriateness or cost-effectiveness, nursing has arrived at an attractive and effective accelerated curriculum for entry to nursing for college graduates. Columbia, Johns Hopkins, Yale, Vanderbilt, the University of Pennsylvania, and other high-quality nursing programs have all adopted similar curricula, and the primary care graduates of these schools have stood up under the scrutiny of policymakers, researchers, and the medical community. After initial professional education, primary care training (three years in medicine, two years in nursing) is similar except that nursing is more focused on primary care skills. Part of this is because graduate medical education funds for primary care residents are provided through hospitals, and the quid pro quo of residency funding is to provide service valuable to hospitals. Therefore, more inpatient care time is built into the three-year residency. Advanced practice nurses, who pay for their primary care training with private after-tax dollars, do not have the same requirement for non–primary care service during their education.

This disparity in primary care training may provide the medical resident with a deeper medical understanding of acutely ill patients. This knowledge enriches and informs primary care and distinguishes the value-added practice of physicians in primary care. Nurses who come directly from their undergraduate nurse training into primary care training have somewhat less experience with acutely ill patients, although their undergraduate hospital-based experiences far outweigh those of medical students. What primary care medical residents learn about acutely ill patients, nurses to some extent cover in their undergraduate clinical experiences.

Although primary care physicians have more critical care skills, the difference in training between the two professions gives nurses the edge in primary care skills. Undergraduate nursing programs (or first-degree nursing programs at the graduate level) focus on many skills fundamental to basic nursing practice. These include the sciences of health education, a six-step intervention, individual risk identification and reduction, and health promotion. Nurses in their first-degree program also engage in a significant clinical experience in community health, learning how to adapt care to noninstitutional settings, how to use and not overwhelm family care potential, and where and how to access public and private sources of care beyond conventional medicine. These experiences and skills underpin and infuse the ultimate primary care practice of a nurse, and this results in a value-added parameter of nursing practice in primary care that distinguishes it from physician-provided primary care. In a system where specialty medicine is increasingly being employed for patients and primary care medicine is increasingly being valued for its preventive, health-promoting, and health-protective measures, the advanced practice nurse becomes the primary care provider of choice.

SPECIALISTS AND PRIMARY CARE

With the rise of the hospitalist, a hospital-based internist or family physician, the primary care physician's knowledge of acute care may be less important. Similarly, more and more specialists are choosing to provide primary care (albeit at specialty prices) to their patients for whom they already provide specialist services. The resulting demand for generalist care therefore may be more and more for the kind of care nurses deliver.

As for specialist physicians providing primary care, their prism deflects patients' symptoms into their specialty first. A cardiologist will perform an echocardiogram stress test, while a gastroenterologist will perform an endoscopy on a patient presenting with the same symptom (Wennberg and Gittelsohn, 1982). A generalist approach is therefore more likely to provide a broader diagnostic net and less likely to narrow the focus prematurely. A generalist approach is also more likely to identify secondary or perhaps other primary conditions by addressing a broader range of possibilities in the early stages of assessment.

Even when a diagnosis has been made and a need for a specialist established, patients require the ongoing involvement of a generalist. Rarely does an individual who is seriously ill have health risks only for the primary condition being treated. Clots form, diabetes spirals out of control, fluids accumulate, electrolytes fluctuate, drug regimens go out of balance, and problems compound. Generalists know the equilibrium that was previously achieved for their patients, and they can be crucial adjuncts to patient health and safety even in the midst of a very focused crisis.

The rise of the hospitalist, further distancing the generalist/primary care provider from acutely ill patients, could place patients at greater vulnerability during hospitalization. Most patients in hospitals today have more than one medical condition, although they may be hospitalized for only one. The necessary comprehensive medical oversight could be lost through the laser focus of a hospitalist, who may know very little about the patient's other conditions, risks for illness, preferences for treatment, need for exercise, and cognitive or emotional impairments—all central factors in successful recovery.

The elderly are particularly at risk for inadequate overall assessments, and not only because of their own fragile health and high risks. An older sick man or woman in the hospital bed may have left a vulnerable spouse home alone or become confused and less physically and emotionally able to resume an independent lifestyle when discharged.

Hospitalists may be a welcome answer for primary care physicians who earn less than specialist physicians. This could be an incentive for primary care physicians to see more office patients rather than cutting big holes in their reimbursement potential by taking precious time to make hospital rounds. While understandable in economic terms, their absence during times of their patients' critical illnesses erodes their authority during times of their patients' relative health, and thereby erodes their effectiveness in achieving optimal outcomes. The influence of clinicians engaged in prevention-oriented therapies will be far greater if they are also centrally engaged in the care and therapies during medical crises. They need the opportunity to say, "I can help you prevent this from ever happening again. I can help you become healthier, but you need to work with me."

NURSE PRACTITIONER REIMBURSEMENT

Advanced practice nurses today have significant and growing authority for providing care. Since the 1997 Balanced Budget Act, Medicare has authorized direct reimbursement for all Part B (physician) services, regardless of site of care, within state scope of practice laws. This authorization provides for direct reimbursement, at 85 percent of physician rates, when the advanced practice nurse has been certified by Medicare. Medicaid has reimbursed advanced practice nurses directly for care in every state for years, again regulated by state practice acts and level of reimbursement, both of which can vary enormously by state. Medicaid reimbursement varies for advanced practice nurses between 50 and 100 percent of physician reimbursement rates.

Before the Balanced Budget Act of 1997, Medicare reimbursed nurses for home care but only for medically necessary services. In a study determining whether home care nurses followed this Medicare policy (medical plan of care, medically necessary care as opposed to supportive management for homebound patients), fewer than half the nurses followed policy (Mundinger, 1983). The reason is that they consciously or unconsciously were making humane, and cost-effective, decisions. One patient, a man living alone, was recovering from a burn on his back, which had essentially healed, caused by a hot shower. The nurse, however, having diagnosed deep depression, kept making visits to get him safely involved with a community mental health agency. Another man, with ulcers related to chronic leukemia, was also healed. But the nurse continued making once-a-week visits, giving the patient's wife her only hour of freedom—the last fragile link that kept her from placing him in a hospice. In each case, the nurse documented wound care that met Medicare guidelines in order to receive reimbursement for the home visit. Perhaps more central to the antihospitalist argument is the woman in this study being seen for a healing staphylococcus wound in her hip following surgery for a fracture. This woman fell while she was visiting her daughter in a city far from her primary care physician. The orthopedist, not knowing her or of her diabetes, treated the staph infection with an antibiotic, and when the infection was resolved told her she could now "stop all your medications." She stopped taking her drug to lower blood sugar levels and antihypertensive medications. Only when the home care nurse queried her "usual medications" was the error rectified. Hospitalists, moving quickly from crisis to crisis, cannot know these central influences in each patient's ability to get well. A fourth patient in the study, hospitalized for an infected gall bladder, signed himself out before surgery because his wife, with Alzheimer's disease, was home alone. Such increasingly fragmented care cries out for a generalist who can be health protective, authoritative, and medically competent.

Commercial insurers have reimbursed advanced practice nurses in a highly uneven fashion for several years. Mental health and midwifery services were the major areas of nursing practice recognized by these payers, but often only in physician shortage areas or at a highly discounted rate, usually for a single individual practitioner and rarely for inpatient care. In the past few years, however, direct reimbursement of advanced practice nurses as a group has increased substantially. Initially, in the early 1990s, a national shortage of primary care physicians was thought to be occurring and was expected to worsen rapidly. Advanced practice nurses were viewed as a way to assuage the shortage. At the same time, the number of uninsured or only partly insured individuals had reached 15 percent of the total population, more individuals than were covered by Medicare. Again, advanced practice nurses were viewed as a solution, especially if they were cheaper to produce and pay than physicians, and if they were willing, as they had been in the past, to devote their practices to the care of the poor and underserved.

Policymakers felt secure in filling these gaps with advanced practice nurses because there was every indication, in both the scientific literature and broad anecdotal evidence, that advanced practice nurses achieved good outcomes and high patient satisfaction. Liberalizing direct reimbursement was an easy policy decision.

COMMERCIAL REIMBURSEMENT: RECOGNITION FOR NURSE PRACTITIONER PRACTICE

With the establishment of the Columbia Advanced Practice Nurse Associates (CAPNA) practice in midtown Manhattan in 1997, the reimbursement system for advanced practice nurses began to broaden to respond to the expressed wishes of all patients, and not just the demand for care of the underserved.

CAPNA was a pioneering effort to see if patients would choose an advanced practice nurse model of primary care even in a setting where there was an oversupply of high-quality doctors and no financial incentive for patients to choose a nurse. In other words, would individuals choose a nurse instead of a physician for primary care simply because of the style and content of the practice? The answer has been a cautious yes. The model built on earlier success with independent practice caring for the underserved.

BUILDING THE SCIENCE FOR NURSE PRACTITIONER VALUE

In 1993, at the request of Presbyterian Hospital at Columbia-Presbyterian Medical Center, School of Nursing faculty were given the opportunity to establish and independently manage two new satellite primary care centers primarily for Medicaid-eligible individuals living in the medical center neighborhood. Two additional identical sites were to be established and managed by primary care physicians. Seeing this as a unique opportunity to compare primary care by physicians and advanced practice nurses, the nursing school asked the hospital to grant hospital admitting privileges to the nurses in the study so that their authority would be identical to that of the physicians. In New York State, nurse practitioners have full prescriptive authority and Medicaid reimbursement at 100 percent of physician fees, and they practice independently within a collaborative framework with a selected physician in their practice specialty. The collaborative arrangement requires the advanced practice nurse to meet quarterly with the physician to discuss patient management generally. No explicit reviews or protocols are required. Most important, the agreement gives the advanced practice nurse a guaranteed responsive consultant when requested.

We sought hospital admitting privileges so that the advanced practice nurses would achieve parity and therefore not be compromised in a comparison of patient satisfaction, utilization (a proxy for costs), or patient outcomes. The medical board approved these privileges for the two-year study period. However, partway through the two years, the board made this a permanent hospital policy in the by-laws for Columbia School of Nursing faculty only. The study had been designed as a randomized controlled trial, and well-respected physicians (including the hospital board president), economists, biostatisticians, and health policy experts served on the external Scientific Advisory Board for the study. The conduct of the evaluation had proved to be a powerful influence in gaining physician support at the medical center.

Two years before the study data were analyzed and reported, the faculty practitioners agreed to expand their services to a commercially insured population. Each practitioner already had full authority for primary care at the medical center; years of experience managing a group of patients, including full prescriptive authority; hospital admitting and comanagement responsibilities; and a deeply held belief that they could practice successfully with a more demanding, if no less needy, population. The only barrier was reimbursement.

Oxford Healthcare was new in New York City and was proud that Columbia had selected it as its preferred provider for university employees; thus, Oxford had developed a particularly strong relationship with Columbia physicians. We believed Oxford might be more open than other payers to consider reimbursing us directly as a full-choice primary care provider for their beneficiaries. It took weeks to secure an appointment, but eventually we had the opportunity to speak to a group of their medical directors, and ultimately they agreed to credential our nurse practitioners.

CAPNA asked that they be listed as primary care providers in Oxford's directory and that Oxford pay them the same primary care rates as physicians. The arguments were as follows. Managed care was being hurt by the wide perception that it limited choice for its beneficiaries. Broadening choice by adding advanced practice nurses to the roster could mitigate that negative view. No beneficiary would be denied an advanced practice nurse, and no one would be forced to have an advanced practice nurse as a primary care provider. Moreover, if Oxford provided that choice as a quality option, and not a lesser service for less money, it would avoid the perception that it was using advanced practice nurses to save money. Similarly, if Oxford were to reimburse CAPNA at a lower rate, then surely it would have to reduce the premiums for those who chose CAPNA practitioners; otherwise, Oxford would appear to be using advanced practice nurses to increase its profits, a policy sure to inflame their beneficiaries.

Finally, the literature already showed that many individuals would change primary care providers based on a deductible difference of only ten dollars. Therefore, if Oxford paid CAPNA less than primary care physicians and patients legitimately paid a lower cost for advanced practice nursing care, this would place CAPNA nurses in direct price competition with physicians, who might respond with anger toward Oxford.

Within weeks of Oxford's agreement with CAPNA, the New York State Medical Association complained aggressively and sent delegates from the New York State Office of Professional Discipline to visit the clinic and investigate whether advanced practice nurses were practicing medicine without a license. The Office of Professional Discipline uncovered no irregularities, the heat abated, the New York State Medical Association withdrew to plot and fume in isolation, and the CAPNA practice began to thrive. As each new payer rate was approved by the Columbia physicians, CAPNA was included at the same rate. There are today eleven commercial payers paying CAPNA and Columbia physicians the same primary care rates.

VALUE-ADDED OUTCOMES OF NURSE PRACTITIONER PRACTICE

The major barrier to paying identical physician or advanced practice nurse rates for primary care was the assumption, since advanced practice nurses came on the scene in 1965, that primary care by nurses was simply a subset of primary care by physicians. The real distinction is far more significant. Although there is a common core of medical competencies shared by physicians and nurse practitioners, there is also a valued-added component of care by physicians and a separate and different value-added component of care provided by nurse practitioners.

While the value-added component from medicine is primarily the deeper understanding of pathology and care of patients with life-threatening or extremely unstable conditions, most would argue that these kinds of patients need to be under the care of a physician specialist rather than a primary care physician. The value-added component that advanced practice nurses bring to primary care, however, is just what patients need from a primary care provider: skills and help in the very areas that no physician is trained to provide.

Payers and physicians have been slow to recognize these differences. Both have long held that the physician is the gold standard in health care, viewed as synonymous with illness care. In fact, payers generally pay only for the illness component. While this ill-conceived limitation is due to the narrow focus of medicine (patients are ill or not ill), it may also be a limitation that serves the financial health of payers. If reimbursement were to freely cover health-related therapies (exercise, diet counseling, stress reduction, smoking cessation, consultation on accessing and using community health resources, and more), payers would have to grapple with several issues.

First, and predictably, costs—and premiums—would rise. Perhaps a savvy group of beneficiaries would pay these additional premiums, at least while they used the extra services, but they might switch to a cheaper payer once they had taken full advantage of the costly initial consultation and health education advice and care. This could mean that disparities in premiums and services would cause episodic switches between payers by beneficiaries, depending on their needs and desires for care and consultation at any one time. This is now seen in traditional managed care Medicare plans. Less predictably, how long would it take for those health-related services to show up as cost reductions by actually improving health? And there is the rub. If Oxford, for example, were to offer more preventive care, the beneficiaries might start to become healthier, but might switch to a cheaper payer just as the positive results began to accrue. What payer wants to make an investment in a competitor's profit? Let us say that all payers bought into paying for preventive care; then every payer would benefit equally from the reduced illness costs. But there are a couple of problems with this model too. What about the 17 or 18 percent of Americans with no insurance or only partial insurance for part of the year? Who assumes their cost of being deprived of health- and illness-preventive services? How do you prevent cream skimming by payers or adverse selection (adverse to payers when a sicker population chooses their plan)? How do you know patients will follow the (expensive) advice and regimens meant to keep them healthier? We know that even sick people fill prescriptions only half the time.

One solution for this problematic situation is to place advanced practice nurses in the primary care role. Trained as experts in illness prevention and health promotion, in the science of health education, and with community-based clinical experiences, they know how to obtain the best—and most cost-effective—results, and they provide this comprehensive constellation of services for the same fee that physicians receive for an illness-only related visit.

This was an influential issue in Columbia's and CAPNA's argument for equal fees with physicians. Because overhead is the same for any quality practice, the only disparity in costs of a practice is the income of the provider. If advanced practice nurses provide longer, more comprehensive services in a primary care visit, then they will see fewer patients a day than will a primary care physician. Fewer patient care visits equal lower income. The argument for equal fees therefore still had the outcome of lower incomes for nurse practitioners. This helped carry the day with physicians, who could not get past their long-held beliefs that doctors are somehow worth more than nurse practitioners. But there is more than politics involved with fee parity. Patients pay no more, and no less, for the differentiated practice of an advanced practice nurse. They are choosing the kind of care they want, not the price they want to pay. And this choice will be powerful in the policy decisions as the health system evolves.

CHRONIC ILLNESS CARE

Recently, a major payer has begun to think about reimbursing nurses for chronic illness care, as well as for the broader category of primary care. The idea is that patients (identified by claims forms) who are high users of care, medications, and hospitalizations due to a diagnosed chronic illness would be offered care (at no deductible) by an advanced practice nurse expert, as well as sustaining the patient's conventional primary care physician and specialist relationships. While this targeted assistance with management of a costly condition might appear to be good for payer and patient alike, the actual logistics probably reduce the benefits. First, most primary care physicians would feel that their care was being questioned and their authority eroded. Specialists may also view chronic illness management as their sphere. Which regimen does the patient follow? Whom does he or she call with a question or symptom? Can patients sort out when to call the chronic illness nurse or the primary care physician or the specialist? Who coordinates three different approaches for the brittle diabetic patient, for example?

While targeted management for chronic illness is valued and cost-effective, it probably works best when incorporated into the comprehensive primary care role. If a patient has an advanced practice nurse as his or her primary care provider, the chronic illness nurse specialist may be irrelevant. If the patient with chronic illness has a physician primary care provider, however, there may be gaps in care—less health education, counseling, home visit assessment and coordination, and individualized risk reduction. It may be that patients with chronic illness are particularly well served by an advanced practice nurse, as opposed to a physician primary care provider.

INDEPENDENT REIMBURSEMENT: AUTHORIZATION FOR DIFFERENTIATED PRACTICE

When advanced practice nurses gain full independent primary care authority, as in the CAPNA model, they are free to provide care within the context of a nursing model, which includes the parameters of cost-effective chronic illness care. When the advanced practice nurse is called in as an adjunct to medical care, to do the subsets of the role that are particular to nursing, the model works less well. Advanced practice nurses need to have authority for the health of the whole person to achieve optimal outcomes.

Physicians often think nursing should just join in and work with them. But because they are not trained as experts in nurse-specific care, physicians cannot fully use advanced practice nurses unless there is joint authority, peer-to-peer decision making, and, perhaps even more powerful, joint accountability.

REORGANIZING AND CLARIFYING NURSING EDUCATIONAL ROLES

Getting to this more mature configuration of health care will be difficult. Breaking down long-held professional expectations (nurses are at fault as well as physicians) about who is in charge is central. Part of the resolution will require painful reorganization within nursing. The profession includes those with a one-year high-school-level program leading to licensed practical nurse licensure, as well as the seven-year education and training of an advanced practice nurse with a graduate degree in a practice specialty. Even then, the best advanced practice nursing graduate programs do not provide training in the fully independent role required to be a true peer in independent or joint practice with a physician. And rarely can someone entering nursing at the most basic level make it to the top level of training and competence.

This ladder system of education does not work for two major reasons: the depth of science needed for each level of practice and the disparity in career aspirations and abilities of incoming students. Because technical practice in a highly supervised environment requires less independent decision making and therefore less depth of knowledge, each succeeding level of practice requires a more comprehensive understanding of even the basics rather than an additive set of skills. Dispensing medications in a structured situation like a hospital requires less knowledge of pharmacology and pathophysiology than an independent nurse primary care provider. For those interested in moving up that career ladder, however, additive courses are not sufficient; a basic and deeper understanding of basic sciences is required.

The issue of nursing education progression, however, is less a problem than the limitations currently posed in terms of who is attracted to the profession in the first place. Although there is great disparity between those who enter a licensed practical nurse or associate degree program and those who enter nursing in a four-year university-level bachelor of science program, the real problem in recruitment is that anyone looking for a fully autonomous career rarely considers nursing at all.

It is the public perception of the intellectual and cultural limitations of nursing that tracks professionally oriented students away from nursing. Those who want an authoritative, independent career in health care prefer medicine. If, however, one is interested in a career with shared and limited responsibility, which still affords an opportunity to provide valued care to sick individuals, while sustaining priority time and energies for other activities, then nursing is the preferred venue. Nursing, however, began to push against this comfortable medical-nursing hierarchy almost forty years ago, and as with any other profound cultural realignment, it has been a troubled transformation. The easy part was the educational advancement in the late 1960s, which included the emerging role of graduate-level advanced practice nurses, especially nurse practitioners and clinical specialists. Despite knowing and understanding more, this new breed of nurse experienced very little increase in authority or economic gain. Physicians and institutional employers were glad to have more nursing knowledge and skill to call on, but they were loathe to change the hierarchy or level of authority of these more expert nurses. Also, because there were so few advanced practice nurses, and still all categorized as "nurses," the public rarely distinguished between novice and expert; certainly, nurses could not be distinguished by authority or pay or title. Although authority for advanced practice nurses is now advancing rapidly, it is happening for the wrong reasons and is probably targeted at the wrong goals.

Advanced practice nurses are not physician substitutes for less critically ill patients. Advanced practice nurses, while holding common core competencies with physicians, have a distinctive practice built on different scientific bases. Armed with that knowledge and engaging in a different practice style, they develop different relationships with their patients and achieve valued outcomes that are less likely to be achieved by physicians.

The expected cascade of nurse primary care providers has not overwhelmed the health care system, for three reasons. Most important, states differ radically in the level of authority they allow advanced practice nurses. This severely hampers development of a national model for educating advanced practice nurses for the highest level of practice.

Second, educational programs lag woefully behind practice, even in the less restrictive states. Although Medicaid and Medicare authorize full-scope practice and commercial insurers are quickly accepting the same broad advanced practice nursing authority, nursing programs have not expanded their curricula to teach these extended skills or the science that underpins broader practice. Part of this gap in education is related to the way faculty participate in conventional schools of nursing.

For decades, faculty taught in the classroom and sent their students to hospital wards for clinical training. In the past thirty years, advanced practice master's degree programs and doctoral degree programs preparing nurse investigators have grown dramatically. The former have focused on site-specific practice—the hospital or the outpatient clinic; rarely was the independent role taught or modeled by faculty practitioners. Now, with that role emerging as a valuable one, schools are largely without faculty who can practice or teach it. Because the expanded nursing role requires cross-site training—emergency department, hospital, outpatient, community-based clinic—and the use of a specialist network, the medical center environment is the richest training ground for independent nurse practitioners. Not inconsequentially, medical centers rarely have a large cohort of generalist physicians, making it far easier for the independent nurse practitioner role to flourish. Less than 1 percent of nursing schools reside in medical centers, whereas 100 percent of medical schools do.

It will be this small, well-located 1 percent of nursing schools that will take the lead in future nursing education advancement. It is unlikely that programs in advanced practice will be able to accommodate the additional training within a marketable master's degree. The single-site training is still needed, and the new training would require 100 credits and may cost $90,000 for a four-year master's degree—hardly competitive or attractive.

THE CLINICAL DOCTORATE IN NURSING

For those who want a health-oriented career (as opposed to one focused on illness resolution), a postbaccalaureate entry into a program that culminates in full authority, with a doctoral degree in nursing, should be established. This would accomplish many important outcomes. First, it would offer a wholly new destination in nursing: an authoritative role with title of doctor. Today, nursing is the only health profession without a doctoral degree in practice (there are doctoral degrees in medicine, dentistry, physical therapy, optometry, and podiatry). Not only does this limit the public view of nursing as a full profession; it powerfully limits the profession's draw for those who want an accountable and independent career.

Second, it would raise the bar of what is expected for a nurse at the highest level of practice. In other words, it would be very clear that new skills and new learning other than existing curricula in advanced practice nursing must be developed.

Third, the development of such a degree would solve a problem unique to nursing: it would be an opportunity to clarify and standardize the level of practice at the highest level. Even now, in the best master's programs preparing advanced practice nurses, credits required may vary by as much as one-third, and clinical experiences and preceptors meet no national standards.

By developing a program for college graduates, the incoming students in both medical and nursing schools, all studying for a doctoral degree in practice, could be true peers from the beginning, erasing the past age, gender, and educational differences between medicine and nursing. This would go far toward erasing the barriers to communication and status and lowering the barriers to the establishment of joint practices. Even with such a program in place, however, three other major issues need to be resolved.

First, state-by-state differences in nurse practice acts must be abolished. The highest level should prevail everywhere, and educational institutions everywhere must teach to provide these competencies for every graduate. Today in states with restrictive practice acts, nursing students cannot learn full-scope practice because their professors cannot practice that way, and their learning is artificially constrained. And yet this same graduate can go to a state with a broader scope of practice laws and gain authority to practice beyond his or her educational experiences. This kind of system is irrational and damages quality.

Second, what about the 100,000 advanced practice nurses with master's degrees already practicing? Do they need to return to school, or are there two levels of advanced practice? Graduates of master's programs are well qualified for site-specific primary care at its highest level: diagnosing and caring for their patients in an ambulatory setting. But when the advanced practice nurse takes on the full scope role, more education is needed. This expanded role means cross-site practice and accountability. It includes admitting and comanaging hospitalized patients, conducting or directing emergency department evaluations, selecting and using specialist referrals independently, knowing how to manage resulting care or diagnostic regimens, and taking calls in a group practice, often triaging or treating patients not personally known to the clinician taking the call.

And third, much more research is needed to verify that advanced practice nurses with this full authority and competency do bring about different, or better, more lasting, and cost-effective outcomes.

The idea of full authority for advanced practice nurses, who are more engaged with their patients and more powerful guides to a better level of health, will be questioned until better outcomes are clearly linked to their practices. The randomized controlled trial conducted in the mid-1990s should help put to rest the fact that advanced practice nurses can provide medically oriented primary care indistinguishable from that provided by primary care physicians (Mundinger and others, 2000). But these advanced practice nurses had admitting privileges, had easy and collegial access to top medical specialists, and more important, had excelled in ambulatory practice for years. This is not the norm for the advanced practice nurse in most practices today.

This one study proves nothing on its own. Its power is the size and rigor of the study and the fact that it confirmed what had been shown in over a hundred smaller, less rigorous studies for over thirty years. The theme is unmistakable.

The CAPNA study—Will patients with an extraordinary level of choice choose a nurse practitioner for primary care?—answered by a cautious yes. The practice is solid and growing; patients stay with the practice; over 80 percent of new patients come by word of mouth. But there are not yet enough people aware of differentiated primary care. In many ways, CAPNA serves those actively seeking a different kind of care: more time, more explanations, more directed help with health improvement, and the few with tragically neglected conditions because the patient so feared a cold clinical encounter with a conventional provider. Not surprisingly, many have a chronic illness, and many have also had several new, and sometimes serious, conditions identified by the practitioners. The patients cannot be simply categorized, but most are remarkably well attuned to health and health care and represent the average Manhattanite: well off financially, well educated, middle-aged, and in a hurry to get into perfect health. It is the last characteristic that distinguishes our client base and may indicate that they recognize that advanced practice nurses offer a differentiated service.

BUILDING A NEW NATIONAL MODEL

One of the reasons the practice has not attracted more patients is the small number of advanced practice nurses, in Manhattan and elsewhere, who aspire to this level of practice and can therefore help market and expand the practice. Individuals seeking a health career often distinguish between the care and cure models; those wishing to be involved in traditional medicine know they are entering a profession that is highly regarded and that gives them clear, independent decision making and authority for diagnosing and treating disease.

Those who are less interested in the authoritative model, and who find the caregiving role profoundly satisfying, may prefer an approach to practice more compatible with conventional nursing. Now, as nursing enters a time of rapidly increasing independent authority, not only are health career choices blurred, but those continuing to seek the less independent role are reluctant to engage in nursing at its most authoritative level. There is not yet the pool of individuals entering nursing from which to recruit for the new roles. There is as yet no broad understanding of what an advanced practice nursing career has to offer, especially to those in high school and college who are contemplating career choices, and therefore very few independent-minded individuals choose nursing. Leaders in the nursing profession will need to distinguish to these individuals what a career in nursing can become, and they will also need to distinguish the different levels of education leading to different levels of practice. A nurse is a nurse is a nurse is a harmful myth. There needs to be a new entry point to nursing to obviate the existing unattractive career path, which forces those seeking a fully independent advanced practice nursing career to first experience so much of the dependent, nonprofessional role.

Second, there is not a critical number of role models for the new practice levels. Expanding regulation has moved much more quickly than the resulting practice and education. Finding those already in nursing who are willing to take on the new roles so that they can mentor students is difficult; those in senior positions rarely entered nursing to establish more advanced practices, and they are reluctant to model them now for tomorrow's nurses. Along the same lines, few nursing faculty practice at all, much less at these new and demanding levels of accountability.

Unlike the site-specific practice for the master's degree–prepared nurse, the new, more independent practices authorized by state practice laws and by payers require cross-site practice. Authority to admit and comanage hospitalized patients, emergency department evaluations, taking calls, choosing and using specialists, and evaluating their advice all take more education and experience, but they also require more primary accountability for treatment and for outcomes, a parameter of practice that has not been associated with nursing and not always valued by those choosing a nursing career. Attracting those who would aspire to the new levels of nursing is a daunting challenge. The nuances of approach that distinguish nursing from medicine, at the zenith of each profession's most independent practice level, are difficult for the uninitiated to ponder. And yet those differences are profoundly responsible for a given individual's success and satisfaction in his or her chosen career.

While the newest level of nursing practice is the most independent, the training required is more multidisciplinary than for the lower levels of nursing independence. The very nature of hospital comanagement requires physician collaboration, as does the use of specialists. This kind of training takes place most effectively at a medical center, and yet very few baccalaureate and graduate nursing schools reside at medical centers. Further constraining the growth of this level of nursing is the paucity of nursing faculty practice at medical centers. Partly because research is a major component of medical centers, and nurse researchers are more likely to be found at medical center nursing schools, there are fewer advanced practice nurses on those faculties. And yet this is where the future practitioners must be trained and learn to work in very high-level collaborations.

It is unlikely that the new level of nursing (essentially *advanced* advanced practice) will catch on without a new distinctive degree. Master's degrees now often require two years of education postbaccalaureate, and students will not be attracted to further master's-level study, nor would that credential hold much meaning to the public or the payers. A new doctor of nursing practice degree is surely the best way to project the level of accomplishment and authority now invested in the higher competencies of cross-site practice. With this advancement, payers, the public, patients, and, most of all, the potential applicants will know what the new career in nursing practice is and demands. Then, and only then, can this new role be fully established and flourish.

References

Donaldson, M. S., Yordy, K. D., Lohr, K. N., and Vanselow, N. A. (eds.). *Primary Care: America's Health in a New Era.* Washington, D.C.: National Academy Press, 1996.

Mundinger, M. O. *Home Care Controversy: Too Little, Too Late, Too Costly.* Rockville, Md.: Aspen, 1983.

Mundinger, M. O., and others. "Primary Care Outcomes in Patients Treated by Nurse Practitioners or Physicians: A Randomized Trial." *Journal of the American Medical Association,* 2000, *283,* 59–68.

Wennberg, J., and Gittelsohn, A. "Variations in Medical Care Among Small Areas." *Scientific American,* 1982, *246,* 120–134.

PART THREE

Reconstructing Primary Care for Patients and Populations

Part Three explores new ideas about how to provide primary care to future populations. In Chapter Eight, Larry Green provides an ecological perspective on the need for primary care. Lewis Sandy and Steven Schroeder suggest in Chapter Nine that current forces in the health care system will create the dissolution of primary care as a single concept, replaced by alignment of providers by economic niche, not role. Arlyss Anderson Rothman and Ed Wagner describe in Chapter Ten the role of primary care in chronic illness management and the chronic care model, which has been used successfully in primary care. In Chapter Eleven, Eric Larson focuses on the role of primary care in caring for the elderly, particularly prevention, long-term care, and home care. Christine Cassel and Beth Demel argue in Chapter Twelve for the importance of training physicians in the basic medical, pharmacological, and psychosocial aspects of palliative care. In Chapter Thirteen, Harold Pincus describes the role of primary care for persons with psychosocial problems and behavioral disorders. In Chapter Fourteen, Michael Weitzman, Jonathan Klein, and Tina Cheng argue that primary care for children differs in fundamental ways from primary care of adults.

CHAPTER EIGHT

Is Primary Care Worthy of Physicians?

An Ecological Perspective

Larry A. Green

Ecology is the study of the relationships of organisms and their environments. Human medical ecology can be understood to include the study of the relationships people have with medical care. One perspective on medical ecology was provided by the 1961 study, "The Ecology of Medical Care," authored by White, Williams, and Greenberg, which quantified where people were in the health care system in an average month. This landmark analysis relied on data from multiple sources and countries, dating from 1928, to make carefully reasoned estimates of the number of adults in an average month receiving health care in particular settings. They concluded that among 1,000 free-living adults, 750 were symptomatic each month, 250 received care from doctors in the office setting, 9 were hospitalized, 5 were referred to a specialist, and fewer than 1 was admitted to an academic medical center (Figure 8.1). Focusing on the adequacy of medical care to meet the needs of all the people, this study challenged

George E. Fryer provided analyses of the National Ambulatory Medical Care Survey and the Medical Expenditure Panel Surveys and with Robert L. Phillips and Tom Miyoshi created the maps in this chapter.

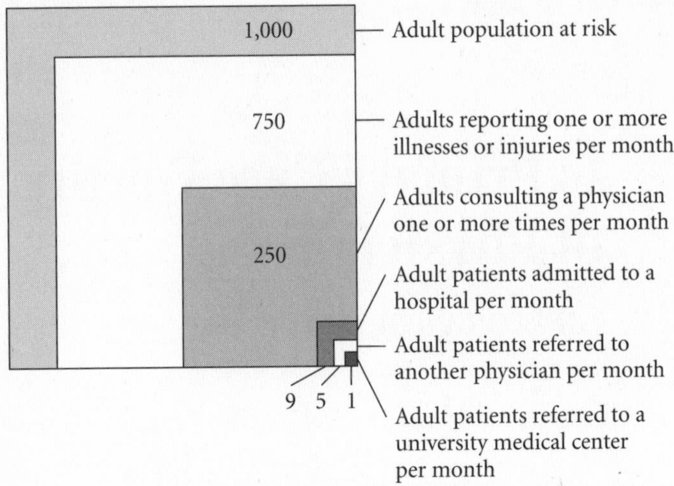

Figure 8.1. The Ecology of Medical Care, 1961

Source: White, Williams, and Greenberg (1961).

the health care enterprise to strike an appropriate balance among the various settings of health care in terms of education, research, and practice. The strong implication was that health policies in the United States overemphasized hospital-based care, and the problems filtered to academic health centers, while relatively neglecting most of the problems that most people have, most of the time.

This study has been replicated and expanded some forty years later, using stronger data sources, all from the United States, and including children as well as adults (Green and others, 2001). This update concluded that in an average month, of 1,000 men, women, and children in the United States, about 800 were symptomatic, 327 considered seeking medical care, 217 visited a doctor, 65 visited a provider of complementary and alternative medicine, 21 visited a hospital outpatient clinic, 14 received health care in their home, 13 visited an emergency department, 8 were hospitalized, and fewer than 1 was hospitalized in an academic medical center (Figure 8.2). Each of these numbers represents unique individuals, not events, and is a portion of 1,000 people "at risk" during an average month.

These renderings of the ecology of medical care provide a framework for thinking about health policy across a range of issues—for example: the organization and financing of health care, the distribution of illness and disease, the choices people make about medical care,

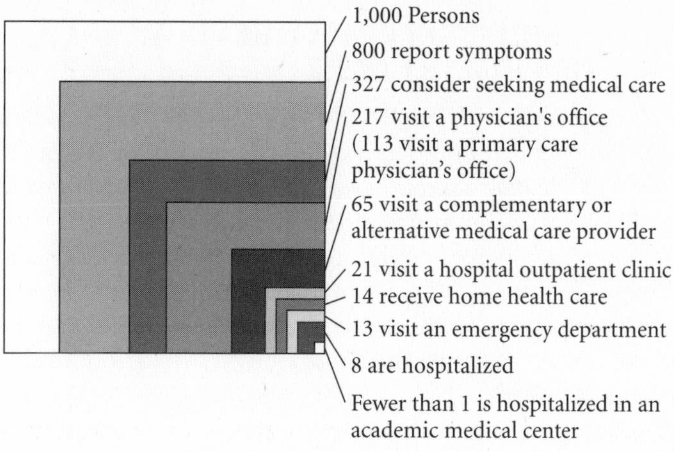

Figure 8.2. The Ecology of Medical Care Revisited, 2000
Source: Green and others (2001).

the interfaces among different components of personal health care, the relationship between public health and medical care, and, the focus of this chapter, the role of primary care. After forty years of nearly tumultuous change in health care and great expansion of knowledge and technology, the similarities between the estimates concerning doctors, hospitals, and academic health center hospitals are provocative. Could the similarities be real and derive from something about the human condition and human behavior that persists and is expressed despite changes in organization and policy? Could it be that interval developments had counterbalancing effects, such as successful reductions in the burden of suffering associated with prevention countered by greater utilization associated with more chronic disease?

Regardless of the explanation of the apparent stability of the estimates over four decades, it is obvious from this population perspective that the bulk of the health care enterprise remains in self-care, primary care, and ambulatory care. The questions of forty years ago about balancing and optimizing health care strategies to meet the needs of all the people are still relevant. The purpose of this chapter is to consider from several perspectives how the nature and role of primary care fit into this ecology of medical care model, particularly to inform considerations of whether primary care is of sufficient importance and complexity to merit the commitment of a physician workforce.

A BRIEF, SELECTIVE REVIEW OF PRIMARY CARE

The term *primary care* is used as if it is precise and widely understood. In fact, it may not be found in dictionaries, and its origins are uncertain. An authoritative definition was developed by an Institute of Medicine (IOM) study committee in 1996: "Primary care is the provision of integrated, accessible health care services by clinicians who are accountable for addressing a large majority of personal health care needs, developing a sustained partnership with patients, and practicing in the context of family and community" (Donaldson, Yordy, Lohr, and Vanselow, 1996, p. 1).

This definition asserts that primary care is a function, achieved in a sustained relationship with those who want and need health care. It is neither a discipline nor a specialty. It is not definable as a list of problems, since by definition all problems can exist in primary care. Like motherhood, primary care cannot be understood only as lists of tasks and services rendered or by the credentials of the person providing a particular service. This function provides and integrates services across all the boxes in the ecology model, for most health care problems, in the context in which the user of health care services lives. Primary care is not the stand-alone solution to all health care problems (Turner and Lain, 2001), but few people can have their health care needs managed optimally without any primary care.

Primary care is known to have salutary effects (Donaldson, Yordy, Lohr, and Vanselow, 1996). When people have continuing access to primary care, treatment occurs before evolution to more severe problems and emergency department use, and hospital admissions decrease. Primary care clinicians use fewer tests and spend less money. Particularly for the poor, access to primary care is associated with improved vision, more complete immunization, better blood pressure control, enhanced dental status, and reduced estimated mortality. Both primary care and subspecialty clinicians fail to achieve preventive service guidelines, but people with a regular source of primary care receive more preventive services. Higher levels of primary care in a geographical area are associated with lower mortality rates, after controlling for important effects of urban-rural difference, poverty rates, education, and lifestyle factors.

Starfield's landmark work (1991, 1992) showed that countries with health systems more oriented toward primary care generally achieved better health status in terms of low birth weight, neonatal mortality, life expectancy, years of potential life lost, with higher patient satisfaction, lower per capita expenditures, and lower medication use. These effects are associated with primary care providing a place where people can bring a wide range of health problems and expect in most instances that their problems will be resolved without referral. Once they are there, an ongoing relationship fosters participation by people in decision making about their own care, opens opportunities for health promotion and disease prevention, and bridges personal health care with family and community needs and circumstances. Thus, after reviewing the evidence about primary care, the Institute of Medicine Study Committee (Donaldson, Yordy, Lohr, and Vanselow, 1996) arrived at the following conclusions:

- Primary care is the logical foundation of an effective health care system because it can address a large majority of the health problems present in the population.
- Primary care is essential to achieving the objectives that together constitute value in health care: high quality of care, including achievement of desired health outcomes; patient satisfaction; and efficient use of resources.
- Personal interactions that include trust and partnership between patients and clinicians are central to primary care.
- Primary care is an important instrument for achieving stronger emphasis on both ends of the spectrum of care: health promotion and disease prevention and the care of the chronically ill, especially among the elderly with multiple problems.

In summary, primary care is important because it provides health care services people want and need, for important problems, in a satisfying manner.

A LOOK AT CURRENT DATA ON PEOPLE WHO GO TO THE DOCTOR

A slight majority of the visits made to physicians' offices in the United States are made to the physician specialties meeting the Institute of Medicine definition of primary care, even though these specialties represent only about one-third of practicing physicians (Table 8.1). The

Number of Visits (rounded)	1997	1998	1999
All physicians	787	829	757
Family physicians/general practitioners	200	202	171
General internists	121	141	136
General pediatricians	92	96	73
Obstetrician/gynecologists	71	84	60

Table 8.1. Visits to Office-Based Physicians in the United States (in millions).

Source: National Ambulatory Medical Care Survey.

most common reasons for visiting primary care physicians and the diagnoses made during these visits during the last five years of the twentieth century in the United States are characterized in six age and sex groupings in Tables 8.2 and 8.3, respectively. The breadth of problems seen in primary care physicians' offices as presented by about 113 individuals per 1,000 per average month, the spectrum of their seriousness, and opportunities for promoting health and preventing disease during these visits are made obvious by these partial listings.

The importance and benefits of having a usual source of care has been documented as illustrated in Table 8.4 (Center for Policy Studies in Family Practice and Primary Care, 2000; Robert Graham Center, 2000). In 1996, 82 percent of Americans had a usual source of health care, and of these, 56 percent named an individual physician, as opposed to an institution, as that source. The distribution by specialty of these physicians identified by people as their usual source of care, was 62 percent family physicians/general practitioners, 16 percent internists, 15 percent pediatricians, and 8 percent some other specialty (Robert Graham Center, 2000).

Another way to understand current primary care in the United States from the perspective of those who visit the physician's office is to examine the care of health problems identified by federal agencies as "priority conditions." These conditions are important because of their threat to life and impact on health status and expenditures. From the Medical Expenditure Panel Surveys (2001), it is possible to identify whom people with priority health conditions indicate as their usual source of care. As shown in Table 8.5, most of these priority conditions affect adults, and these people usually identify the primary care physicians caring for adults as their usual source of care. Of course, people could claim a usual source of care but not go see the physician, preferring to go elsewhere or being referred to specialty rather than

	Female		Male	
Age Group	**Reason**	**Visits**	**Reason**	**Visits**
Under age 15	Well baby examination	127.54	Well baby examination	118.25
	Cough	94.49	Cough	100.69
	General medical examination	86.24	General medical examination	90.44
	Fever	82.87	Fever	86.54
	Sore throat	52.89	Earache	50.14
	Earache	50.24	Sore throat	46.33
	Nasal congestion	38.35	Nasal congestion	34.22
	Head cold, upper respiratory infection	31.88	Skin rash	29.34
	Skin rash	31.63	Head cold, upper respiratory infection	27.45
	Vaccination/immunization	17.65	Ear symptoms NOS	20.98
Ages 15–24	Sore throat	81.08	Sore throat	103.11
	General medical examination	62.25	General medical examination	70.89
	Routine prenatal examination	61.56	Cough	64.35
	Cough	45.26	Sports/camp physical exam	35.15
	Headache	28.81	Skin rash	25.44
	Abdominal pain NOS	24.09	Head cold, upper respiratory infection	20.92
	Skin rash	21.84	Back pain, ache, discomfort	20.12
	Head cold, upper respiratory infection	21.68	Headache	18.87
	Sports/camp physical exam	19.78	Required school physical exam	18.63
	Earache	18.53	Nasal congestion	18.48
Ages 25–44	General medical examination	53.20	General medical examination	64.27
	Cough	43.08	Cough	41.42
	Sore throat	42.61	Sore throat	40.78
	Headache	30.43	Back pain, ache, discomfort	34.64
	Routine prenatal examination	26.29	Follow-up visit NOS	26.41
	Back pain, ache, discomfort	26.28	Low back pain, ache, discomfort	23.23
	Head cold, upper respiratory infection	20.67	Skin rash	20.34
	Earache	18.51	Headache	19.85
	Skin rash	17.88	Chest pain NOS	18.55
	Follow-up visit NOS	17.32	Blood pressure check	17.92
Ages 45–64	General medical examination	86.82	General medical examination	103.75
	Hypertension	39.67	Hypertension	43.33
	Cough	37.81	Follow-up visit NOS	40.58
	Follow-up visit NOS	35.27	Cough	36.55
	Blood pressure check	28.89	Blood pressure check	33.21
	Back pain, ache, discomfort	25.97	Diabetes mellitus	32.48
	New/renewed medication NOS	24.51	Back pain, ache, discomfort	27.59
	Headache	21.63	New/renewed medication NOS	23.98
	Sore throat	17.85	Chest pain NOS	23.76
	Diabetes mellitus	17.33	Head cold, upper respiratory infection	17.11
Ages 65–74	General medical examination	94.99	General medical examination	106.42
	Follow-up visit NOS	53.98	Follow-up visit NOS	50.42
	Hypertension	46.51	Hypertension	47.46
	Cough	42.09	Cough	33.03
	Blood pressure check	37.31	Blood pressure check	30.49

Table 8.2. Most Frequent Reasons for Visits by Patient Gender and Age Group to the Offices of U.S. Primary Care Physicians, 1995–1999 (per 1,000).

	Female		Male	
Age Group	Reason	Visits	Reason	Visits
	Diabetes mellitus	30.11	Diabetes mellitus	28.32
	New/renewed medication NOS	23.88	Chest pain NOS	20.08
	Back pain, ache, discomfort	19.53	Knee pain, ache, discomfort	17.86
	Vertigo-dizziness	18.48	Skin rash	16.18
	Knee pain, ache, discomfort	17.61	New/renewed medication NOS	16.08
75 and over	General medical examination	95.55	General medical examination	102.65
	Follow-up visit NOS	66.17	Follow-up visit NOS	73.24
	Hypertension	42.72	Hypertension	29.30
	Cough	35.47	Cough	27.67
	Blood pressure check	34.41	Vertigo-dizziness	27.02
	Vertigo-dizziness	23.73	Diabetes mellitus	26.37
	Diabetes mellitus	19.73	Shortness of breath	21.95
	Back pain, ache, discomfort	19.26	Blood pressure check	9.82
	New/renewed medication NOS	19.14	Back pain, ache, discomfort	18.18
	Leg pain, ache, discomfort	16.24	General weakness	17.03

Table 8.2. Most Frequent Reasons for Visits by Patient Gender and Age Group to the Offices of U.S. Primary Care Physicians, 1995–1999 (per 1,000), Cont'd.

Note: NOS = not otherwise specified.

Source: National Ambulatory Medical Care Survey.

primary care settings for their care. The specialty of physicians whom patients with these conditions actually visit can be determined by analyzing the National Ambulatory Medical Care Survey. As seen in Table 8.6, the care of these priority conditions is shared across many specialties, with the primary care physicians typically providing a majority of visits across the spectrum of priority conditions, with cancer being a notable exception. These data confirm that integrating care for people with these important conditions is possible through the offices of primary care physicians.

A geographical perspective can also inform the ecology of medical care by depicting relationships between people living in particular jurisdictions and health care. Access to primary care physicians can be represented by mapping primary care health professions shortage areas, as shown in Figure 8.3. This figure confirms that the United States has not yet provided adequate access to primary care for substantial portions of the country. A measure of the U.S. reliance on primary care physicians for service can be portrayed by simulating the effects that withdrawal of primary care physicians of various specialties would have on the designation of specific counties as whole county shortage areas (Fryer, Green, Dovey, and Phillips, 2001). The

	Female		Male	
Age Group	**Diagnosis**	**Visits**	**Diagnosis**	**Visits**
Under age 15	Routine child health exam	212.82	Routine child health exam	210.15
	Otitis media NOS	97.35	Otitis media NOS	109.99
	Acute upper respiratory infection NOS	90.10	Acute upper respiratory infection NOS	91.68
	Acute pharyngitis	37.93	Acute pharyngitis	34.35
	Chronic sinusitis NOS	24.83	Chronic sinusitis NOS	25.46
	Viral infection NOS	23.84	Chronic bronchitis NOS	24.51
	Asthma NOS	19.78	Asthma NOS	24.15
	Chronic bronchitis NOS	18.66	Viral infection NOS	19.98
	Acute tonsillitis	17.33	Acute tonsillitis	14.80
	Gastrointeritis NOS	13.73	Gastroenteritis NOS	12.89
Ages 15–24	Acute upper respiratory infection NOS	57.03	Acute upper respiratory infection NOS	58.97
	Normal prenatal exam	38.95	Acute pharyngitis	49.35
	Routine medical exam	37.23	Routine child health exam	47.01
	Acute pharyngitis	37.09	Routine medical exam	41.99
	Chronic sinusitis NOS	33.24	Medical exam, administrative purpose	39.36
	Routine child health exam	27.71	Chronic sinusitis NOS	36.39
	Asthma NOS	24.86	Chronic bronchitis NOS	34.67
	Pregnancy, incidental	21.77	Asthma NOS	19.35
	Chronic bronchitis NOS	20.20	Gastroenteritis NOS	14.48
	Medical exam, administrative purpose	19.37	Acute tonsillitis	14.04
Ages 25–44	Chronic sinusitis NOS	42.90	Hypertension NOS	7.46
	Acute upper respiratory infection NOS	42.07	Acute upper respiratory infection NOS	34.96
	Routine medical exam	28.12	Chronic sinusitis NOS	31.91
	Hypertension NOS	26.94	Routine medical exam	29.67
	Chronic bronchitis NOS	23.74	Chronic bronchitis NOS	28.09
	Depression NOS	22.20	Acute pharyngitis	20.33
	Acute pharyngitis	1.60	Type 2 diabetes	17.14
	Normal prenatal exam	21.28	Allergic rhinitis	14.64
	Allergic rhinitis NOS	19.28	Health exam–group survey	13.75
	Obesity NOS	19.23	Asthma NOS	13.20
Ages 45–64	Hypertension NOS	94.71	Hypertension NOS	117.76
	Type 2 diabetes	44.19	Type 2 diabetes	63.67
	Acute upper respiratory infection NOS	25.14	Routine medical exam	25.56
	Chronic sinusitis NOS	4.23	Acute upper respiratory infection NOS	25.25
	Chronic bronchitis NOS	20.03	Chronic bronchitis NOS	20.65
	Routine medical exam	18.24	Chronic sinusitis NOS	16.09
	Urinary tract infection NOS	14.84	Coronary artery disease	16.03
	Obesity NOS	13.67	Hypercholesterolemia	15.65
	Osteoarthritis NOS	13.40	Hyperlipidemia NOS	13.53
	Hyperlipidemia NOS	13.13	Allergic rhinitis NOS	11.20
Ages 65–74	Hypertension NOS	127.67	Hypertension NOS	124.94
	Type 2 diabetes	52.68	Type 2 diabetes	66.22
	Chronic bronchitis NOS	22.66	Coronary artery disease	37.39
	Osteoarthritis NOS	22.57	Chronic obstructive lung disease	32.15

Table 8.3. Most Frequent Diagnoses by Patient Gender and Age Group in the Offices of U.S. Primary Care Physicians, 1995–1999 (per 1,000).

	Female		Male	
Age Group	Diagnosis	Visits	Diagnosis	Visits
	Acute upper respiratory infection NOS	21.91	Chronic bronchitis NOS	25.71
	Chronic obstructive lung disease	18.65	Routine medical exam	17.39
	Coronary artery disease	17.65	Acute upper respiratory infection NOS	16.49
	Urinary tract infection NOS	17.36	Hyperlipidemia NOS	16.40
	Chronic sinusitis NOS	16.96	Hyperplasia of prostate	15.53
	Hyperlipidemia NOS	15.56	Congestive heart failure	15.35
Age 75 and over	Hypertension NOS	134.42	Hypertension NOS	95.10
	Type 2 diabetes	50.17	Type 2 diabetes	62.59
	Coronary artery disease	31.74	Congestive heart failure	34.69
	Congestive heart failure	28.47	Coronary heart disease	34.63
	Osteoarthritis NOS	22.18	Chronic obstructive lung disease	32.99
	Arthropathy NOS	15.97	Osteoarthritis NOS	16.83
	Chronic bronchitis NOS	15.57	Chronic bronchitis NOS	14.58
	Urinary tract infection NOS	15.27	Atrial fibrillation	14.52
	Chronic obstructive lung disease	13.55	Hyperplasia of prostate	14.19
	Acute upper respiratory infection NOS	11.33	Acute upper respiratory infection NOS	12.93

Table 8.3. Most Frequent Diagnoses by Patient Gender and Age Group to the Offices of U.S. Primary Care Physicians, 1995–1999 (per 1,000), Cont'd.

Note: NOS = not otherwise specified.

Source: National Ambulatory Medical Care Survey.

geographical portrayal of what would be the status of U.S. counties without their primary care physicians, at the end of the twentieth century, is shown for general pediatricians, general internists, and family physicians in Figures 8.4, 8.5, and 8.6, respectively. These maps illustrate the large, current role filled by these primary care physicians and provide another way of thinking about health care services that would be required if physicians abandoned primary care.

In summary, when the relationships people now have with their health care system are examined from a primary care perspective, there is evidence that:

- People need primary care, and many seek it out every month.
- Primary care provides and integrates services for most health care problems that people bring to the health care system, and these problems are an unorganized mix of important and not-so-important problems.

	Have Usual Source of Care	Do Not Have Usual Source of Care
Had difficulty obtaining care	11%	17%
Did without needed care	6	12
Had a doctor visit	75	39
Admitted to a hospital	8	4
Purchased a prescribed medicine	70	38
Children		
Had DPT immunization	97	90
Had MMR immunization	92	82
Had polio immunization	96	85
Had hepatitis B immunization	80	73
Adults		
Had influenza immunization	30	13
Blood pressure check	83	56
Cholesterol check	51	23
General examination	52	28
Women: Had Pap smear	60	47
Women: Had mammogram	51	29
Men: Had prostate exam	36	10

Table 8.4. Examples of Impact of Having a Usual Source of Care: Percentage of U.S. Population.

Note: DPT = diphtheria, pertussis and tetanus. MMR = measles, mumps, and rubella.

Source: Based on the 1996 Medical Expenditure Panel Surveys (2001).

Condition	Family Practice/ General Practitioner	General Internal Medicine	General Pediatrics	All Others
Atherosclerotic cardiovascular disease	56%	31%	0.0%	14%
Stroke	56	34	0.9	9
Hypertension	63	28	0.2	8
Diabetes	67	23	0.6	10
Cancer	60	26	2.3	11
Chronic obstructive pulmonary disease	62	22	5.4	11
Asthma	58	15	20.8	6
Anxiety/depression	62	20	7.0	11

Table 8.5. Distribution by Specialty of the Usual Source of Care for People with Selected Conditions and a Physician as That Usual Source.

Source: Based on 1996 Medical Expenditure Panel Surveys (2001).

Condition	Family Practice/ General Practitioner	General Internal Medicine	General Pediatrics	All Others
Atherosclerotic cardiovascular disease	27%	30%	0.4%	43%
Stroke	36	22	0.0	42
Hypertension	43	38	1.0	18
Diabetes	37	31	0.2	32
Cancer	7	13	1.0	79
Chronic obstructive pulmonary disease	41	43	1.1	15
Asthma	28	28	0.2	44
Anxiety/depression	25	13	1.2	60

Table 8.6. Distribution by Physician Specialty of Office Visits by Which Selected Conditions Were the Primary Diagnosis.

Source: Based on 1996 National Ambulatory Medical Care Survey.

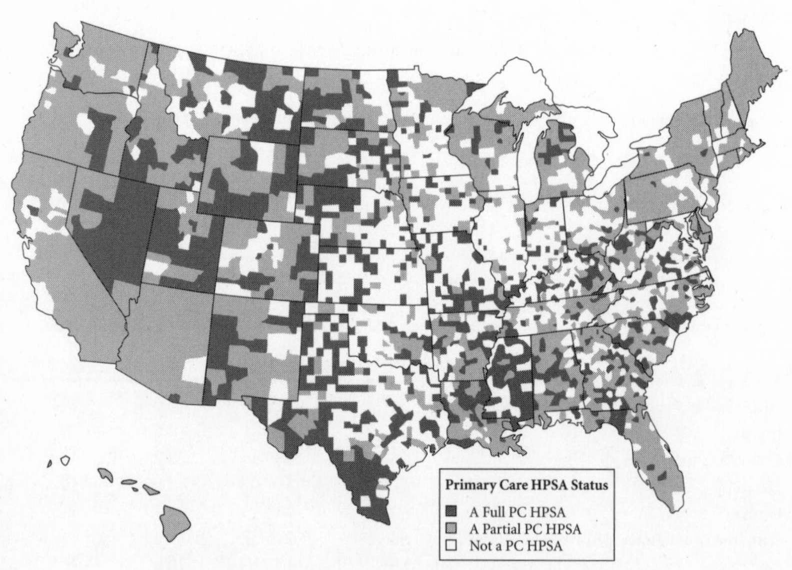

Figure 8.3. Primary Care Health Professions Shortage Areas, by County, 1999

Note: HPSA = health professions shortage area; PC = primary care.

Source: Original analyses done at the Robert Graham Center, Washington, D.C., in 2001.

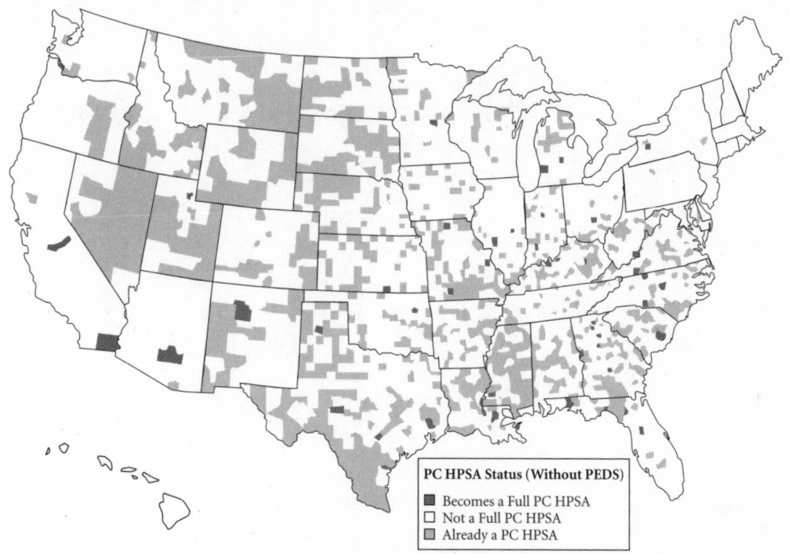

Figure 8.4. Simulation of Whole County Primary Care Health Professions Shortage Areas Without General Pediatricians, 1999

Note: HPSA = health professions shortage area;
PC = primary care; PEDS = general pediatricians.

Source: Original analyses done at the Robert Graham Center, Washington, D.C., in 2001.

- Primary care has important, positive effects that are important to people and governments and would be missed if not provided.
- Health care systems with strong primary care perform better than those without strong primary care systems.
- Primary care provides an organizing focus, a medical home, and a starting place for people that permits intelligent organization of health care services.
- Primary care provides opportunities for clinical prevention.
- Primary care accepts any problem and copes with comorbidity that afflicts many people.
- In an average month, more people receive care in primary care physicians' offices than any other professional health care setting.

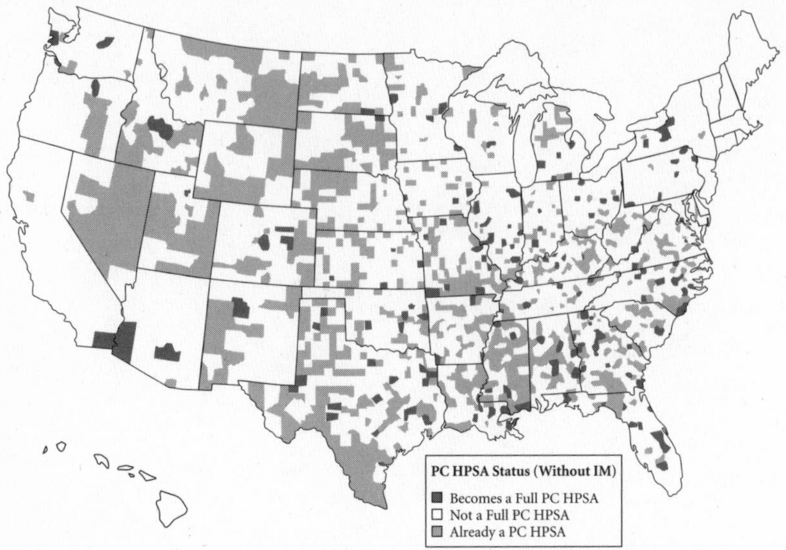

Figure 8.5. Simulation of Whole County Primary Care Health Professions Shortage Areas Without General Internists, 1999

Note: HPSA = health professions shortage area; PC = primary care; IM = general internists.

Source: Original analyses done at the Robert Graham Center, Washington, D.C., in 2001.

- Primary care physicians treat people with priority conditions.
- Primary care physicians are the usual source of care for many people.
- If physicians abandon primary care, there will be a lot of work for someone else to do.

A BRIEF, FORWARD LOOK AT HEALTH CARE

An imminent shift from old ways of thinking and delivering health care toward a new world of health care occurring in the information age has been glimpsed and characterized (Institute of Medicine, 2001). Care based on visits (the boxes of 217, 65, 21, 14, 13 in the ecology model) will adapt to care based on continuous healing relationships, including the boxes of 1,000, 800, 327, 8, and 1. Instead of professional autonomy sequestered in a single box driving variability, care will be

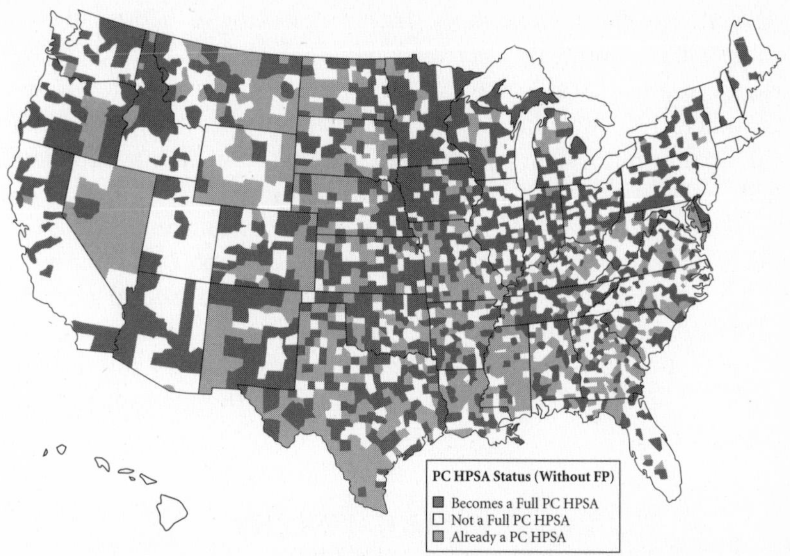

Figure 8.6. Simulation of Whole County Primary Care Health Professions Shortage Areas Without Family Physicians, 1999

Note: HPSA = health professions shortage area; PC = primary care; FP = family physicians.

Source: Original analyses done at the Robert Graham Center, Washington, D.C., in 2001.

customized according to the needs and values of patients, in whatever ecology box they enter. Patients, more than professionals, will be the source of control of care, and not just in the box of 800. Information will cease being a mere record; knowledge will be shared and flow freely across health care, work, and home settings; and decisions will be based less on training and experience and more on evidence. Thus, the same database will be useful and accessible in each of the ecology boxes, and authority and power previously based on controlling information will be diminished, and authority based on understanding may expand.

Avoiding harm will become a property of the entire health care system, a requirement in every box; and secrecy will yield to the necessity of transparency in health care services, cutting across all the ecology boxes. The future system will not just react to demands and needs; it will anticipate needs, making a medical home for every person even more necessary, perhaps connecting the boxes of 217 and

327 with the entire population. Instead of seeking reductions in cost, waste will be continually decreased, perhaps by locating services in the right box and guaranteeing reliable interfaces between each box and the others, reducing unnecessary redundancy. Rather than professional roles trumping system performance, cooperation among clinicians will be the priority—in every one of the boxes.

Such a vision invites integration, the primary care function, as defined. Thus, the future of primary care and its impact on improving people's lives depends heavily on how its place is constructed in evolving health care systems. Given the nature and role of primary care as it has evolved so far, it is likely that the future sufficiency and sustainability of new health care systems depend in part on the adequacy of primary care.

IS PRIMARY CARE WORTHY WORK FOR PHYSICIANS?

This question is being asked now, in part, because multiple initiatives focused on medical schools to strengthen primary care (examples are the Robert Wood Johnson Foundation's Generalist Physician Initiative and the Health Resources and Service Administrations Interdisciplinary Generalist Curriculum Program) have not succeeded. Despite programs such as these, medical students' interest in primary care has waned, possibly because of the effects of managed care, student debt, and persistent social forces that steer medical students away from primary care (Dwinnell and Adams, 2001).

Meanwhile, measurements of the performance of U.S. health care have been disturbing, with the World Health Organization (WHO, 2000) ranking the United States at thirty-seventh overall, fifteenth using the WHO Index weighted to reward responsiveness, and seventy-second when the system is evaluated from the perspective of disease-adjusted life expectancy. These rankings reach a level of embarrassment when juxtaposed to the world-leading expenditures in the United States for personal health care services, whether calculated as total amount, per capita amount, or percentage of gross domestic product (World Health Organization, 2000; Heffler and others, 2001).The growing outcome gap raises further concerns about people excluded from health care or neglected while others may be overserved (Farmer, 2001). New calls for access to high-quality health care for everyone are being made, identifying as basic features automatic and affordable health insurance coverage, easy access to services, patient-responsive care, and a commitment to quality improvement (Davis, Schoen, and Schoenbaum, 2000). This situation certainly looks complicated enough to merit a bit of attention from physicians. And the problems themselves, though not solvable by primary care alone, seem to require primary care for their solution.

The lengthy and demanding educational and training processes required of physicians result in a highly selected minority of individuals who become physicians. Certainly not the only human resources of great importance in health care, physicians are a precious and influential resource to a society, not to be squandered on insignificant endeavor. It can be argued that the extraordinary preparation of physicians is of particular value when the depth and breadth of their training and experience are necessary to respond to problems and provide services that people need and want. There is no codified list of these problems and services that make it clear when a physician is needed or not. Indeed, one of the most important functions of physicians is to answer the question, "Is a doctor needed here?" This diagnostic and prognostic question is among the most complex decisions in health care. It is constantly present in daily primary care practice. Is there someone other than a physician better suited to make this decision and the other complex decisions required to integrate personal health care across the various ecology boxes?

CONCLUSION

From the perspective of an ecological model of health care, there is a large need and demand by people for primary care. Evidence about primary care confirms that it is a distinct and complex enterprise that is central to the medical enterprise. Doubts about the role of physicians in primary care should be replaced by a firm resolve to engage physicians in the further design and implementation of health care to ensure effective primary care for everyone. Absent superb primary care, a high-performance health care system is likely to elude the United States.

References

Center for Policy Studies in Family Practice and Primary Care. "The Importance of Having a Usual Source of Health Care." *American Family Physician,* 2000, *62,* 477.

Davis, K., Schoen, C., and Schoenbaum, S. C. "A 2020 Vision for American Health Care." *Archives of Internal Medicine,* 2000, *160,* 3357–3362.

Donaldson, M. S., Yordy, K. D., Lohr, K. N., and Vanselow, N. A. (eds.). *Primary Care: America's Health in a New Era.* Washington, D.C.: National Academy Press, 1996.

Dwinnell, B., and Adams, L. "Why We Are on the Cusp of a Generalist Crisis." *Academic Medicine,* 2001, *76,* 707–708.

Farmer, P. "The Major Infectious Diseases in the World—To Treat or Not to Treat?" *New England Journal of Medicine,* 2001, *345,* 208–210.

Fryer, G. E., Green, L. A., Dovey, S. M., and Phillips, R. L. Jr. "The United States Relies on Family Physicians Unlike Any Other Specialty." *American Family Physician,* 2001, *63,* 1669.

Green, L. A., and others. "The Ecology of Medical Care Revisited." *New England Journal of Medicine,* 2001, *344,* 2021–2025.

Heffler, S., and others. "Health Spending Growth Up in 1999; Faster Growth Expected in the Future." *Health Affairs,* 2001, *20,* 193–203.

Institute of Medicine. Committee on Quality of Health Care in America. *Crossing the Quality Chasm: A New Health System for the Twenty-First Century.* Washington, D.C.: National Academy Press, 2001.

Medical Expenditure Panel Surveys. Rockville, Md.: Agency for Healthcare Research and Quality, Mar. 2001. Microfiche. [http://meps.ahrq.gov/].

National Ambulatory Medical Care Survey. Annual. [ftp://ftp.cdc.gov/pub/Health Statistics/NCHS/Datasets/NAMCS/].

Robert Graham Center. "The Importance of Primary Care Physicians as the Usual Source of Healthcare in the Achievement of Prevention Goals." *American Family Physician,* 2000, *62,* 1968.

Starfield, B. "Primary Care and Health: A Cross-National Comparison." *Journal of the American Medical Association,* 1991, *266,* 2268–2271.

Starfield, B. *Primary Care: Concept, Evaluation, and Policy.* New York: Oxford University Press, 1992.

Turner, B. J., and Lain, C. "Differences Between Generalists and Specialists. Knowledge, Realism, or Primum Non Nocere?" *Journal of General Internal Medicine,* 2001, *16,* 422–424.

White, K. L., Williams, T. F., and Greenberg, B. "The Ecology of Medical Care." *New England Journal of Medicine,* 1961, *265,* 885–892.

World Health Organization. *The World Health Report 2000. Health Systems: Improving Performance.* Geneva: World Health Organization, 2000.

CHAPTER NINE

Primary Care in a New Era

Disillusion and Dissolution?

Lewis Sandy
Steven Schroeder

If you're so smart, why aren't you rich?

For decades, health policy experts have bemoaned the specialty domination of the U.S. health care system. Rather than building our health care system based on "provision of integrated, accessible health care services by clinicians who are accountable for addressing a large majority of personal health care needs, developing sustained partnerships with patients, and practicing in the context of family and community" (Donaldson, Yordy, Lohr, and Vanselow, 1996, p. 1), the organization and financing of our health care system continues to emphasize technologically oriented specialty care.

While this in itself is unremarkable, given the long-standing pro-specialty biases in our payment and medical education systems (Schroeder and Showstack, 1978; Showstack, Blumberg, Schwartz, and Schroeder, 1979), what is perhaps more surprising is that primary care seems more precarious than ever before, even as forces thought to promote it continue to strengthen. For example, the vast majority of both privately employed and Medicaid populations are in managed care.

Managed care, with its emphasis on cost-effective care for populations, was envisioned by many as a major stimulus to promote primary care. Medical school curricula have evolved to place greater emphasis on early exposures to patients, longitudinal clinical experiences, and clinical clerkships with community-based physicians, all of which are thought to increase interest in primary care. And indeed, graduating medical student interest in primary care is significantly higher now than a decade ago.

Yet those of us concerned about primary care feel not a sense of satisfaction or positive momentum but foreboding, concern, and even dread. Primary care residency matches were down 3.8 percent in 2001, the fourth straight year of decline (Greene, 2001). Graduating medical student interest in generalism declined from 40 percent in 1997 to 32 percent in 2000 (Association of American Medical Colleges, 2000; see Figure 9.1). Primary care physicians feel beleaguered, and evidence of a primary care backlash is emerging among students and medical school faculty.

We suggest that the current dilemmas in primary care stem from two fundamental issues: the unintended consequences of forces thought to promote primary care and the "disruptive technologies of care" that attack the very function and concept of primary care itself. We suggest that these forces, in combination with tiering in the health insurance market, could create the dissolution of primary care as a single concept, replaced by alignment of providers by economic niche, not role.

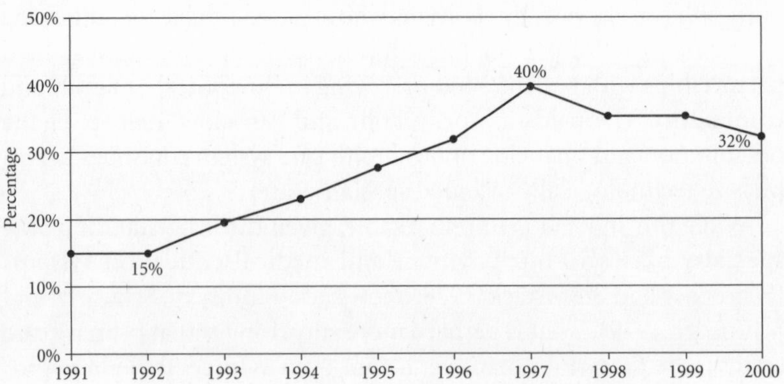

Figure 9.1. Interest in Generalist Specialties Among Graduating Medical Students, 1991–2000

Source: Association of American Medical Colleges (1997, 2000a, 2000b).

THE ASSAULT ON PRIMARY CARE

Much of the current concern with primary care is driven by those very forces that had been thought to be friendly to it: managed care and medical education reform. The growth of managed care, particularly capitation, would, the theory went, create major incentives for primary care; increase income, status, and reputation; and create new provider incentives for broad, comprehensive, and cost-effective care. Medical education reform, with an emphasis on early patient care experiences and curriculum changes broadening the worldview beyond biomedical science, would also promote primary care.

In reality, what happened was the worst of both worlds for primary care. Although managed care as an insurance product dominated the market, the reality of payment policy perpetuated essentially a discounted fee-for-service financing system. Although preferred provider organizations (PPOs) are well known for their discounted fees, even so-called health maintenance organizations (HMOs) pay predominantly fee for service. As a result, in 1999, the average physician derived only 17 percent of revenues from capitation (Center for Studying Health System Change, 1998–1999). Thus, neither enhanced income nor incentives for cost-effective care came to pass as a result of managed care. The gap between primary care physicians' income and that of specialists has widened over the past two decades in the absence of relative changes in specialty workload. In short, the technology-intensive biases of fee-for-service payment continue to penalize physicians with less resort to technology (Figure 9.2).

Nonetheless, consumer and provider anger over gatekeeper arrangements and highly publicized limitations on care in HMOs created a managed care backlash, within which primary care was swept up.

Moreover, the second-order effects of managed care created new challenges and promoted disruptive technologies for primary care. As described by Christensen, Bohmer, and Kenagy in their widely cited article, "Will Disruptive Innovations Cure Health Care?" (2000), "disruptive" innovation in a field occurs from below when less expensive approaches enable a product or service to be delivered faster, better, or cheaper. They cite, for example, the fact that nurse practitioners can provide primary care services for most people at less cost than physicians. And indeed, managed care promoted the growth of nurse practitioner and physician assistant programs to enhance the productivity of physician practice, but also in some markets (with fewer scope of practice regulations) to offer a more cost-effective form of primary

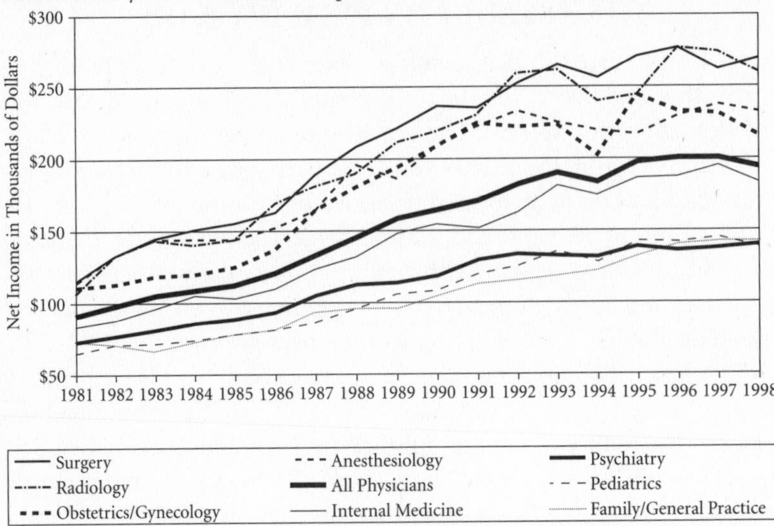

Figure 9.2. Mean Annual Physician Net Income After Expenses and Before Taxes, 1981–1998

Note: In real dollars.

Source: American Medical Association, 2001.

care itself. From 1992 to 1997, this group of health professionals doubled, and further growth is anticipated (Cooper, Laud, and Dietrich, 1998; see Figure 9.3).

Furthermore, proponents favoring growth of this workforce segment asserted that these providers could offer care equivalent to primary care physicians (Mundinger, 2000). This "technical equivalence" argument between physicians and nurses (and also between internal medicine and family practice) has created the impression among some that primary care is a simple, intellectually thin field of practice. The growth of schools of osteopathy, whose graduates dominantly enter primary care practice, provided further ammunition for the intellectual critics of primary care.

Second, managed care created the need for hospitals and medical groups to become more efficient in inpatient care, giving rise to the hospitalist movement (Schroeder and Shapiro, 1999). While the debate continues on the virtues of hospitalists, there is no question that the hospitalist movement created an alternative pathway for internists interested in a broad practice that crosses subspecialty boundaries. By

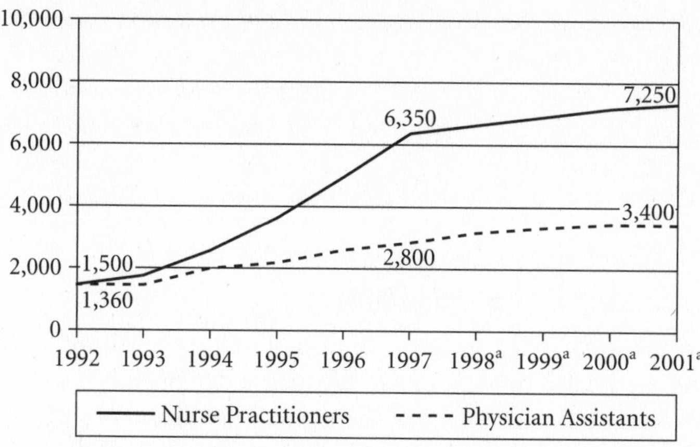

Figure 9.3. Number of Nonphysician Clinical Graduates: Physician Assistants and Nurse Practitioners, 1992–2001

[a]Projected.

Source: Cooper, Laud, and Dietrich (1998).

1999, 65 percent of internists had hospitalists in their community (Auerbach, 2000), and the hospitalist movement is projected to grow significantly (Lurie, 1999).

Most devastating, the policy promise that primary care could increase quality and reduce health care costs was not supported by evidence. Some studies noted that primary care providers were not regularly superior in the delivery of secondary preventive services (Chen, 2000), and research continued to show that, not surprisingly, specialists are more current in their practices than primary care physicians are (Solomon, 1997). (Interestingly, no studies have questioned how well specialists perform in comparison with generalists outside the specialist's own domain.) Managed care's use of discounts and the health insurance underwriting cycle succeeded in moderating health care costs in the mid- to late 1990s, an important object lesson suggesting that market forces independent of primary care can attack cost inflation (Ginsburg, 1999).

Primary care fared scarcely better within the walls of academe. Although many medical schools revised their overt curricula to create a greater balance between generalism and specialism, the "hidden" curriculum that serves to powerfully socialize learners continued to promote subspecialty training and tertiary care. The population-based approaches of the best managed care organizations, some of which worked in partnership with academic health centers, were overshadowed by more aggressive health plans with limited interest in social mission (Firshein and Sandy, 2001). As a result, student and resident interest in primary care, which increased in the mid-1990s in response to perceived greater opportunity, regressed in the late 1990s when those perceptions underwent revision.

Primary Care Circa 2003: Supply Exceeds Demand

In our view, these forces have combined with the unique dynamics among the health professions to create greater primary care supply than demand. For physicians, the growth in the overall number of physicians has led the Council on Graduate Medical Education and other policy bodies to the new view that no significant shortage of primary care providers currently exists (Council on Graduate Medical Education, 1999). For nonphysician primary care providers, the promise of prestige and access to reimbursement has resulted in dramatic growth in the supply of nurse practitioners and physician assistants providing primary care (Hogan, Ginsburg, and Gabel, 2000). Nurses in particular may find the troubled landscape of primary care a relative nirvana when compared with the problems facing regular hospital nursing practice. Indeed, nurse practitioners and physician assistants have been quite successful in securing access to public and private reimbursement (see Table 9.1). These nonphysician providers, in turn, are augmented by both a wide variety of other health providers providing alternative medicine and by specialists providing principal care to their patients with a single chronic condition.

	Medicaid Reimbursement	Private Insurance Mandates[a]	Medicare Reimbursement
Nurse practitioners	48 states	29 states	Yes
Physician assistants	49 states	3 states	Yes

Table 9.1. Reimbursement of Nurse Practitioners and Physician Assistants, 1998.

[a]Number of states that have enacted mandates requiring private insurers to offer the services of various nonphysician clinician disciplines.

Source: Cooper, Henderson, and Dietrich (1998).

Unfortunately, this increase in aggregate supply has done little to mitigate the shortage of primary care in rural, inner-city, and low-income areas. There is little evidence that provider supply is diffusing to health professions shortage areas. Rather, providers remain concentrated in higher-income communities.

Excess Supply Meets Tiered Demand

In order to understand how primary care will operate in a new era, it is important to consider how the health insurance market will evolve over the next decade. Currently, the majority of those with private health insurance are in loose managed care arrangements, such as open network HMOs and PPOs. These arrangements, while meeting employer and employee demands for wide choice and "kinder, gentler" managed care, offer little prospect of reining in costs over the long haul. Their predominant cost control mechanism is discounting fee-for-service reimbursement to providers. Indeed, after several years of moderation in health care costs, by 2000, both health insurance premiums and underlying costs were increasing at nearly double-digit rates (Hogan, Ginsburg, and Gabel, 2000).

Although predictions are hazardous, most analysts believe employees will gradually assume a greater burden of cost sharing over time and that should the economy go into recession and the labor market loosen (as now seems likely), employees will face far greater cost sharing and will have to pay a significant premium for the open access to wide networks that many currently enjoy (Cookson, 2001; Swartz, 2001).

One could reasonably predict that lower-income workers would increasingly "tier" into tightly managed HMOs, while higher-paid workers would prefer to pay for greater flexibility. Preliminary evidence suggests that this is already occurring. Gabel, Hurst, Whitmore, and Hoffman (1999) found that workers in high-wage firms tend to enroll in PPOs and point-of-service-type HMOs, while low-wage firms tend to offer traditional HMO coverage. This tiering, predicted some time ago by Reinhardt (1996), has become the common wisdom among health care futurists (Grosel, Hamilton, Koyano, and Eastwood, 2000).

Similarly, among Medicaid beneficiaries, state budgetary pressures increased the percentage of Medicaid recipients in managed care from 10 percent in 1991 to 56 percent in 2000 (Center for Medicare and Medicaid

Services, 1997, 2000). At the same time, more and more state Medicaid programs are migrating from primary care case management (PCCM) managed care, with loose controls on utilization, to tightly managed care, through either capitation or tight network design. Consequently, PCCM managed care declined from 31 percent of all Medicaid managed care in 1995 to only 18 percent in 2000 (Center for Medicare and Medicaid Services, 1995–2000).

As this tightening of the system for middle- and low-income groups occurs, other dynamics are in play for the well-off. The affluent, particularly empowered aging baby boomers, will demand not only free choice of provider but also the highest level of customer service. Already, some practices offer a "medical concierge" service where physicians are only a cell phone away and always on call; others offer integrative medical practices, which combine traditional Western medicine with acupuncture, massage therapy, aromatherapy, and other adjunctive treatments. (How Medicare responds to this pressure is a major wild card, discussed below.)

In summary, the health insurance and patient markets for those under age sixty-five will in all likelihood begin to divide into three tiers. The top tier will be the affluent, with full coverage or the ability to pay out of pocket. The middle tier will be the middle- or upper-middle-class employee with some choice but significant cost sharing; the bottom tier will encompass low-income workers, Medicaid, and the uninsured.

Medicare: Tiering's Wild Card

Although the evidence strongly suggests greater tiering in both the private health insurance market and Medicaid, Medicare remains the "800 pound gorilla," with Medicare policy often driving the entire industry. Medicare managed care grew significantly in the mid-1990s, driven by consumer demand for coverage of prescription drugs. Recently, however, Medicare HMOs have complained of inadequate reimbursement and have begun to leave certain markets. Policy changes to encourage Medicare managed care enacted as part of the Balanced Budget Act of 1997 did not work as intended, and enrollment in Medicare HMOs declined from a peak of 6.1 million in 1999 to 5.6 million as of May 2001 (Mathematica Policy Research, 2001). Most Medicare beneficiaries remain in the fee-for-service system, using supplemental (medigap) insurance paid by individuals or as part of a retiree health benefit. To the extent that Medicare remains static, its non-tiered, fee-for-service-oriented approach would provide countervailing force against tiering.

It is unlikely, however, that Medicare will remain in its current form over the long haul. First, pressures exist to expand the Medicare benefit to include prescription drug coverage and cover the near-elderly uninsured. Second, both government and market-oriented policy experts believe Medicare requires revamping to move from a structure modeled on 1960s health insurance benefits and financing to one that supports introduction of practices to improve quality and control costs (Reischauer, Butler, and Lave, 1997).

Although no one can reliably predict Medicare's future, the most likely future direction of Medicare reform will be in the general direction outlined by the 1999 Bipartisan Commission on the Future of Medicare. The commission, although failing by one vote to achieve a supermajority needed to make an official recommendation to Congress, had a majority in favor of a premium support model, in which the government would pay a fixed, risk-adjusted premium to plans as part of a competitive bid program. Under this approach, if Medicare beneficiaries choose plans more costly than the premium, they would pay out of pocket (Oberlander, 2000). Although many challenges, both political and technical, face Medicare reform, the commission's views clearly indicate a consensus to moving Medicare toward greater use of competitive markets and then creating greater price sensitivity among consumers. Both of these forces, if actualized, would increase the likelihood of significant tiering in our health care system.

PRIMARY CARE IN A TIERED MARKETPLACE

If the marketplace does evolve in this fashion, the function and approach of primary care could vary significantly by tier. In each tier, the epidemiology of disease and risk, the expectations of the provider, and the supporting financial incentives and drivers will vary. These variations will begin to splinter primary care itself in terms of both what is done and who does it. As this occurs, the very concept of primary care faces the prospect of dissolution, replaced by allegiance to an economic niche.

Upper-Tier Primary Care: The Full-Service Broker

For those in the upper tier, primary care will be just another service. Just as the affluent engage the services of their accountant, stockbroker, and personal trainer, they will engage health professionals in the same manner and expect the same level of service. As affluent baby boomers age, they will spend some their earned and inherited wealth to bypass the usual hassles of medical care practice. They will expect to reach their physician by cell phone, fax, e-mail, or the Internet. They will expect their provider to provide them with syntheses of information culled from the Internet and to arrange their visits to a preferred subspecialist. The medical concierge will grow as a niche, most likely as an adjunct service to high-end single- or multispecialty groups. Physicians and coalitions of health professionals and others will begin to offer comprehensive wellness programs, building off current executive physical fitness programs and lifestyle programs such as Canyon Ranch.

These providers will think of primary care as predominantly a service, not a profession. They will be continually thinking about how to enhance both service and revenues. One could envision attempts to brand these programs or develop franchises. Most likely, high-end specialty practices will begin to add primary care as a wraparound, loss-leader service.

Although teams will deliver this kind of primary care, it will be a unique kind of team, which consists not only of health professionals but also others who specialize in wellness and mind-body issues. It might include personal life coaches, fitness trainers, and even financial advisers, in addition to health professionals. Furthermore, there is no assurance that physicians will become leaders of this niche; nurse practitioners, physician assistants, and entrepreneurs will all stake a claim in this lucrative segment.

Middle-Tier Primary Care: Responsive Advocate or Diffident Bureaucrat?

This tier will most dramatically feel the tug between retaining classic concepts of professional autonomy and obligation to the patient versus accommodating to the bureaucratic reality of contemporary medical practice. These strains can already be observed in large multispecialty groups and prepaid group practices. Many primary care providers will be attracted to this tier if history is any guide. They will want to provide high-quality comprehensive care, coordination, and continuity. Yet they will also be attempting to maintain their income and preferred work style, while continually struggling with demands placed on them by insurers, regulators, and patients. They will be asked by demanding patients to provide the same level of service as in the upper tier, without commensurate reimbursement. In many markets, they will be asked to return to the gatekeeper role of the traditional HMO. To adapt to these tensions, the more innovative will explore new team arrangements for care, group visits, or some forms of technology assistance. New services will spring up to help relieve some of the burden on these providers. For example, providers can now buy a practice newsletter off the shelf, adding some customized information for their practice. Providers may "outsource" their e-mail and telephone queries from patients, using existing nurse triage services, essentially buying a full-time answering service. Physician Web site companies will offer a range of services, competing with vendors supplying electronic medical record systems and hand-held prescription writing devices.

As they practice day to day, month to month, fighting with indifferent insurance companies and attempting to satisfy demanding patients, burnout and loss will be close to the surface for many physicians. Some will find renewal in new developments in their practice such as technology enhancements or in building communications skills. Others will become diffident bureaucrats, going through the motions, but seeking satisfaction in family and outside interests, viewing medicine more as a job than a calling.

For these physicians, primary care will be a continual struggle. Some will successfully adapt to the challenge; others will burn out. This group will remain, however, most strongly connected to their identity—as primary care providers. Where else do they have to go?

Lower-Tier Primary Care: The Community-Oriented Primary Care Advocate

As second-tier physicians struggle to meet personal and professional goals, low-income patients will find access to the second tier increasingly difficult. In some markets, the uninsured will find few resources outside community health centers and public health departments; in others, the safety net will be a broader web of institutions. Nonetheless, even with insurance coverage, low-income populations in most locales will become concentrated in provider organizations such as safety net hospitals and existing community health centers. This trend has already begun. In Medicaid managed care, for example, competition among commercial plans has given way to the bulk of care being provided by safety net–sponsored HMOs, with competition giving way to cooperation between Medicaid agencies and these HMOs (Hurley, 2000).

Primary care in these tiers will increasingly be thought of as a social mission. Physicians entering this tier will have no illusion as to their income possibilities and will be attracted to the possibility of community-oriented primary care and their role as social advocates. Providers in this tier will become less connected to primary care and more aligned with advocacy movements for social justice. They will join Health Care for All, not the American College of Physicians.

Furthermore, these physicians will begin to bridge the conceptual and practical gaps between medicine and public health. Working with vulnerable populations, they will readily observe the impact that community, social, and economic factors play in the health of their patients, and they will work at the community level with public health advocates on issues of violence, substance abuse, lack of economic opportunity, and racism.

Clearly, these physicians will find the practice of primary care different from that of physicians in higher tiers. Their organizations will have far greater public than private financing, and their incomes will be lower. The teams needed to provide care in this tier will be broader in scope and function, including not only health professionals but also community health advocates, community organizers, and local community leaders.

IMPLICATIONS FOR PRIMARY CARE

As the marketplace evolves into more segmented tiers, those who practice will increasingly begin to align with their economic niche, not their specialty domain. For example, an upper-tier wellness practice will have more in common with an upper-tier cardiology group than with a lower-tier COPC practice. Thus, whatever current solidarity exists within and among primary care disciplines will begin to erode over time. Accelerating this will be greater income stratification within primary care, with the greatest income growth naturally occurring in the upper tier. Even now, the gap between primary care and specialty care may be growing (Salsberg, 2001).

How will this income stratification influence primary care practice? First, financial incentives will increase for physicians to occupy a place in the upper tier. At present, income from primary care is driven predominantly by practice design and productivity, not by economic niche served. As this shifts, however, current and newly forming primary care practices will realize that their choice of stratum makes a major difference in income.

If this occurs, a new kind of war for talent may emerge in primary care, particularly between the first and second tiers. The most aggressive physicians (especially those armed with the right skill set) will occupy a position in the upper tier, and those unsuccessful at finding a spot will need to downshift into the second tier. This emergence of a class distinction in primary care will erode solidarity further.

Second, increased consumerism and market stratification will continue to escalate health care costs, which could both help and hurt primary care. For the affluent, nothing but the best will do, and many will shift upmarket to specialists. For many others, however, who are facing economic consequences at the point of service (due to increased copays and coinsurance), generalists could provide lower-cost and more comprehensive advice regarding medical decision making (for example, as to whether the patient really needs a positron emission tomography scan).

How will each of the primary care disciplines in medicine fare? Each will face unique challenges. For family medicine, its orientation to families and communities will lead it to populate the middle and lower tiers, although a few will take their discipline's holistic approach to the upper-tier wellness market. For general pediatrics, those who wish to occupy the top-tier niche will need to develop novel ways to provide the level of service expected and a sustainable business model for practice. For example, upper-tier pediatricians may begin to bill for telephone consultation, but also send nurses to the schools and soccer fields in affluent communities.

In our view, general internal medicine faces the most daunting challenges for the future. The analytic background of most general internists is suited to complex medical diagnosis and treatment, not to a marketplace with economic stratification. While patients with complex, chronic illness will be concentrated in the middle and lower tiers, few internal medicine residencies have developed a training model for practice in either a bureaucratic organization or a distressed community. Some upper-tier internists will develop and market their acumen as advisers for and analytics around complex areas of medical decision making and effectively partner with others who will deliver high-end service. Many patients in the upper tier will eschew the traditional primary care functions as outmoded paternalism, preferring instead to be "captain of their own ship" and make their own decisions. Although the aging of the population will increase the population base for general internal medicine, general internists will also be competing with specialists for these patients. Indeed, falling age-specific disability rates suggest that healthy aging could be better for plastic surgeons than for internists (Salsberg, 2001). In order to survive and even thrive, general internists in the middle and lower tiers will need to develop competencies and practice styles much closer to family medicine, since family medicine's training model, which emphasizes family and community context and a biopsychosocial model of care, is more congruent with this tier's practice realities. Another niche for general internists will also be the management of multiple, complex, chronic conditions, a practice that will blur the specialty boundary between general internal medicine and geriatrics.

IMPLICATIONS FOR THE FUTURE

If these predictions about the future organization and financing of care come to pass and if the primary care response is anything like the forecast outlined here, then clear implications for the immediate future exist. First, how managed care evolves will have a major impact on the future of primary care. If managed care returns to a tightly managed gatekeeping model and retains its bureaucratic, low-customer-service ethos, then primary care will continue to be tarred by its brush. Learners will not be enthused about practicing under the conditions they see, and dispirited providers will actively dissuade new entrants to the field. Given this, we can expect medical student interest in primary care to drop to the 20 percent level seen in the early 1990s, without the subsequent opportunity bump offered by managed care growth in the mid- to late 1990s.

If, however, managed care principles and practices evolve into forms more acceptable to patients, either through consumer pressure, regulation, or changes in payment policy, the middle tier will look much more promising. Providers could see the opportunity to use advanced information technology to rationalize their practices and make better use of their time and energy. Primary care could even have a bit of a renaissance if the promise of information technology to streamline mundane tasks such as billing, charting, and forwarding information through complex systems becomes reality.

Given the magnitude of these forces on primary care, this analysis suggests that primary care policy should concern itself less perhaps with workforce issues and more with macrolevel organization and financing. A new consortium (or an existing one such as the Primary Care Organizations Consortium) might begin analyzing the impact that Medicare reform, Health Insurance Portability and Accountability Act regulations, Patient Bill of Rights, or HMO lawsuits will have on primary care.

Second, serious consideration should be given to the existing training model and departmental structure of general internal medicine and family practice. While some have called for the unification of general internal medicine and family practice, creating a single generalist division, others may want to develop a more coordinated model of training while retaining the distinctive competencies and cultures of each discipline.

For all primary care providers, however, we see five major challenges embodied in this forecast. First, current training in primary care does not provide the requisite skills for effective practice in any of the tiers we describe. Major training enhancements in communications skills, information technology, working in teams, prevention, and behavior change counseling will be needed (Yedidia, Gillespie, and Moore, 2000).

Second, and more fundamental, for primary care to survive as a construct in a new era, greater attention is needed for the essential core values of primary care. As we have outlined, the functions of primary care will vary by economic tier. If primary care is to have relevance as a concept for the future, perhaps its overarching focus should be on values and ethos, not solely on functions, since these functions will vary significantly in the future. Just as all of medicine has sought to unify the profession by focusing on core values of professionalism, primary care may need to do the same.

Third, this analysis suggests the need to consider primary care as a function that could be delivered by specialty physicians, not just the generalist specialties. Perhaps a new organization such as the "Society for Primary Care Practice," open to any specialty, should be developed.

Fourth, general internal medicine, and its relationship to primary care and to internal medicine, requires further thought. The underlying conceptual basis of general internal medicine, wherein the parent discipline of internal medicine is applied to the primary care of adults, is not tracking with either the changing marketplace for medical care or the evolution of internal medicine and the rise of the hospitalist movement.

Finally, like most other ideas, primary care is a concept that must continue to have demonstrated utility—to the public, the health professions, and health care. The future segmentation of the market suggests that unless fundamental changes in training, acculturation, and professional development of those who practice primary care occur, as a concept it will be swept away by economic, demographic, and social forces.

References

American Medical Association. *Physician Socioeconomic Statistics, 2000–2002.* Chicago: American Medical Association, 2001.

Association of American Medical Colleges. *Medical School Graduation Questionnaires: All School Reports, 1997.* Washington, D.C.: Association of American Medical Colleges, 1997. [http://www.aamc.org/data/gq/allschoolreports/1997.pdf].

Association of American Medical Colleges. *Medical School Graduation Questionnaires: All School Reports, 2000.* Washington, D.C.: Association of American Medical Colleges, 2000a. [http://www.aamc.org/data/gq/allschoolreports/2000.pdf].

Association of American Medical Colleges. *AAMC Graduation Questionnaires: All School Reports, 1984–2000.* Washington, D.C.: Association of American Medical Colleges, 2000b. [http://www.aamc.org/data/gq/allschoolreports/1997.pdf].

Auerbach, A. D. "Physician Attitudes Toward and Prevalence of the Hospitalist Model of Care: Results of a National Survey." *American Journal of Medicine,* 2000, *109,* 648–653.

Center for Medicare and Medicaid Services *Medicaid Managed Care Enrollment Report: Summary Statistics as of June 30, 1995–June 30, 2000.* Baltimore, Md.: Center for Medicare and Medicaid Services, 1995–2000.

Center for Medicare and Medicaid Services. *1997 Medicaid Managed Care Enrollment Report.* Baltimore, Md.: Center for Medicare and Medicaid Services, 1997.

Center for Medicare and Medicaid Services. *2000 Medicaid Managed Care Enrollment Report.* Baltimore, Md.: Center for Medicare and Medicaid Services, 2000.

Center for Studying Health System Change. *Community Tracking Study Physician Survey, 1998–1999.* Washington, D.C.: Center for Studying Health System Change. Data file. [www.hschange.org].

Chen, J. "Care and Outcomes of Elderly Patients with Acute Myocardial Infarction by Physician Specialty: The Effects of Comorbidity and Functional Limitations." *American Journal of Medicine,* 2000, *108*(6), 460–469.

Christensen, C. M., Bohmer, R., and Kenagy, J. "Will Disruptive Innovations Cure Health Care?" *Harvard Business Review,* Sept.-Oct. 2000, pp. 102–111.

Cookson, J. P. "Outlook for Health Care Trends." Report prepared for the Council on the Economic Impact of Health System Change Conference, Waltham, Mass., Jan. 11, 2001. [http://www.sihp.brandeis.edu/council/pubs/spending/Cooksonpaper.htm].

Cooper, R. A., Henderson, T., and Dietrich, C. L. "Roles of Nonphysician Clinicians as Autonomous Providers of Patient Care." *Journal of the American Medical Association,* 1998, *280,* 795–802.

Cooper, R. A., Laud, P., and Dietrich, C. "Current and Projected Workforce of Nonphysician Clinicians." *Journal of the American Medical Association,* Sept. 2, 1998, pp. 788–794.

Council on Graduate Medical Education. *COGME Physician Workforce Policies: Recent Developments and Remaining Challenges in Meeting National Goals.* Bethesda, Md.: U.S. Department of Health and Human Services, Mar. 1999.

Donaldson, M. S., Yordy, K. D., Lohr, K. N., and Vanselow, N. A. (eds.). *Primary Care: America's Health in a New Era.* Washington, D.C.: National Academy Press, 1996.

Firshein, J., and Sandy, L. G. "The Changing Approach to Managed Care." In S. L. Isaacs and Knickman, J. R. (eds.), *To Improve Health and Health Care 2001: The Robert Wood Johnson Anthology.* San Francisco: Jossey-Bass, 2001.

Gabel, J., Hurst, K., Whitmore, H., and Hoffman, C. "Class and Benefits at the Workplace." *Health Affairs,* May–June 1999, *18,* 144.

Ginsburg, P. "Tracking Health Care Costs: Long-Predicted Upturn Appears."

Center for Studying Health System Change issue brief. Nov. 23, 1999.

Greene, J. "Primary Care Matches down Again: Fourth Year of Decline Worries Some." *AMA News,* Apr. 9, 2001. [http://www.ama-assn.org/sci-pubs/amanews/pick_01/prse0409.htm].

Grosel, C., Hamilton, M., Koyano, J., and Eastwood, S. (eds.). *Health and Health Care 2010: The Forecast, the Challenge.* San Francisco: Jossey-Bass, 2000.

Hogan, C., Ginsburg, P. B., and Gabel, J. "Tracking Health Care Costs: Inflation Returns." *Health Affairs,* Nov.–Dec. 2000, *19,* 217.

Hurley, R. E. "Partnership Pays: Making Medicaid Managed Care Work in a Turbulent Environment." Center for Health Care Strategies Working Paper, May 2000.

Lurie, J. D. "The Potential Size of the Hospitalist Workforce in the United States." *American Journal of Medicine,* 1999, *106,* 441–445.

Mathematica Policy Research. *Early Experience Under Medicare + Choice: Final Summary Report.* Washington, D.C.: Mathematica Policy Research, Dec. 14, 2001. [http://www.mathematica-mpr.com/PDFs/earlyfinalsumm.pdf].

Mundinger, M. O. "Primary Care Outcomes in Patients Treated by Nurse Practitioners or Physicians: A Randomized Trial." *Journal of the American Medical Association,* 2000, *283*(1), 59–68.

Oberlander, J. "Is Premium Support the Right Medicine for Medicare?" *Health Affairs, 19*(5), 2000, 84.

Reinhardt, U. E. "Rationing Health Care: What It Is, What It Is Not, and Why We Cannot Avoid It." *Baxter Health Policy Review,* 1996, *2,* 63–99.

Reischauer, R. D., Butler, S., and Lave, J. R. (eds.). *Medicare—Preparing for the Challenges of the Twenty-First Century.* Washington, D.C.: National Academy of Social Insurance, 1997.

Salsberg, E. S. "Observations on the Physician Marketplace." Presentation at Physician Workforce Colloquium, Association of the American Medical Colleges, May 31, 2001, Washington, D.C.

Schroeder, S. A., and Shapiro, R. "The Hospitalist: New Boon for Internal Medicine or Retreat from Primary Care?" *Annals of Internal Medicine* (Supplement), 1999, *130,* 382–387.

Schroeder, S. A., and Showstack, J. A. "Financial Incentives to Perform Medical Procedures and Laboratory Tests: Illustrative Models of Office Practice." *Medical Care,* 1978, *16,* 289–298.

Showstack, J. A., Blumberg, B. D., Schwartz, J., and Schroeder, S. A. "Fee-for-Service Physician Payment: Analysis of Current Methods and Their Development." *Inquiry,* 1979, *16,* 230–246.

Solomon, D. H. "Costs Outcomes and Patient Satisfactions by Provider Type for Patients with Rheumatic and Musculoskeletal Conditions: A Critical Review of the Literature and Proposed Methodologic Standards." *Annals of Internal Medicine,* 1997, *127*(1), 52–60.

Swartz, K. "Rising Health Care Costs and Numbers of People Without Health Insurance." Prepared for the Council on the Economic Impact of Health System Change Conference, Waltham, Mass., Jan. 11, 2001.

Yedidia, M. J., Gillespie, C. C., and Moore, G. T. "Specific Clinical Competencies for Managing Care: Views of Residency Directors and Managed Care Medical Directors." *Journal of the American Medical Association,* 2000, *284*(9), 1093–1098.

CHAPTER TEN

Chronic Illness Management in Primary Care

Arlyss Anderson Rothman
Edward H. Wagner

An estimated 99 million Americans live with a chronic illness (Hoffman, Rice, and Sung, 1996). That is the good news and the bad news, as the saying goes. Through improved knowledge and treatment of chronic illness, people are living longer with chronic diseases. The number of Americans who must live with chronic illness, however, is increasing rapidly along with the longevity of our population. Meeting the needs of this population is one of the major challenges facing the American health care system. To date, we have not done enough. Dozens of studies, surveys, and audits have revealed that sizable proportions of chronically ill patients have not received effective therapy and do not have optimal disease control (Wagner and others, 2001b).

Chronic illness care is highly variable and largely organization or provider specific. Organizations that have tackled improving chronic illness care have done so to control costs and improve quality and have commonly developed specific disease management programs that focus on one disease (for example, diabetes, congestive heart failure, or hypertension), ignoring the fact that over 50 percent of patients with one chronic disease have another (Partnership for Solutions, 2002). The complexity of chronic illness care exposes the weakest link in health care: coordination of care. It is within this arena that the interface between chronic illness care and primary care may be most germane.

Primary care has been defined in many ways, and the definition developed by the Institute of Medicine in 1996 is most highly recognized (Donaldson, Yordy, Lohr, and Vanselow, 1996): primary care is "the provision of integrated, accessible health care services by clinicians who are accountable for addressing a large majority of personal health care needs, developing a sustained partnership with patients, and practicing in the context of family and community" (p. 33). The unique features of primary care (accessibility, longitudinality, comprehensiveness, and coordination) would seem to be well suited to chronic disease management (Hiss, 1996). Theoretically, a system with a strong primary care base and a small group of specialists for consultation in cases of high complexity or acuity would seem ideal. However, our system of primary care has fallen short in many areas, and our system of specialty care has expanded in numbers, length of interaction, and territory, and in many specialty areas it competes directly with primary care for patients as opposed to a referral-and-consultation relationship.

While studies demonstrate little difference in overall health outcomes between care provided by generalists or specialists in the management of many chronic illnesses, a major debate in health care policy continues as to whether our national system is based on a primary care foundation or a specialty care model. Although this debate has been audible for over thirty years, and countless federal and state programs have addressed the need to educate and train primary care physicians, most newly minted physicians choose specialty careers. The foundation of the system, although important in theory, may in fact become academic as individual health care organizations and the workforce that is available to them determine the delivery of chronic illness services. Although our own bias leans toward a primary care–based system, it is clear that substantial improvements must occur before that would be the most attractive approach to the challenge of chronic illness management.

This chapter analyzes the delivery of chronic illness care in a variety of models, explores a conceptual model for improving chronic illness care in the future, and identifies obstacles to improvement.

WHY PRIMARY CARE?

The managed care movement of the late 1990s has elevated the words *primary care* and *primary care provider* (PCP) to household status. Most consumers are able to identify whether they have a PCP and who that person is. The role that the PCP plays in each individual's health care varies widely and may range from ordering laxatives and completing referral authorizations, to coordinating an interdisciplinary team and managing a broad spectrum of care. Primary care is broadly accepted as being the first step in care, as well as having care-coordinating responsibilities. Although generally positive, both of these functions have come under criticism as gatekeeping in response to increasingly managed care.

In looking to the future of chronic illness management, determining an appropriate location in the system that would serve as a home to chronic illness management is a critical step. We propose that primary care is not only a logical choice from a systems perspective but also the preferred choice of patients. One rationale for managing chronic illness in primary care is Suttons's law: it is where the patients are. More than 90 percent of American diabetic patients, for example, receive their care in primary care (Hiss, 1996). Approximately 58 percent of all office visits in 1999 were to the patient's primary care provider, and about half of all visits were to physicians in the primary care specialties of general and family practice, internal medicine, and pediatrics (Cherry, Burt, and Woodwell, 2001). For patients over sixty-five years of age, physician visit rates have risen 22 percent from 1985 levels—from 485 to 592 visits per 100 persons—and much of this increase was seen in visit rates to internal medicine physicians (Cherry, Burt, and Woodwell, 2001). From a patient perspective, the primary care provider is an easy and familiar access point for care.

Another rationale for situating chronic illness management in primary care is the critical importance of coordination of care for persons with chronic disease. Although the concept of coordination has suffered from the gatekeeper backlash, having a provider or possibly a team of providers familiar with the whole patient and his or her family and able to communicate and coordinate medical activities is theoretically of great value in managing long-term illness. One could argue that without coordination of care, the goal of comprehensiveness, and ultimately quality, could not be achieved. However, given the demands of everyday primary care practice, major structural reforms are needed to facilitate change rather than relying on individual provider effort.

The clinical epidemiology of major chronic diseases also suggests a central role for primary care. First, major chronic diseases such as diabetes and arthritis present a broad spectrum of severity, ranging from modest biochemical or physiological derangements requiring little intervention to devastating illness requiring sophisticated, complex therapies. The large majority of patients tend to occupy the less severe end of this spectrum. Second, the majority of adults with major chronic diseases have more than a single chronic condition. For example, over half of patients with type 2 diabetes have concurrent hypertension, and another one-third or more will have clinically apparent coronary artery disease. Third, for the majority of patients with the most prevalent chronic illnesses, the pharmacological regimens involve a limited number of widely used and relatively nontoxic agents. Fourth, expertise with behavioral change and self-management support is central to successful management. These characteristics of the diseases and their treatment provide strong arguments for care to be coordinated by generalists with practices that can provide strong behavioral and self-management support. This characterizes most conceptions of modern primary care practice.

While the consumer and epidemiological arguments favor primary care as the base for chronic disease management, current performance argues otherwise. A probable majority of Americans with major chronic illnesses are not receiving appropriate or effective management (Wagner and others, 2001b). The consequences are prevalences of poor disease control, exacerbations, and complications that far exceed what is possible with appropriate care. The Institute of Medicine (2001) has described this difference between care as usual and appropriate care as the "quality chasm." In fairness to primary care, most of these studies of the quality of chronic illness care have made no distinctions about sources of care or the specialty of their primary provider. The few comparative studies of primary and specialty care, described more fully below, make it clear that the quality chasm pertains to both.

Thus, there is a dilemma and much debate. Primary care would appear to be the logical home for most patients with major chronic illnesses based on consumer preference and epidemiological grounds, but the lackluster performance of primary care must give pause. We can do a lot better. Although there is potential within primary care to address all of these areas, it will take some major changes in the organization and financing of care to improve the quality of chronic illness care. A little tinkering around the edges is unlikely to strengthen primary care and chronic illness care within it, but more substantive redesign of our systems hold promise (Institute of Medicine, 2001).

ALTERNATIVES TO PRIMARY CARE

Specialty Care

The specialty literature is replete with articles and editorials urging the shift of the care of the chronically ill from primary to specialty care. The empirical argument for such a shift can be found in the growing body of evidence demonstrating that specialists are more knowledgeable about the management of conditions associated with their specialty, more aware of guidelines delineating such management, and more likely to use tests and medications in accord with guidelines (Harrold, Field, and Gurwitz, 1999; Donohoe, 1998). Evidence also suggests that specialists more quickly change practice in accord with new developments. It has been more difficult for investigators to demonstrate differences in clinical and health status outcomes by specialty. This body of evidence might well support the argument that chronically ill patients will do better receiving their care from a specialist.

Arguments against such a shift include the relative paucity of evidence suggesting that the increase in knowledge- and guideline-associated prescribing practices of specialists translates into better clinical and health status outcomes. The evidence about specialty differences in diabetes care may be instructive. One important study demonstrated minimal differences in the care of diabetics between specialists and generalists when both were practicing in typical practice settings such as health maintenance organizations (HMOs) or private practice (Greenfield and others, 1995). Conversely, endocrinologists practicing in the context of specialized diabetes clinics with access to a full range of multidisciplinary resources provided substantially better care and achieved far better disease control than did generalists in the same area (Verlato and others, 1996; Ho and others, 1997). These differences strongly support the importance of the practice environment or practice system in determining the nature of care and its consequences.

Arguments opposing the shift of chronic illness care from generalists to specialists include concerns about the receipt of preventive care, the care of comorbid conditions outside the specialty focus, and cost. Some evidence does in fact suggest that specialists are less likely than generalists to provide preventive services (Rosenblatt and others, 1998) unless they are directly related to their specialty; for example, obstetricians and gynecologists are more likely to provide clinical breast exams, mammograms, and Pap smears (MacLean and others, 2000). Because of the frequent co-occurrence of chronic illnesses, the care of comorbid conditions plays a major role in chronic illness care. We were unable to identify any evidence that compares the performance of generalists and specialists in the management of comorbid conditions that are outside the particular specialty focus of the specialty group under study. Redelmeier, Tan, and Booth (1998) found that Ontario patients with diabetes, emphysema, and severe mental disorders were less likely than patients without these conditions to receive lipid-lowering medications, treatment for arthritis, or estrogen replacement therapy. These data suggest that there may well be deficiencies in the care of comorbid conditions, but the study did not provide evidence about whether the specialty of the primary caregiver made a difference.

Several commentators have suggested that shared care between primary care physician and specialist may produce the best outcomes (Greenfield, 1999; Nash and Nash, 1997). For example, Katon and others (1999) tested a shared care model for the management of patients with major depression. Alternating care between psychiatry and primary care led to substantial increases in the proportion of patients receiving appropriate therapy and the incidence of recovery from a major depressive episode. Lafata and others (2001) studied the care of diabetes in the Henry Ford Health System. They found that diabetic patients who had visits with both primary care and endocrinology were more likely to receive appropriate diabetes-related preventive care, as well as general preventive care services such as pneumococcal vaccination, mammography, and Pap smear. Parenthetically, they also found that patients who exclusively received care from endocrinology were somewhat more likely to receive diabetes-related preventive health services but somewhat less likely to receive general preventive health services. Willison and others (1998) found that HMO patients with acute myocardial infarction cared for by generalists with cardiology consultation were more likely to receive guideline-directed care than were patients treated by generalists alone. Focused and appropriate involvement of specialists in the care of selected patients with chronic disease would appear to be an area worthy of further study.

Disease Management

The high costs of care for major chronic illnesses and the deficiencies in usual medical care have been viewed as a business priority and opportunity. In a recent review, Bodenheimer (2000) estimated that over two hundred commercial disease management firms now offer services for patients with major chronic illnesses. In California, of seventy-one health care organizations studied, all suggested that disease or case management interdisciplinary teams were developed to decrease costs and increase quality (Anderson Rothman, 2000). Most often, these services are provided in a carve-out model in which the disease management organization or program provides focused educational and clinical services for patients with a given condition, with service generally limited to that condition. Programs vary in the extent to which the primary care practice team is informed and participates in decision making. Published evidence of the effectiveness of these programs remains scant, although unpublished testimonials are generally glowing. Because cost containment is the primary market driver for disease management carve-outs, these organizations tend to focus on the highest-cost end of a spectrum of patients with the condition of interest. As a result, they should benefit from regression to the mean. Disease management carve-outs threaten continuity and coordination of care, and anecdotal reports suggest that such concerns may be founded. Carving out the care of a particular condition often has the pernicious effect of limiting interest in or resources for improving the primary care of patients with other conditions. Careful study of this issue is urgently needed.

HOW TO IMPROVE CHRONIC ILLNESS CARE IN PRIMARY CARE

In our view, the extensive rhetoric and posturing on both sides of the generalist-specialist debate misses the point. In the words of one commentator, "There are not enough specialists (nor financial resources) for every individual with asthma to be cared for by a pulmonologist, or every patient with depression to be followed a psychiatrist. Thus, more attention should be paid to minimizing quality of care differences for the more common illnesses, eliminating those deficiencies in the provision of preventive care common to all physicians, . . . improving the referral process for patients with complicated conditions . . . , and promoting co-management and a teamwork approach" (Donohoe, 1998, p. 1604). The issue then is to identify the factors associated with the generally substandard chronic illness and preventive care being provided by practices of all specialties.

Is the problem cognitive—that is, are many primary care practitioners simply unaware of effective interventions—or does the root of the problem lie elsewhere? The previously cited literature on specialty differences in knowledge and use of effective treatments suggests that knowledge gaps may play a role. But disease control and other outcomes fall far short of what is possible even when primary chronic disease care is delivered by specialists. If unawareness or unfamiliarity with effective therapies were the principal explanation for poor quality, one might expect more bimodal distributions of quality ratings. Instead, the variation in chronic illness care and outcomes from patient to patient within individual practices generally exceeds the variation from practice to practice (Katon and others, 2000; Hofer and others, 1999). These findings strongly suggest that even knowledgeable practice teams have difficulty providing optimal care consistently to all of their patients. One factor may be the value that the medical profession gives to the individualization of therapy, a major argument made by those resisting the imposition of guidelines. This attitude persists despite the fact that most randomized trials of treatment, which constitute the evidence base for modern practice, use standardized treatment protocols for all patients with certain clinical characteristics.

Although some of the variation is clearly patient related, we believe that this inconsistency is principally a function of the organization and orientation of primary care practice, regardless of the specialty of the primary caregiver. The essential structure and operation of primary care practice has changed little over the past decades, despite the dramatic demographic shifts that have aged the patient population, and the equally dramatic progress in the clinical and behavioral management of most major chronic diseases. Primary care systems were and continue to be organized to react to acute illnesses. Attention is focused on the efficient definition of the problem, the exclusion of more serious alternative diagnoses, and the prompt initiation of treatment, usually in the form of drug prescriptions. The patient's role is largely passive. Since the time horizon is short and the focus is on immediate problem resolution, there has been little urgency to provide more than cursory patient education or develop computer tracking systems or organized approaches to follow-up. As a consequence, the care of chronic illnesses is often a poorly connected string of episodes determined by patient problems.

In contrast, optimal chronic disease management ensures that people with chronic illness have the confidence and skills to manage their condition, the most appropriate treatments for optimal disease control and prevention of complications, a mutually understood care plan, and careful, continuous follow-up. This requires a longitudinal and preventive orientation manifested by well-designed, planned interactions between practice team and patient in which the important clinical and behavioral work of modern chronic illness care gets done predictably (Wagner, Austin, and Von Korff, 1996). The evidence for many chronic conditions suggests that the typical problem-oriented visit is a barrier to such care, a barrier made worse by recent organizational demands to see more patients. Thus, the acute care–oriented medical care system often fails to meet the needs of persons with chronic illness because it has been designed to respond to a different type of health problem.

What characterizes effective chronic illness care? First, the chronically ill person has a primary care practice team that organizes and coordinates his or her care. Whether led by generalist physician, nurse practitioner, or medical subspecialist, this team ultimately optimizes patient outcomes through a series of interactions with the patient (and family) during which they:

- Elicit and review data concerning patient perspectives and other critical information about the course and management of the condition.
- Help patients set goals and solve problems for improved self-management.
- Adjust therapy to optimize disease control and patient well-being.
- Ensure follow-up.

We look at each of these interactions more closely:

• *Elicit and review data concerning patient perspectives and other critical information about the course and management of the condition.* To manage chronic disease effectively, providers need up-to-date information about the patient. Most practices do not have standardized or organized approaches to collecting, summarizing, and reviewing this information. Patient reports of their self-management efforts, symptoms, and ability to function are critical considerations in the adjustment of therapy, and the effective management of many chronic conditions requires regular clinical assessments of disease severity or examinations for early evidence of exacerbations or complications. In traditional medical practice, such data are collected sporadically and accumulated in unorganized clinical notes that must be reviewed at the time of a patient interaction. Successful efforts to improve chronic illness care routinely collect key patient data through the use of standardized assessment tools and systematic data collection methods, summarize the information, and use it to plan care.

- *Help patients set goals and solve problems for improved self-management.* Traditional patient education emphasizes knowledge acquisition, and didactic counseling and classes are the norm in medical practice. Mounting evidence indicates that although such interventions may increase knowledge, they are almost invariably unsuccessful in changing behaviors or improving disease control and other outcomes (Norris, Engelgau, and Narayan, 2001). More recent theoretical and empirical research has shifted the focus from the patient's knowledge of the disease and its treatment to his or her confidence (self-efficacy) and skills in managing the condition—that is, self-management (Von Korff and others, 1997). The interventions that have emanated from this research give primacy to the patient's and family's role in managing the condition, as manifest in a self-management treatment or action plan. Effective self-management interventions help patients set limited goals for improving their management of their illness, arrive at a plan, identify barriers to reaching their goals, and support their efforts to overcome the barriers. The objective of such interventions, whether individual or in groups, personal or electronic, is to provide patients with a strategy and tools for effectively handling the multiple challenges of chronic disease and the confidence that they can do so. Ideally, routine medical care reinforces self-management through continuous involvement in collaborative goal setting, planning, and problem solving (Von Korff and others, 1997).
- *Adjust therapy to optimize disease control and patient well-being.* The effective control of most chronic diseases requires appropriate medical therapy as well as competent self-management. We now have highly efficacious drugs and surgical procedures for most major

chronic conditions and proven protocols for their implementation. Most protocols recommend the intensification of therapy (higher dosage, new or additional drugs, possible surgery) if appropriately taken treatment at the previous level fails to achieve optimal disease control. Studies of usual medical care in several chronic diseases have found that poorly controlled patients often are receiving inappropriate medication or inadequate dosages of appropriate drugs (O'Connor, 2001; Unutzer and others, 2000). Arriving at effective therapy requires that providers regularly assess indicators of disease severity (for example, depressive or asthmatic symptoms), adjust treatment according to disease severity and evidence-based protocols, and closely follow up for evidence of better disease control or adverse effects. This may be daunting in practices that are not organized to do so (O'Connor, 2001).

- *Ensure follow-up.* Holman and Lorig (2000) have described the features of chronic illness that distinguish it from acute medical problems. One is its long time span. A second is its undulating, somewhat unpredictable course. The different time horizons and fluctuating courses of many chronic illnesses require regular, planned interactions between caregivers and patients to ensure optimal disease control. A recent IOM report, *Crossing the Quality Chasm* (2001), described this as a "continuous healing relationship" and argued for the increased use of methods of interaction other than face-to-face visits. The use of the telephone, for example, allows for more intensive yet cost-efficient follow-up of chronically ill patients and has been associated with improved outcomes in a variety of chronic diseases. These calls, whether made by a physician, nurse, trained counselor, or nonprofessional, can accomplish some or all of the tasks characteristic of productive interactions outlined above. More intensive follow-up can also be provided by outreach workers, and more efficient forms of visits such as group or cluster visits can be used. Use of e-mail or the Internet to maintain contact with patients is under study.

SYSTEM CHANGES SUPPORTIVE OF MORE EFFECTIVE CHRONIC ILLNESS CARE

Ensuring the routine performance of these critical tasks in the management of major chronic illnesses has proved to be extremely difficult in current primary care practice. The literature strongly suggests the need for multifaceted, interconnected changes to the organization and functioning of the practice. We have been impressed that system changes that lead to improvements in the process and outcomes of chronic disease care are similar from condition to condition. To illustrate, consider care for diabetes and for depression, two seemingly different conditions that have been the subject of the largest volume of quality improvement research in primary care.

A recent Cochrane Collaborative review examined forty-one studies of interventions to improve diabetes performance in primary care (Renders and others, 2001). Most demonstrated some degree of improvement in care processes such as hemoglobin A1c testing or the performance of retinal or foot examinations. A few studies showed significant improvements in indicators of disease control such as HbA1c, blood pressure, or lipid levels. The interventions that resulted in the largest positive changes tended to be multifaceted, with interventions in four areas: activities directed at changing provider behavior, changes to the organization of practice, information systems enhancements, and educational or supportive programs directed to patients. The greater the number of these four areas involved in the intervention, the more successful it appeared to be. Of particular interest, the only interventions that achieved improvements in patient outcomes such as glycemic control were those that had a strong patient-oriented component. No specific intervention if used alone led to major improvements in the quality of chronic illness care. The importance of patient educational and supportive interventions found in the Cochrane diabetes review is consistent with the growing body of literature demonstrating that chronic disease interventions that have a positive impact on patient well-being generally include systematic efforts to increase the knowledge, skills, and confidence of patients to manage their condition.

Recent reviews of research to improve the care of depression in primary care practice have come to conclusions remarkably similar to those for diabetes (Callahan, 2001; Von Korff and others, 2001). For example, Callahan (2001) concluded that "achieving guideline-level therapy requires the substantial participation of an informed and motivated patient working in concert with a health care team and health care system designed to care for chronic conditions" (p. 772). Based on their reviews of the research, Callahan and Von Korff and colleagues each propose multicomponent models for depression care that include system changes directed at activating the care system, the providers, and the patients and families. Callahan's proposed system (2001) depends on trained multidisciplinary primary care teams guided by guidelines, performance feedback, and other decision support. Practice systems must have access to resources for providing targeted education, support for self-management, patient monitoring, and outreach. Von Korff and colleagues (2001) propose the use of the quite similar chronic care model, described below.

Because multicomponent system change interventions are most effective, the Cochrane diabetes reviewers (Renders and others, 2001) urged that future research should "evaluate *reproducible complex interventions and encourage replications of using the same model*." One of us (E.W.) and colleagues had independently arrived at the need for a model to guide efforts to improve diabetes care at Group Health Cooperative (Hofer and others, 1999; Wagner, 1995; McCulloch, Price, Hindmarsh, and Wagner, 1998). Based on the literature, interventions were initially tried in a variety of areas—registries, guidelines, patient education—but without an overall vision for the optimal care system. The chronic disease improvement literature strongly suggested that changing process and outcomes in chronic illness required multicomponent interventions that change the prevailing clinical system. We then attempted to categorize the components of those interventions that had been shown to influence the quality of care, specify the features within each component associated with better outcomes, and suggest how the components interact to influence patients, providers, and their interactions to produce better care. Our first attempts tried to categorize the practice enhancements that improved patient outcomes (Wagner, Austin, and Von Korff, 1996):

Guidelines—the use of explicit plans and protocols

Practice redesign—the reorganization of practice teams, visits, and follow-up systems to meet the needs of patients

Patient education—systematic attention to the information and behavioral change needs of patients

Expert system—increased provider training and decision support through guidelines, interaction with specialists, and other tools

Information—information systems that support population-based care, and provider reminders and feedback

This preliminary scheme was reviewed by an international group of advisers who provided suggestions for model improvement (Wagner and others, 1999). Based on their suggestions, expert systems and guidelines were combined with other interventions to improve provider expertise under a new rubric: decision support. The advisers also suggested that resources in the surrounding community are often important to improving care for chronically ill patients and that improvement efforts should include the development of linkages to key community-based services. They felt that overarching organizational factors like leadership, incentives, and quality improvement strategies have a major influence on the structure and functioning of practices and their care. Finally, many advisers viewed the original framework or model as incomplete because it did not indicate how organizational characteristics and practice system enhancements translated into improved care processes and better outcomes. Based on these suggestions, a revised version of the model was sent back to the advisers for a second review. The ensuing comments led to the current chronic care model, shown in Figure 10.1 (Wagner, 1998a; Wagner and others, 1999, 2001a, 2001b).

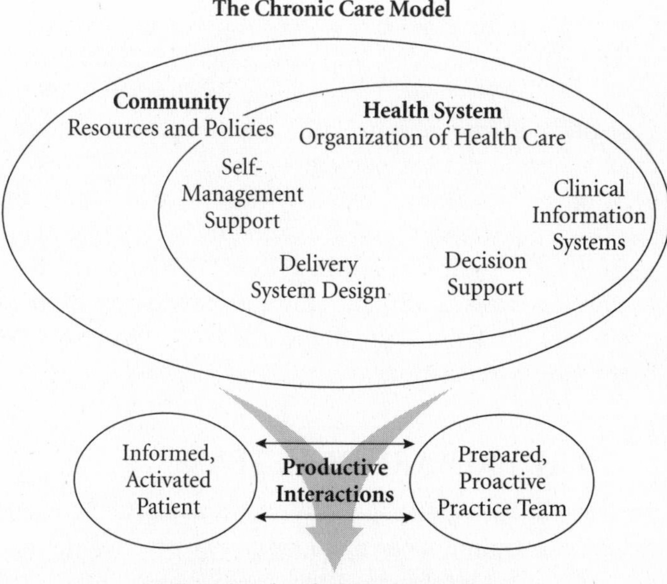

Figure 10.1. The Chronic Care Model

Most chronically ill individuals interact frequently with the medical care system. But those interactions often do not result in effective treatment: they are not consistently producing the assessments, support for self-management, optimization of therapy, and follow-up productive of good outcomes. Interactions are likely to be more productive if patients are active, informed participants in their care. Patients must have the information, skills, and confidence to make best use of their involvement with their practice team. And practice teams must have the necessary expertise, information, time, and resources to act, rather than just react, to ensure effective clinical and behavioral management. The challenge is to create a delivery system that promotes productive interactions by informing and activating patients and ensuring that practice teams are prepared and proactive.

The chronic care model (CCM) considers the health system as part of the larger community and the practice as a part of one or more health organizations. Effective chronic illness management requires an appropriately organized delivery system linked with necessary resources available in the broader community. The CCM represents the enhancements to the organization and its practices that contribute to productive interactions between providers and patients. Effective self-management support and links to patient-oriented services (such as exercise programs, hospital chronic disease resources, support groups) in the community (community resources) help patients and families cope with the challenges of managing their chronic illness. Well-functioning practice teams use planned interactions with patients to ensure appropriate clinical and behavioral management and follow-up (delivery system design). Clinical decisions are aided by clear protocols and sufficient expertise (decision support) and access to timely patient and practice information (clinical information system). Making the necessary changes in these areas is difficult, if not impossible, without strong leadership, appropriate incentives, and effective improvement strategies (health care organization).

THE PRIMARY CARE TEAM

Effective chronic disease management is a team effort. Physicians have neither the time, training, nor memory capacity to ensure that every chronically ill patient receives essential care (Wagner, 2000). It requires more than a physician to ensure that assessments are completed, patient self-management supported, protocols adhered to, and patients carefully monitored. Teams must be stable and organized to do the work (Taplin and others, 1998). The delegation to nonphysician team members of responsibility for key tasks in chronic illness care (such as ensuring the completion of disease severity questionnaires or ordering protocol-driven laboratory procedures) increases the likelihood of completion. New skills appear to be required as well. Several studies have shown that nonphysician professionals such as nurses or pharmacists skilled in modern self-management support and adjustment of therapy by protocol may be critical components of effective chronic disease care (Wagner, 1998b, 2000). These clinical case managers are unavailable to most primary care practices, but traditional practice team members such as nurses, receptionists, and medical assistants can be trained to do aspects of the clinical case management function. For example, investigators have demonstrated improved outcomes through the use of nonprofessionals and computerized telephone systems to monitor patients with arthritis (Weinberger and others, 1993), diabetes (Piette, Weinberger, Kraemer, and McPhee, 2001), and depression (Simon, Von Korff, Rutter, and Wagner, 2000). In these instances, standardized assessments were performed and evidence of any difficulties referred immediately to the physician or a nurse case manager.

BARRIERS TO IMPROVING CHRONIC DISEASE MANAGEMENT IN PRIMARY CARE

Incomplete Chronic Disease Management Education

Current clinical training fails to equip physicians and other health professionals with either the knowledge or tools to create or improve practice systems and approaches that produce optimal care. Few medical schools or continuing-education programs prepare their trainees to be practice team leaders and practice system improvers or to expose them to optimally functioning primary care systems. The focus is instead on biotechnological developments in therapy that may or may not be real advances. Also, the shift from traditional didactic patient education to collaborative self-management support is relatively new, and few nurses and other health professionals have been trained accordingly.

Inertia

Inertia is the property of matter by which it remains at rest or in uniform motion in the same straight line unless acted on by some external force. Primary care practices are in constant motion, which is linear in the sense that it is always directed at completing the clinical work of the day safely and successfully. Optimal chronic disease care necessitates planning, team meetings, reviewing data, and arranging linkages with people and resources—the sort of work that is the first to be postponed in the heat of the busy practice day. This inertia of busy practice leads to the commonest response to efforts to improve chronic disease management: "We don't have the time." But we do not allow busy surgeons to forgo scrubbing on particularly hectic days. Physical inertia can be overcome by external force. Some of the potential external forces that might overcome practice inertia may be at the level of policy (such as performance indicators or reimbursement) or the health care organization (such as quality improvement approaches or motivated leadership).

Optionality

Chronic disease improvement efforts will be successful only if the medical care experience of the average patient in the system changes. For example, Solberg and colleagues (2001) found that only 12 percent of relevant patients were exposed to a well-designed new approach for primary care patients with depression even in practices that participated in its design and testing. And of sixty-one medical groups in California, only half are using any sort of interdisciplinary team in caring for diabetes or other chronic disease, although these teams clearly improve outcomes (Anderson Rothman, 2000). If enhancements are optional and do not fundamentally change the structure and function of the delivery system, practice inertia tends to maintain the status quo for most patients. Health professionals understandably resist attempts to limit their choices, but embedding care enhancements based on sound evidence into routine practice should not be viewed as a threat to professional autonomy. The chronic disease quality chasm will close only when the majority of patients experience a primary care system designed to meet their needs.

Financial Disincentives

Limited reimbursement, adverse selection, and other financial issues are often cited as key barriers to chronic care improvement. The recent Institute of Medicine *Quality Chasm* report (2001) dealt with the financial issues in detail. Their recommendations are for policy changes that would promote and reward improved quality by reimbursing nontraditional services proven to be effective in improving the care of chronically ill patients (such as self-management support, group visits, and electronic or telephonic follow-up), protecting organizations from attracting high-cost, chronically ill patients and supporting investments in infrastructure. For some parts of the health care system, there are disincentives associated with better care (for example, reductions in admissions for hospital-based systems) that will go away only with large-scale restructuring of the health system. In our quality improvement experience, financial disincentives appear to be more influential with administrative leaders than with clinicians.

Ineffective Implementation Strategies

Difficulties in implementing effective practice changes have prevented motivated organizations from realizing gains in the quality of chronic illness care. Improvement approaches that were early adaptations from industrial quality improvement (QI), despite their conceptual elegance, have proven unsuccessful in changing care in several trials (Goldberg, 2000). Some interpreted these early adaptations of industrial QI as "a process that specifically prohibits 'leaping to solutions' [which] . . . must leave open the possibility of poorly conceived remedial actions" (Brown and others, 2000). As a result, some chronic disease QI interventions did in fact produce "improvements" that were unlikely to alter practice and did not (Goldberg and others, 1998). Other QI efforts apparently failed because the organizational leadership was not supportive of promising improvement strategies (Brown and others, 2000). More intensive improvement approaches that use evidence-based change ideas, rapid-cycle change testing, and careful measurement of goal attainment may afford the best chance of success. Several hundred organizations have used this QI approach and the chronic care model to improve their care of patients with various chronic diseases. Early results are promising (Wagner, 2000). But even these will fail unless the improvement process receives strong organizational support (Solberg and others, 2001).

Unsupportive Leadership

In our work with organizations attempting to improve their care, lack of leadership support may be the single most trenchant barrier to success (Wagner and others, 2001b). Front-line clinicians and administrators can design and test changes to the practice and the care of patients, but they need support and access to resources that only senior leaders of medical groups and health plans can supply.

CONCLUSION

Demographic shifts are escalating the number of persons with chronic illness, and most are receiving the bulk of their medical care from generalist primary care practices. While the rationale for keeping the nucleus of care for the average chronically ill patient in primary care is compelling, the consistent findings of generally substandard care across multiple chronic conditions have spurred proposals that care be shifted to specialists or a growing disease management industry. Published evidence to date does not indicate any clear superiority of these alternatives to primary care, but support for primary care is likely to erode if chronic illness care does not improve. A rapidly growing body of health services research evidence has identified the fundamental problem as a mismatch between the needs of chronically ill patients and typical care systems. Some useful models and specific interventions to change delivery systems are emerging. System change is made difficult by barriers intrinsic to practice and in the environment, but it can be accomplished with supportive organizational leadership and the use of effective improvement methods.

References

Anderson Rothman, A. L. *Interdisciplinary Health Care Teams: An Organizational Structural Adaptation to Environmental Change.* San Francisco: School of Nursing, University of California, 2000.

Bodenheimer, T. "Disease Management in the American Market." *British Medical Journal,* 2000, *320*(7234), 563–566.

Brown, J. B., and others. "Controlled Trials of CQI and Academic Detailing to Implement a Clinical Practice Guideline for Depression." *Joint Commission Journal on Quality Improvement,* 2000, *26*(1), 39–54.

Callahan, C. M. "Quality Improvement Research on Late Life Depression in Primary Care." *Medical Care,* 2001, *39*(8), 772–784.

Cherry, D. K., Burt, C. W., and Woodwell, D. A. *Statistics DoHC: National Ambulatory Medical Care Survey: 1999 Summary. Advance Data from Vital and Health Statistics.* Hyattsville, Md.: National Center for Health Statistics, 2001.

Donaldson, M. S., Yordy, K. D., Lohr, K. N., and Vanselow, N. A. (eds.). *Primary Care: America's Health in a New Era.* Washington, D.C.: National Academy Press, 1996.

Donohoe, M. T. "Comparing Generalist and Specialty Care: Discrepancies, Deficiencies, and Excesses." *Archives of Internal Medicine,* 1998, *158*(15), 1596–1608.

Goldberg, H. I. "Continuous Quality Improvement and Controlled Trials Are Not Mutually Exclusive." *Health Services Research,* 2000, *35*(3), 701–705.

Goldberg, H. I., and others. "A Randomized Controlled Trial of CQI Teams and Academic Detailing: Can They Alter Compliance with Guidelines?" *Joint Commission Journal of Quality Improvement,* 1998, *24*(3), 130–142.

Greenfield, S. "The Next Generation of Research in Provider Optimization." *Journal of General Internal Medicine,* 1999, *14*(8), 516–517.

Greenfield, S., and others. "Outcomes of Patients with Hypertension and Non-Insulin Dependent Diabetes Mellitus Treated by Different Systems and Specialties: Results from the Medical Outcomes Study." *Journal of the American Medical Association,* 1995, *274*(18), 1436–1444.

Harrold, L. R., Field, T. S., and Gurwitz, J. H. "Knowledge, Patterns of Care, and Outcomes of Care for Generalists and Specialists." *Journal of General Internal Medicine,* 1999, *14*(8), 499–511.

Hiss, R. G. "Barriers to Care in Non-Insulin-Dependent Diabetes Mellitus: The Michigan Experience." *Archives of Internal Medicine,* 1996, *124,* 146–148.

Ho, M., and others. "Is the Quality of Diabetes Care Better in a Diabetes Clinic or in a General Medicine Clinic?" *Diabetes Care,* 1997, *20*(4), 472–475.

Hofer, T. P., and others. "The Unreliability of Individual Physician 'Report Cards' for Assessing the Costs and Quality of Care of a Chronic Disease." *Journal of the American Medical Association,* 1999, *281*(22), 2098–2105.

Hoffman, C., Rice, D., and Sung, H. Y. "Persons with Chronic Conditions: Their Prevalence and Costs." *Journal of the American Medical Association,* 1996, *276*(18), 1473–1479.

Holman, H., and Lorig, K. "Patients as Partners in Managing Chronic Disease: Partnership Is a Prerequisite for Effective and Efficient Health Care." *British Medical Journal,* 2000, *320*(7234), 526–527.

Institute of Medicine. Committee on Quality of Health Care in America. *Crossing the Quality Chasm: A New Health System for the Twenty-First Century.* Washington, D.C.: National Academy Press, 2001.

Katon, W., and others. "Stepped Collaborative Care for Primary Care Patients with Persistent Symptoms of Depression: A Randomized Trial." *Archives of General Psychiatry,* 1999, *56*(12), 1109–1115.

Katon, W., and others. "Are There Detectable Differences in Quality of Care or Outcome of Depression Across Primary Care Providers?" *Medical Care,* 2000, *38*(6), 552–561.

Lafata, J. E., and others. "Provider Type and the Receipt of General and Diabetes-Related Preventive Health Services Among Patients with Diabetes." *Medical Care,* 2001, *39*(5), 491–499.

MacLean, C. H., and others. "Quality of Care for Patients with Rheumatoid Arthritis." *Journal of the American Medical Association,* 2000, *284*(8), 984–992.

McCulloch, D. K., Price, M. J., Hindmarsh, M., and Wagner, E. H. "A Population-Based Approach to Diabetes Management in a Primary Care Setting: Early Results and Lessons Learned." *Effective Clinical Practice,* 1998, *1*(1), 12–22.

Nash, D. B., and Nash, I. S. "Building the Best Team." *Annals of Internal Medicine,* 1997, *127*(1), 72–74.

Norris, S. L., Engelgau, M. M., and Narayan, K. M. "Effectiveness of Self-Management Training in Type 2 Diabetes: A Systematic Review of Randomized Controlled Trials." *Diabetes Care,* 2001, *24*(3), 561–587.

O'Connor, P. J. "Organizing Diabetes Care: Identify, Monitor, Prioritize, Intensify." *Diabetes Care,* 2001, *24*(9), 1515–1516.

Partnership for Solutions. *Chronic Conditions: Making the Case for Ongoing Care.* Baltimore, Md.: Johns Hopkins University, 2002.

Piette, J. D., Weinberger, M., Kraemer, F. B, and McPhee, S. J. "Impact of Automated Calls with Nurse Follow-Up on Diabetes Treatment Outcomes in a Department of Veterans Affairs Health Care System: A Randomized Controlled Trial." *Diabetes Care,* 2001, *24*(2), 202–208.

Redelmeier, D. A., Tan, S. H., and Booth, G. L. "The Treatment of Unrelated Disorders in Patients with Chronic Medical Diseases." *New England Journal of Medicine,* 1998, *338*(21), 1516–1520.

Renders, C. M., and others. "Interventions to Improve the Management of Diabetes in Primary Care, Outpatient, and Community Settings: A Systematic Review." *Diabetes Care,* 2001, *24*(10), 1821–1833.

Rosenblatt, R. A., and others. "The Generalist Role of Specialty Physicians: Is There a Hidden System of Primary Care?" *Journal of the American Medical Association,* 1998, *279*(17), 1364–1370.

Simon, G. E., Von Korff, M., Rutter, C., and Wagner, E. "Randomised Trial of Monitoring, Feedback, and Management of Care by Telephone to Improve Treatment of Depression in Primary Care." *British Medical Journal,* 2000, *320*(7234), 550–554.

Solberg, L. I., and others. "A CQI Intervention to Change the Care of Depression: A Controlled Study." *Effective Clinical Practice,* 2001, *4*(6), 278–280.

Starfield, B. *Primary Care: Balancing Health Needs, Services, and Technology.* New York: Oxford University Press, 1998.

Taplin, S., and others. "Putting Population-Based Care into Practice: Real Option or Rhetoric?" *Journal of the American Board of Family Practice,* 1998, *11*(2), 116–126.

Unutzer, J., and others. "Care for Depression in HMO Patients Aged Sixty-Five and Older." *Journal of the American Geriatric Society,* 2000, *48*(8), 871–878.

Verlato, G., and others. "Attending the Diabetes Center Is Associated with Increased Five-Year Survival Probability of Diabetic Patients: The Verona Diabetes Study." *Diabetes Care,* 1996, *19*(3), 211–213.

Von Korff, M., and others. "Collaborative Management of Chronic Illness." *Annals of Internal Medicine,* 1997, *127*(12), 1097–1102.

Von Korff, M., and others. "Improving Depression Care: Barriers, Solutions, and Research Needs." *Journal of Family Practice,* 2001, *50*(6), E1–E5.

Wagner, E. H. "Population-Based Management of Diabetes Care." *Patient Education and Counseling,* 1995, *26*(1–3), 225–230.

Wagner, E. H. "Chronic Disease Management: What Will It Take to Improve Care for Chronic Illness?" *Effective Clinical Practice,* 1998a, *1*(1), 2–4.

Wagner, E. H. "More Than a Case Manager." *Annals of Internal Medicine,* 1998b, *129*(8), 654–656.

Wagner, E. H. "The Role of Patient Care Teams in Chronic Disease Management." *British Medical Journal,* 2000, *320*(7234), 569–572.

Wagner, E. H., Austin, B. T., and Von Korff, M. "Organizing Care for Patients with Chronic Illness." *Milbank Quarterly,* 1996, *74*(4), 511–544.

Wagner, E. H., and others. "A Survey of Leading Chronic Disease Management Programs: Are They Consistent with the Literature?" *Managed Care Quarterly,* 1999, *7*(3), 56–66.

Wagner, E. H., and others. "Quality Improvement in Chronic Illness Care: A Collaborative Approach." *Joint Commission Journal on Quality Improvement,* 2001a, *27*(2), 63–80.

Wagner, E., and others. "Improving Chronic Illness Care: Translating Evidence to Action." *Health Affairs,* 2001b, *20*(6), 64–78.

Weinberger, M., and others. "Cost-Effectiveness of Increased Telephone Contact for Patients with Osteoarthritis: A Randomized, Controlled Trial." *Arthritis and Rheumatism,* 1993, *36*(2), 243–246.

Willison, D. J., and others. "Consultation Between Cardiologists and Generalists in the Management of Acute Myocardial Infarction: Implications for Quality of Care." *Archives of Internal Medicine,* 1998, *158*(16), 1778–1783.

CHAPTER ELEVEN

Reconstructing Primary Care of the Elderly

Eric B. Larson

Primary care in the United States is at an important crossroads. In the wake of dramatic growth of the subspecialties of medicine, primary care by the end of the 1960s had become virtually nonexistent in most medical schools. In the early 1970s, visionary leaders led a rebirth of primary care in the United States. They received support from foundations and some state legislatures, whose elected members and their constituents saw the need for well-trained generalists to provide primary, first contact care, as well as ongoing and preventive care and continuity of care for the population at large. By the last decade of the twentieth century, primary care departments were an evident and, typically, a vital component of U.S. medical schools. Residency programs in family medicine, general internal medicine, and general pediatrics that were established, for the most part, in the 1970s had expanded and produced a well-trained cadre of generalist physicians (Roberg, 1988; Roback and Mason, 1977; Grumbach, 1999; Larson, 2001).

Coincident with the rise of primary care, the ascendancy of the randomized clinical trial (Cochrane, 1972), along with the so-called therapeutic revolution, provided increasingly effective therapies and preventive strategies for primary care physicians and their patients. High-quality clinical research also allowed clinicians to deliver care with much greater precision than in the past (Larson and Sheffield, 1997; Sheffield and Larson, 1996).

The last quarter of the century witnessed steadily increasing news coverage of medical advances, culminating in aggressive direct-to-consumer advertising of drug advances. This, along with the dramatic growth in medical therapeutics, has expanded public awareness and public expectations of benefit from medical care (Millenson, 1997).

Over the last quarter of the twentieth century, as the primary care movement gained momentum, the United States experienced the well-known demographic shift toward an older population. The therapeutic revolution has, arguably, benefited elderly patients more than any other group. Care of persons with common chronic diseases, like hypertension, ischemic heart disease, asthma, diabetes, and peptic ulcer disease, among many others, is better today than it has ever been. Chronic diseases are more prevalent among older persons. In addition, more people are living longer (Hoyert, Kochanek, and Murphy, 1999), and more people are living with chronic diseases for longer periods of time (Manton and Gu, 2001; Manton, Corder, and Stallard, 1997; Manton, Stallard, and Corder, 1995).

Thus, we seem to have an ideal situation in which primary care and, in particular, primary care of older adults, should be thriving. There are more practitioners with better training and better therapeutic tools to offer their patients. These patients have more information, many are better educated, and they certainly have higher expectations than in the past. Older persons arguably have the most to gain from therapeutics, a phenomenon noted in recent reviews of medical advances (Sheffield and Larson, 2001).

Unfortunately, the situation is not entirely rosy. Many practitioners are dispirited (Grumbach, 1999; Larson, 2001), especially primary care practitioners with fifteen to twenty years of experience whose practices have aged with them and who provide care for large numbers of older patients. Managed care is conceptually attractive for primary care physicians interested in providing a broad range of care, especially for the management of chronic diseases. However, the promise of managed care has generally not been realized in the wake of complex political and market forces (Robinson, 2001). In the more competitive marketplace that has emerged since the demise of Clinton-inspired health care reform, health care expenditures have shifted to pharmaceutical firms and equipment suppliers and away from providers. Among providers, primary care physicians are increasingly disadvantaged, especially in fee-for-service medicine, and many are leaving practice. Coincidentally, there has recently been declining interest in primary care residencies.

Today's market forces and the presence of tens of millions of uninsured have made it particularly challenging to provide continuity of primary care. There is increasing evidence that access to services in general, and especially, access to continuity of primary care services, is a mounting problem for patients, especially those with chronic disease (Millman, 1993; Billings, Anderson, and Newman, 1996; Kozak, Hall, and Owings, 2001).

A recent study of avoidable hospitalizations points out some of the problems. In its 1993 report, *Access to Health Care in America* (Millman, 1993), the Institute of Medicine (IOM) recommended that the prevalence of avoidable hospitalization be used to monitor access to health care services, especially for vulnerable groups.

Avoidable hospitalizations are associated with lack of access to timely and effective ongoing care, especially for persons with chronic diseases and for vulnerable populations. To date, only a few longitudinal analyses are available. Previous studies have shown rising avoidable hospitalization rates in low-income areas in New York City from 1982 to 1993 (Billings, Anderson, and Newman, 1996) and increasing rates of avoidable hospitalizations for uninsured and Medicaid-covered children in selected states from 1990 to 1995 (Friedman, Jee, Steiner, and Bierman, 1999). A national study (Kozak, Hall, and Owings, 2001) shows that the rate of hospitalization (Figure 11.1) for avoidable conditions increased from 2.2 million in 1980 to 3.7 million in 1998 and from 5.9 percent of all hospitalizations in 1980 to 11.5 percent of all hospitalizations in 1998. Hospitalizations for other conditions declined during the same period. Avoidable hospitalizations increased, particularly for persons over age sixty-five (Table 11.1). The rate increases also were progressively greater with advancing age over sixty-five.

Interestingly, at the beginning of the 1970s, when the effects of the Great Society projects and the recently introduced Medicare program were perhaps most evident, access was not the major reason for "deficient" ambulatory care in the elderly in a national study based on the national Health and Nutrition Examination Survey (HANES) data (Heller, Larson, and LoGerfo, 1984). Today, I suspect access to care

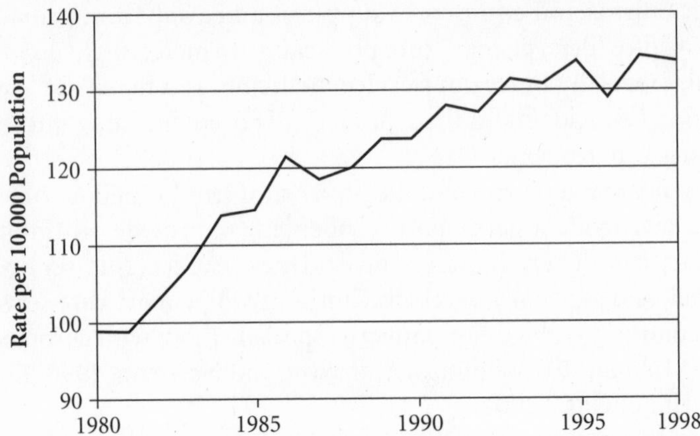

Figure 11.1. Rates of Avoidable Hospitalization, 1980–1998

Source: Kozack, Hall, and Owings (2001).

would be the predominant reason for substandard quality, not some failure of physician practice or delivery systems, as we concluded then.

Lack of access is the single biggest challenge to providing elderly patients with adequate primary care. Patients lacking access to primary medical care, much less ongoing medical care for a chronic condition, will not receive adequate care. At best, care will be episodic; at worst, it will be limited to emergency medical and hospital services, services that are currently overwhelmed by the added costs of this stopgap care. Given that chronic disease is impoverishing and also places persons at risk for lack of insurance coverage or inadequate coverage, vulnerable persons with chronic disease experience something like double jeopardy when it comes to care access and ability to sustain ongoing doctor-patient relationships. As a consequence, they may generally forgo the substantial benefits of recent medical advances in improved chronic disease care.

Changes in insurance coverage also undermine continuity of primary medical care. There is an increasing tendency for patients to change insurance coverage. Younger patients and families are affected, often because their employer changes the plans available to them. Older persons change coverage as supplemental plans come and go and because plans change their cost and benefit structure. A recent report (Cunningham and Kohn, 2000) stated that one in six patients changes insurance coverage each year. In many communities, a change in insurance coverage means changing providers. These changes can

Payment Source	1980	1990	1998	Tests for Trends, 1980–1998
Under age 65				
Medicaid	7.0%	9.4%	9.8%	+
Other government	5.5	8.9	11.4	+
Private insurance	4.1	6.8	7.5	+
Self-pay	5.1	9.4	11.6	+
Other Sources	4.2	7.3	7.5	+
Age 65 and older				
All Medicare	9.6	15.0	15.9	+
Medicare and Medicaid	13.3	20.9	20.4	+
Medicare and private insurance	8.3	14.1	15.7	+
Medicare only	9.9	14.7	15.4	+

Table 11.1. Percentage of Hospitalizations for Avoidable Conditions, by Source of Payment, 1980–1998.

Note: Tests for trends are based on percentages for all years (1980–1998). A plus sign indicates an increasing trend, significant at the 0.05 level.

Source: Kozack, Hall, and Owings (2001).

be particularly devastating to the elderly, the disabled, and persons with chronic disease.

Providers and provider groups can play a major role in undermining the continuity of the primary doctor-patient relationship. Examples are numerous, but generally they share a common feature: they typically relate to chronic undervaluing of so-called cognitive services. For example, providers are increasingly likely to refuse to accept managed care coverage, especially managed Medicare, and other insurance plans because of their inadequate fee schedules. These changes frequently occur literally overnight, casting adrift large numbers of their patients. Even public institutions like mine (the University of Washington Medical Center) have increasingly abandoned capitated commercial insurance plans due to high risk exposure.

In addition, physician provider groups, especially those with large programs in internal medicine and ambulatory pediatrics, have closed their doors in cities large and small across the country (Larson, 2001). Hospital networks have abandoned primary care clinics and networks they established in anticipation of managed competition because they experienced continued financial loss and saw no relief in sight. In all of these situations, ongoing doctor-patient relationships are disrupted, a disruption that is particularly harmful to patients with chronic disease.

One indicator of the consequences of disrupted doctor-patient relationships might be emergency room (ER) use. Rosenblatt and colleagues at the University of Washington recently examined the effect of the doctor-patient relationship on ER use in the elderly (Rosenblatt and others, 2000). Using 1994 data, they noted that 18 percent of elderly persons have one or more ER visits per year. Persons with principal care physicians were less likely to use the ER, regardless of disease category. Based on a referent odds ratio of 1.0, persons with a generalist principal care physician (PCP) had an (adjusted) odds ratio for ER use of 0.47; persons with a specialist PCP had an (adjusted) odds ratio of 0.58. They concluded that the presence of a continuous relationship with a physician reduces ER use. They went on to state, "This study suggests that, in disrupting a sustained relationship between one patient and one doctor, something of value is destroyed, with increased emergency department use an indicator of that disruption" (Rosenblatt and others, 2000, p. 101).

In summary, the challenge of providing continuous primary care, especially for elderly patients and those with chronic disease, is quite different than it was twenty-five to thirty years ago. The United States currently has a well-trained cadre of primary care physicians with a far more effective therapeutic toolkit for the increasing numbers of patients who enter old age, especially those with chronic disease. However, access to primary care services is poor to nonexistent for a large portion of the population. Market forces are causing primary care clinics and practices to be closed. Practitioners themselves disrupt primary care relationships when they drop certain insurance plans. I believe this highly unstable situation is just beginning to result in growing published evidence that due to lack of primary care services, the elderly and other persons with chronic disease are experiencing increased levels of avoidable hospitalizations and potentially avoidable ER service use. Practitioners and patients can likely recount anecdotes of everyday shortcomings leading to bad outcomes. I believe we will see more evidence and hear more anecdotes of the consequences of disrupted patient care relationships until more fundamental changes, including reconstructing primary care, occur.

PATTERNS OF MEDICAL CARE OF ELDERLY PERSONS

Contexts of Care

Descriptions of medical care of elderly persons often emphasize contexts of care. Care can be viewed as occurring across a continuum. As a hospital medical director, I could view this continuum as stretching from hospitalization for stroke, to rehabilitation on a subacute ward, to convalescence in a nursing home, to continued care at home, and finally, to return to care in an office (Rubinstein, 2003).

By contrast, that continuum can be viewed, and in my judgement and from the perspective of most elderly persons should be viewed, in the opposite direction, beginning in primary care (including ongoing care and preventive care) and spanning a spectrum of sites. The spectrum might lead eventually, but not necessarily or not even in most cases, to institutional care.

In fact, most older persons live in a home or apartment and have most of their encounters with physicians in their offices or clinics. A 1991 study from Agency for Health Care Policy and Research attempted to construct a diagrammatic movement pathway for the U.S. population through the health care system (Denson, 1991). This is shown as a simplified version for one thousand persons aged seventy-five and older in Figure 11.2. According to this survey, in any given year, 87 percent of persons age seventy-five will see a physician, 34 percent will be hospitalized, 8.5 percent will enter a nursing home, and 8.5 percent will die.

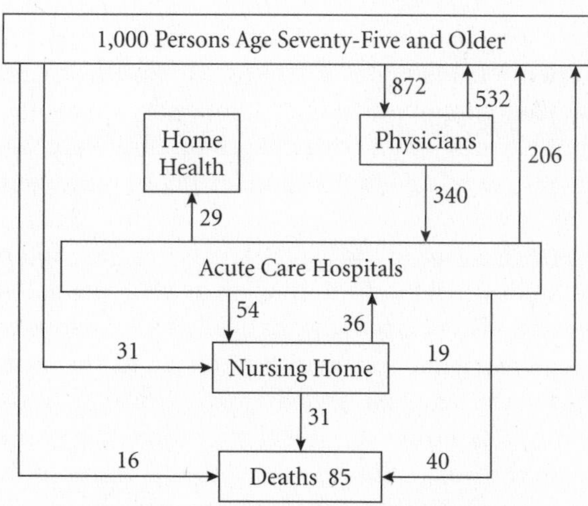

Figure 11.2. Movement of the Elderly Population Through the U.S. Health Care System

Source: Rubinstein, L. Z. "Contexts of Care." In C. K. Cassel and others (eds.), *Geriatric Medicine: An Evidence-Based Approach.* (4th ed.) New York: Springer, 2003. © 2003 Springer-Verlag. Used by permission of the publisher.

Two features of this figure are particularly relevant to thinking about the primary care of older persons. First, physician contacts are overwhelmingly the most common. Persons over age sixty-five had an average of 10.4 physician contacts per year, of which 65 percent occurred in a physician's office or in a clinic. In national data, persons seventy-five and older had 12.3 physician contacts per year (Rubinstein, 2003). In a health maintenance organization (HMO), visit frequencies are likely slightly higher than average and increase with age. Visits experienced by a control group selected for studies (McCormick and others, 1995) of health care utilization among Alzheimer's disease patients are instructive. The population (which was likely healthier than an average population), with a mean age of seventy-seven at entry, received 13.7 visits per year in the two years prior to enrollment and 16.3 visits per year two years after enrollment. Approximately 60 percent of visits were to primary care physicians. (Interestingly, 75 percent of visits of Alzheimer's disease patients were to primary care physicians.) Thus, visits to physicians and, in some settings, to primary care physicians are common.

The second feature of Figure 11.2 is the complexity of movement among many of these services. The movement among services is a particular challenge to patients and families. Failure in the so-called handoff can have disastrous consequences, especially as a source of medical error, jeopardizing patient safety. Inefficiencies are particularly common as patients transfer from site to site and from provider to provider in many communities. In addition, elderly patients, especially those without family or an advocate, can figuratively slip through cracks and crevices related to the complexities of movement between services.

The system displayed in the Figure 11.2 is dynamic and plastic and at times responds dramatically to changes in Medicare policy changes. The system can also respond dramatically to a curious mixture of Medicare, regulatory, and free-market forces. In recent years, the market described in the figure has seen dramatic growth in long-term care services, especially home care services, followed by an exodus of providers—in the wake of losses related to the Balanced Budget Act. This has occurred coincidentally with the unleashing of the forces I described earlier, which have so disrupted continuity of care and patient-physician relationships. Thus, most U.S. communities have experienced dramatic changes in the way patients move through the health care system, thereby adding to the complexity of providing care to an elderly population.

Amid all this complexity, the overall pattern of health care use of the elderly since the advent of Medicare in the United States has been one of consistent growth. In particular, this growth has occurred at a greater rate than for the population under age sixty-five. Displayed graphically in Figure 11.3 (Lubitz and others, 2001), the growth is dramatic across all groups but especially in the oldest old (age eighty-five and older). Amid the growth, there has been a shift toward a more complex mix of services, leading to relatively less growth in the dominant sector of hospital services. Medicare spending for hospital services, as a percentage of total spending, decreased from 70 percent in 1967 to 49 percent in 1998. The shift away from hospital services is even more marked for persons over age eighty-five (77 percent of total spending in 1967 to 46 percent in 1998). Per capita Medicare spending has risen the most for the oldest old, an increase that is entirely attributable to a greater rate of growth in Medicare-covered postacute services (home health, skilled nursing facilities, and hospice).

Outcomes of Care

Coincident with growth of Medicare, the health of the elderly has improved, as measured by gains in longevity and functional status. Life

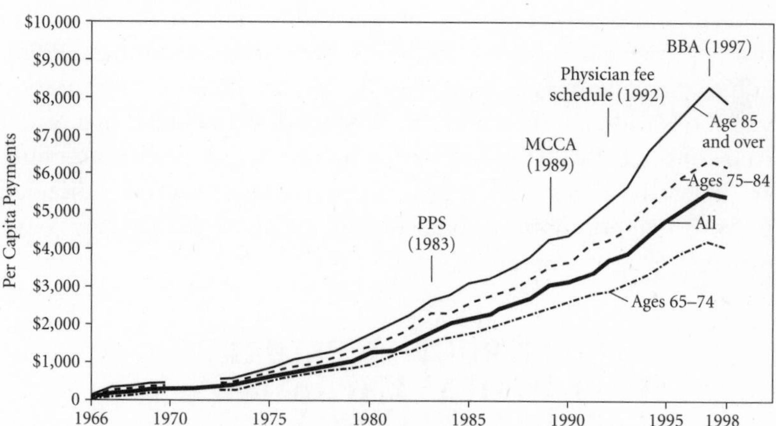

Figure 11.3. Medicare per Capita Payments, by Age Group, 1966–1998

Note: Data for 1970–1972 included total per capita payments for persons age sixty-five and older. Data by age group were not available.

PPS: prospective payment system. MCCA: Medicare Catastrophic Coverage Act. BBA: Balanced Budget Act.

Source: Lubitz and others (2001).

expectancy at age sixty-five increased from 14.3 years in 1960 to 17.8 years in 1998. The chronically disabled elderly declined from 24.9 percent of elderly persons in 1982 to 21.3 percent in 1993 (Lubitz and others, 2001).

What we see is a population of elderly persons whose functional status has been improving (Manton and Gu, 2001; Manton, Corder, and Stallard, 1997; Manton, Stallard, and Corder, 1995; Lubitz and others, 2001). This population is receiving increasing numbers of restorative procedures like coronary angioplasties, coronary artery bypass grafts, total joint replacements, and carotid endarterectomies, especially compared with time trends for similar procedures in those under age sixty-five.

While the elderly overall are functioning at higher levels and living longer than in the past, there is also an absolute and continual increase in the number of frail persons who have survived to more advanced old age (Hoyert, Kochanek, and Murphy, 1999; Manton and Gu, 2001). Especially as one reaches age groups of eighty, eighty-five, and older, frailty from chronic illnesses, and especially cognitive impairment due to Alzheimer's disease, becomes particularly prevalent and noteworthy. The prevalence of persons with dementing illnesses increases dramatically with age, from 12.7 percent of those aged eighty to eighty-four, to nearly 30 percent of persons eighty-five to eighty-nine, to 50 percent of persons between ninety and ninety-four, and nearly 75 percent of those over ninety-five (Graves and others, 1996). Lubitz and colleagues from the Health Care Financing Administration and the National Center for Health Statistics concluded in a recent study of three decades of health care use by the elderly, "Our findings are suggestive of a steady or growing percentage of severely disabled persons in a population whose overall average health status is improving" (Lubitz and others, 2001, p. 29).

RECONSTRUCTING PRIMARY CARE WITH AN EMPHASIS ON CARE OF THE ELDERLY

I believe that efforts to meet the care needs of older persons represent a great opportunity for reconstructing primary care. The current marketplace is best characterized as in disarray (Grumbach, 1999; Institute of Medicine, 2001). In fact, the recent IOM report, *Crossing the Quality Chasm* (2001), argues that the system is so dysfunctional it needs to be reconstructed.

Previously, I described the ongoing threats to doctor-patient relationships, especially to the ability of doctors and patients to sustain continuity of care. One of the consistent mantras of the primary care movement has been that continuity-of-care relationships are essential to good medical care and produce the best outcomes for patients (Branch, 2000). Perhaps the strongest force that attracts students and trainees to primary care and patients to primary care physicians is the opportunity to have an ongoing relationship between doctor and patient—for patients and doctors to know one another and through personal knowledge and application of professional knowledge and skill for patients to benefit.

We also have increasing evidence that access to care, and especially access to primary care, has measurable benefits (Larson, 2001; Institute of Medicine, 2001). Evidence ranges from studies describing factors associated with avoidable hospitalization (Billings, Anderson, and Newman, 1996; Kozak, Hall, and Owings, 2001; Friedman, Jee, Steiner, and Bierman, 1999) and ER visits (Rosenblatt and others, 2000), to benefits in the management of chronic diseases, and to everyday anecdotes about the personal losses and bad outcomes that patients, especially elderly patients with chronic diseases, experience when they "lose" their doctor.

We also find ourselves with a system where the most frequent care that elderly patients receive is a physician's care (Denson, 1991). At the same time, that system is one in which the care is occurring in an increasing variety and number of sites and from ever more differentiating types of providers (Rubinstein, 2003). Physicians are now differentiated into not only traditional organ specialists but also site-specific generalists (hospitalists, emergency medicine physicians, nursing home practitioners, officists). Nonphysician providers provide care to older patients, usually based on the organizations they work for (nursing homes, home health care, infusion services, hospice, respite). None of these generalist, nonprimary care providers embrace continuity of care over the long term as a defining characteristic of their profession. In most cases, their relationship with a patient (or client) is time limited and based on an episode that urgently and often passively (not by choice) creates an encounter leading to a brief therapeutic relationship. That relationship is usually valued but can be quite isolated—even unconnected or disconnected to prior care. This disconnectedness or unconnectedness is usually not preferred by older persons, especially those with chronic, complex diseases. Handoffs are notoriously difficult, and they are not without risk to patients (Kohn, Corrigan, and Donaldson, 1999). In the absence of good information exchange, which is rare and especially challenging in older patients with complex histories, inefficiencies and unnecessary resource consumption are the rule, not the exception.

Those persons most at risk to suffer from a system in disarray are those with chronic diseases, including the frail elderly. The highest risk is likely experienced by persons with limited access to care, particularly persons without access to ongoing care.

RECONSTRUCTING PRIMARY CARE FOR THE ELDERLY: TEN RECOMMENDATIONS

Do we face a choice between two extremes in caring for older persons: care based on continuity of care versus care based on fragmentation into site-specific, chronic-condition-specific, discontinuous care, which may even include nontraditional (complementary) providers? Is a synthesis desirable or even possible?

My answer to these admittedly hyperbolic questions is straightforward: reconstructing primary care for elderly persons begins with an endorsement that the best care will be based on a primary care model that emphasizes and is designed to promote continuity of care.

Since both my personal experience and conventional wisdom support the position that most patients, and especially older patients, prefer a system based on an ongoing personal relationship between a physician and a patient, why don't we have this? What must be done to accomplish such a reconstruction?

I believe there are at least ten critical steps to reconstruct primary care, and in particular, primary care of the elderly, based on this model:

1. *Achieve universal access to health care, especially to primary medical care in the United States.* The IOM report, *Crossing the Quality Chasm* (2001), is correct. We need to "build . . . a system that is more equitable and meets the needs of all Americans without regard to race, ethnicity, place of residence or socioeconomic status including . . . 43 million people who currently lack health insurance" (p. 35).

Although my topic is care of the elderly, who presumably have access through Medicare, the gaps that occur in our system ultimately cut across all age groups. They reflect a society that is willing to accept inadequacies in medical care and subsequent injustices in the world's wealthiest nation. Any serious attempt to improve health in the United States must acknowledge that solutions that do not include universal access will be suboptimal.

2. *Endorse that the best system of care of elderly persons is based on a primary care model.* This is not as trivial as it sounds. We need to create public and professional alliances that support availability and high-quality primary care relationships as essential to good health care. Most public-professional partnerships have emerged around advocacy for specific diseases (Alzheimer's disease, breast cancer) or to solve shortcomings in contemporary care (such as hospice, end-of-life care). Where are the voices that advocate for primary, ongoing medical care of elderly persons (Covinsky, 2000)? These voices have not emerged from the geriatric movement, and to date, not much has been heard from organized primary care or other organized advocacy groups like the American Association for Retired Persons or the foundations.

I contend that just as state legislators, whose citizens were facing an absence of generalist physicians in the 1960s, helped launch the U.S. primary care movement, a public-professional partnership is needed to advocate for care of the elderly based on primary care.

3. *Embrace consumerism and choice.* Consumerism is a rising force in health care. In the elderly, the related concepts of self-efficacy and active participation in medical care are associated with better outcomes for both successful aging and chronic disease management. Managed care, although initially it seemed attractive to primary care physicians (Goodson and others, 2001), was unsuccessful because, among other things, it failed, and still fails, to address the uniquely American desire of many persons to be choice-driven consumers (Robinson, 2001). In older persons, primary care physicians can provide valuable direction and expertise to address contemporary desires to consume a wide range of health care—from complementary and alternative medicine to an increasing array of traditional care options and end-of-life choices. The primary care provider can be particularly valuable, assuming there are no conflicts of interest. That is, primary care providers are presumably advocating for their patients' and the population's best interests (Goodson and others, 2001). Consumerism and choice are best addressed in a context where patients and physicians have stable, trusting, empowering relationships and enjoy continuity of care (Covinsky, 2000).

4. *Use information technology to link the disparate parts of our system. Locate ownership in the primary care provider and in individual patients and families and other caregivers.* Information technology will revolutionize how health care and health information are exchanged and stored. Currently, however, even with electronic medical records (EMRs) and within EMRs, accessing and using highly detailed, complex care information that develops over time is extremely challenging to both patients and providers. Information exchange as patients, usually older patients, move through sites of care within a complex system (Rubinstein, 2003; Denson, 1991) is particularly troublesome and a source of error and inefficiency (Branch, 2000; Kohn, Corrigan, and Donaldson, 1999). I predict that patient information will eventually assume its rightful place and become property that is owned by and in the possession of patients. The primary care physician or principal care physician should also have access to this information and should have it in a form that can be efficiently viewed and used. The best solution would be for patients and their primary care provider to co-own, manage, organize, and modify over time the equivalent of a lifetime medical record together. I predict this will lead to better patient and doctor-patient satisfaction, more efficient care, and better outcomes. Chip technology makes this possible today, but organizing and interpreting will best be accomplished within a continuing physician-patient partnership.

5. *Embrace the rising tide of consumerism and patient activism, and embrace self-care and patient education.* A separate aspect of the rising tide of consumerism involves patient activism, patient self-care, and the long-standing interest in patient education. This phenomenon has particular relevance as we look to the future: baby boomers begin to turn sixty-five in 2010. Today's seniors are the best educated of all time (Federal Interagency Forum on Aging Related Statistics, 2000), and baby boomers, especially those born in the United States, will be even better educated. Even now, over 90 percent of boomers who come to the University of Washington Medical Center as newly referred patients to cancer surgical specialists have consulted the Internet (D. Byrd, personal communication, July 24, 2001). Ever more convincing evidence is emerging indicating that patients do better, are more satisfied with their care, and will likely require less care for chronic diseases when they actively participate in their care (Larson, 1997). Better understanding obviously helps, but it may not be sufficient. Primary care physicians can use existing tools, work with teams organized around a specific condition, and generally be the force that integrates and con-

solidates the whole patient. Many of these self-management programs will be disease specific and require integration. As this style of care becomes more widespread and diffuses beyond demonstration efforts, it should naturally diffuse into the everyday practice of primary care, especially in older patients.

6. *Aggressively seek out, develop, and use technology that will bring care to where the patient is, with or without the physical presence of the provider.* Traditionally, modern physicians have expected patients to come to them for service. As technology advanced, patients and physicians increasingly came together around imaging, treatment, and various other technologies that are in fixed locations and considered essential to good care. Most recently, with wireless communication, miniaturization, and availability of remote control technology, there are increasing opportunities for persons to receive more care in their homes and at a distance from major centers (Institute of Medicine, 2001). This may occur with or without the actual presence of a provider. I believe these trends offer marvelous opportunities for patients and doctors. I know anecdotally of one oncologist who designed and arranged (for himself) a bone marrow transplant for a solid organ tumor, during which he never required hospitalization and which mostly occurred in his vacation home (primarily because the transplant was not covered by his health insurance). Such patient-enabling technology should be particularly helpful for older persons, especially those who are frail and mostly homebound, and will ideally be developed in the context of ongoing doctor-patient relationships.

7. *Increase training and skill levels of primary care practitioners in ongoing management of chronic diseases and principles of geriatric care.* It is virtually self-evident that chronic disease management is important for care of older persons. The issue of whether a primary care physician will provide that care or whether it will be parsed out among various subspecialists is less self-evident. Nevertheless, it is self-evident that generalists need to be well trained and up-to-date to provide effective care of patients with chronic disease (Larson, 2001). My belief is that primary care physicians, if well trained and up-to-date, are best suited to handle the vast majority of care of patients with chronic diseases. That care should be characterized by adherence to standard tenets of geriatrics, including a focus on functional assessment and functional well-being, and not be just disease based; awareness and appropriate use of teams or providers from other disciplines, especially for persons with complex problems; rehabilitation and "prehabilitation"

to maintain or enhance functional well-being; attention to end-of-life care issues; and familiarity with major geriatric syndromes like dementia, delirium, and frailty. Care of such patients can be time-consuming and complicated. However, if a physician has the skill set and interest, I believe such care is more likely to be efficient and done well in the context of an ongoing, trusting, and informed relationship—that is, the continuing primary care physician-patient relationship (Branch, 2000).

8. *Reform payment systems to reimburse primary care practitioners fairly compared with their peers in other specialties and in such a way that captures many unfunded activities critical to ongoing primary care.* Probably the biggest challenge facing primary care today is the inadequate payment levels for the core services of primary care. It is now so well known that this is a bad business enterprise that we at the University of Washington Medical Center have been informed by various financial consultants and auditors that bond raters will regularly downgrade hospitals and medical enterprises on the basis of the presence and extent of their efforts in primary care. Increasingly, primary care is about evaluation, information exchange, so-called cognitive services, and prescription of medications and services. Current payment levels favor procedures, use of devices, and complex diagnostic procedures. Economic incentives drive providers to provide more noninvasive diagnostic services and, if anything, fewer primary care services. Virtually all of the recommendations I have made are not viable for practitioners or institutions that wish to develop them in today's fee-for-service, non–managed care setting.

Primary care will need to have markedly increased and radically changed reimbursement systems if the field is to survive (Larson, 2001). Primary care physicians will likely need to be reimbursed more like attorneys: some will be paid on salaries as in-house or corporate employees, but most will be paid for the value of their skills and knowledge on a time expenditure basis. Skills and knowledge have value. Primary care services will never be encouraged if they are viewed only as a necessary entry point, a "front door" (in the same way that mayonnaise is a loss leader at Costco) leading to downstream referrals or consumption of more highly reimbursed services. I am also skeptical about the viability of a system where primary care physicians need to earn their income based on control and management of labs, diagnostic, or other services (Robinson, 2001). Ultimately, primary care needs to be reimbursed for its intrinsic value, which is considerable in the management of older patients and chronic diseases.

9. *Bring a generalist perspective to research and problem solving in geriatrics.* A recent issue of the *Journal of General Internal Medicine* had three articles on issues primarily affecting older patients: functional decline after hospitalization, end-of-life decision making, and impaired drivers (Covinsky, 2000). The accompanying editorial describes these as examples of pressing issues that defy typical disease-oriented approaches and that "have not been adequately studied . . . in part because academic geriatrics has not been sufficiently influenced by generalist approaches." Covinsky (2000) concludes, "Increasing the number of generalists who think about old people, and increasing the number of geriatricians who think like generalists, will significantly advance the care of older patients" (p. 674).

10. *Celebrate and accept that patients and doctors want to create and sustain meaningful relationships with each other.* In this era of increasing skepticism related to widespread publicity about medical errors, a health care system that suffers from a quality chasm, and untimely and tragic deaths of persons in medical research, we need to remember that the practice of medicine is still an intensely personal experience for both patients and doctors (Branch, 2000; Eisenberg, 2001). Institutional leaders along with everyday folks need to remind each other that relationships are not only what most people want but are also important to achieving the best possible patient-valued outcomes. As Charles Odegaard, a medieval historian and president emeritus of the University of Washington, wrote in his remarkable 1986 essay in the form of a letter, "Dear Doctor": "What we need above all now is a greater bond of faith and trust between patient and doctor, sufferer and healer, which is accommodated with whatever health care institutional arrangements emerge in our society. . . . Doctor, the future of the doctor-patient relationship is still very importantly in the hands of your professional colleagues and of yourself, as is the welfare of patients and the future of the professional of medicine" (p. 113).

References

Billings, J., Anderson, G. M., and Newman, L. S. "Recent Findings on Preventable Hospitalization." *Health Affairs,* 1996, *15,* 239–249.

Branch, W. T. Jr. "Is the Therapeutic Nature of the Patient-Physician Relationship Being Undermined?" *Archives of Internal Medicine,* 2000, *160,* 2257–2260.

Cochrane, A. L. *Effectiveness and Efficiency: Random Reflections on Health Services.* London: Nuffield Hospital's Provincial Trust, 1972.

Covinsky, K. E. "Bringing a Generalist Approach to the Problems of Older Patients." *Journal of General Internal Medicine,* 2000, *15*(9), 673–674.

Cunningham, P. J., and Kohn, L. "Health Plan Switching: Choice or Circumstance?" *Health Affairs,* 2000, *19,* 158–164.

Denson, P. M. *Tracing the Elderly Through the Health Care System.* Washington, D.C.: Agency for Health Research and Quality, 1991.

Eisenberg, L. "Good Technical Outcome, Poor Service Experience: A Verdict on Contemporary Medical Care?" *Journal of the American Medical Association,* 2001, *285*(20), 2639–2641.

Federal Interagency Forum on Aging Related Statistics. *Older Americans 2000: Key Indicators of Well-Being.* Hyattsville, Md.: National Center for Health Statistics, 2000.

Friedman, B., Jee, J., Steiner, C., and Bierman, A. "Tracking the Children's Health Insurance Program with Hospital Data." *Medical Care Research and Review,* 1999, *56,* 440–455.

Goodson, J. D., and others. "The Future of Capitation: The Physician Role in Managing Change in Practice." *Journal of General Internal Medicine,* 2001, *16,* 250–256.

Graves, A. B., and others. "Prevalence of Dementia and Its Subtypes in the Japanese-American Population of King County, WA: The KAME Project." *American Journal of Epidemiology,* 1996, *144,* 760–771.

Grumbach, K. "Primary Care in the United States—The Best of Times, the Worst of Times." *New England Journal of Medicine,* 1999, *341,* 2008–2010.

Heller, T. A., Larson, E. B., and LoGerfo, J. P. "Quality of Ambulatory Care of the Elderly: An Analysis of Five Conditions." *Journal of the American Geriatric Society,* 1984, *32*(11), 782–788.

Hoyert, D. L., Kochanek, K. D., and Murphy, S. L. "Deaths: Final Data for 1997." In *National Vital Statistics Report* (vol. 47, no. 19). Hyattsville, Md.: National Center for Health Statistics, 1999.

Institute of Medicine. Committee on Quality of Health Care in America. *Crossing the Quality Chasm: A New Health Care System for the 21st Century.* Washington, D.C.: National Academy Press, 2001.

Kohn, L., Corrigan, J., and Donaldson, M. *To Err Is Human: Building a Safer Health System.* Washington, D.C.: National Academy Press, 1999.

Kozak, C. J., Hall, M. J., and Owings, M. F. "Trends in Avoidable Hospitalization, 1980–1998." *Health Affairs,* 2001, *20,* 225–232.

Larson, E. B. "Successful Aging: An Overview." *Western Journal of Medicine,* 1997, *167,* 204–205.

Larson, E. B. "General Internal Medicine at the Crossroads of Prosperity and Despair: Caring for Patients with Chronic Diseases in an Aging Society." *Annals of Internal Medicine,* 2001, *134,* 997–1000.

Larson, E. B., and Sheffield, J.V.L. "Update in General Internal Medicine." *ACP Journal Club,* 1997, *127,* A14–A15.

Lubitz, J., and others. "Three Decades of Health Care Use by the Elderly, 1965–1998." *Health Affairs,* 2001, *20*(2), 19–32.

Manton, K. G., Corder, L., and Stallard, E. "Chronic Disability Trends in Elderly United States Populations: 1982–1994." *Proceedings of the National Academy of Sciences USA,* 1997, *94,* 2593–2598.

Manton, K. G., and Gu, X. "Changes in the Prevalence of Chronic Disability in the United States Black and Nonblack Population Above Age 65 from 1982 to 1999." *Proceedings of the National Academy of Sciences USA,* 2001, *98,* 6354–6359.

Manton, K. G., Stallard, E., and Corder, L. "Changes in Morbidity and Chronic Disability in the U.S. Elderly Population: Evidence 1982, 1984, and 1989 National Long Term Care Surveys." *Journals of Gerontology Series B: Psychological Sciences and Social Sciences,* 1995, *50,* S194–204.

McCormick, W. C., and others. "The Effect of Diagnosing Alzheimer's Disease on Frequency of Physician Visits: A Case-Control Study." *Journal of General Internal Medicine,* 1995, *10,* 187–193.

Millenson, M. L. *Demanding Medical Excellence: Doctors and Accountability in the Modern Age.* Chicago: University of Chicago Press, 1997.

Millman, M. (ed.). *Access to Health Care in America.* Washington, D.C.: National Academy Press, 1993.

Odegaard, C. E. *Dear Doctor: A Personal Letter to a Physician.* Menlo Park, Calif.: Henry J. Kaiser Family Foundation, 1986.

Roback, G., and Mason, H. K. *Physician Distribution and Licensure in the U.S., 1975.* Chicago: American Medical Association, 1977.

Roberg, N. "Internal Medicine in the 1930s." *Journal of the American Medical Association,* 1988, *260,* 3645–3646.

Rosenblatt, R. A., and others. "The Effect of the Doctor-Patient Relationship on Emergency Department Use Among the Elderly." *American Journal of Public Health,* 2000, *90,* 97–102.

Robinson, J. C. "The End of Managed Care." *Journal of the American Medical Association,* 2001, *285*(20), 2622–2628.

Rubinstein, L. Z. "Contexts of Care." In C. K. Cassel and others (eds.), *Geriatric Medicine: An Evidence-Based Approach.* (4th ed.) New York: Springer, 2003.

Sheffield, J.V.L., and Larson, E. B. "General Internal Medicine Update: Information Clinicians and Teachers Need to Know." *Journal of General Internal Medicine,* 1996, *11,* 613–621.

Sheffield, J.V.L., and Larson, E. B. "Update in General Internal Medicine." *Annals of Internal Medicine,* 2001, *135*(4), 269–277.

CHAPTER TWELVE

Palliative Care and Primary Care

Opportunities for Cooperation and Improvement

Christine Cassel
Beth Demel

Palliative care is the comprehensive management of patients' physical, psychological, social, spiritual, and existential needs. It can be part of the treatment of any person for whom a patient-centered approach, pain and symptom control, family involvement, and compassionate care are needed. Palliative care should be practiced throughout the scope of any serious illness, not only at the end of life, and can be received along with active treatment. With today's medical technology, no one should suffer unavoidably.

In 1997, the Robert Wood Johnson Foundation funded the Last Acts project designed to educate the public, policymakers, and health care professionals on issues surrounding end-of-life care. The following Precepts of Palliative Care, developed by the Last Acts Palliative Care Task Force, affirm a vision of better care:

We gratefully acknowledge the support of the Robert Wood Johnson Foundation and the thoughtful intellectual contributions of Albert L. Siu, R. Sean Morrison, and Diane E. Meier.

- Respecting patient goals, preferences, and choices
- Comprehensive caring
- Using the strengths of interdisciplinary resources
- Acknowledging and addressing caregiver concerns
- Building systems and mechanisms of support

PAST TRENDS IN PALLIATIVE CARE IN THE UNITED STATES

Why, at the beginning of the twenty-first century, do we need a grassroots movement to help us learn something as basically human as how to die? We need to relearn death because people today die differently than our forebears did: we tend to die older, of different causes, and in different environments. In 1900, people often died at home, surrounded by family. Physicians routinely comforted the dying and their families. In the past century, medical and public health advances have almost doubled the average life expectancy, from less than fifty years to nearly eighty (Rowe and Kahn, 1998). People who die in old age tend to experience a long period of functional decline before death and thus require intensive caregiving and well-coordinated medical care. As medical advances allowed us to delay death, we moved death out of the home and into institutions. Today, although most people say they would prefer to die at home, 75 percent die in institutions (56 percent in the hospital and 19 percent in nursing homes) (National Center for Health Statistics, 1999).

In the United States, we became so caught up in our ability to cure disease that our health care system forgot that death is inevitable. When Medicare was enacted in 1965, it was largely intended to reduce the financial burden of episodic, acute hospital stays on families.

The origins of palliative care as a medical movement in the United States date back to the early 1970s, when Dame Cicely Saunders gave a lecture at Yale University about caring for dying patients. Her talk stimulated the Yale community to start a hospice program, and the first hospice in the United States was established in Connecticut in 1974 (Bosanquet, 1999). Medicare established a hospice benefit in 1983 in an attempt to remember death and reduce costly inpatient hospital stays at the end of life. Hospice was seen as an alternative to use when life-prolonging options had been exhausted. The Medicare hospice benefit is available only to patients whose doctors are willing to certify they have a life expectancy of six months or less, who agree to receive only palliative care, and who have a full-time primary caregiver.

Despite its good intentions, the hospice benefit does not help everyone; it remembers only certain types of death.

Hospice in the United States works well for people with fairly predictable diseases, especially end-stage cancer. At least 60 percent of hospice enrollees have a cancer diagnosis (Bosanquet, 1999; National Hospice Organization, 1999). Hospice is less helpful for people with less predictable diseases, like heart disease, or diseases with a long period of decline, like Alzheimer's.

Recent history of the palliative care movement in the United States has been driven largely by Medicare funding. When Congress approved the Medicare hospice benefit, it dramatically altered how and where hospice care is provided. The number of hospice admissions immediately increased; by 1985, 40 percent of people dying of cancer were enrolled in hospice. Because the Medicare hospice benefit emphasizes home care, hospices that had been built around an inpatient model changed the way they operated, shifting their emphasis to home care in order to qualify for Medicare reimbursement. As Herbert Lukashok of Albert Einstein College of Medicine writes, "By providing a hospice benefit under Medicare, the government has, in effect, defined what a hospice is" (Bosanquet, 1999, p. 39).

Medicare did more than define hospice when it limited hospice eligibility to a certain type of dying patient—one with a home, a caregiver, and a terminal diagnosis with an easily predicted disease course. The government also determined who would likely receive end-of-life palliative care and who would not. Medicare's hospice eligibility rules have curtailed the development of a broader palliative care movement in the United States, and until very recently few palliative care programs emphasized treatment of pain and other symptoms in conjunction with attempts to cure disease.

Medicare's hospice eligibility rules have led to a decreased length of hospice stay; too many patients do not enter hospice until their final days, when opportunities to reap maximum benefit have been lost. Because of the six-month rule, hospices may hesitate to accept patients until death is clearly imminent to avoid being charged with Medicare fraud or abuse. With many diseases, it is impossible for physicians to feel confident predicting death within six months. Similarly, the six-month prognosis and the requirement to stop life-prolonging efforts have the implication of giving up, something neither doctors nor their families are comfortable doing.

The Medicare hospice benefit was a good step toward a public acknowledgment that people die and that care for the dying is a valuable part of health care. We now need to expand hospice to enable more people to receive excellent end-of-life care, and we need to apply the precepts of palliative care to all care, not just care at the end of life. Inspiring clinicians around the country have begun to accomplish these goals; some have documented their experiences in *Pioneer Programs in Palliative Care: Nine Case Studies* (Robert Wood Johnson Foundation and Milbank Memorial Fund, 2000).

Unfortunately, too few patients receive adequate end-of-life palliative care. The Study to Understand Prognoses and Preferences for Outcomes and Risks of Treatments (SUPPORT) documented the type of care dying patients in teaching hospitals preferred and how closely their wishes were followed. The study found that patients' wishes were frequently not followed and that pain was common. Half the patients able to communicate in the last three days of life said they were in severe pain. These findings demonstrated the need for hospitals and health systems to pursue a higher standard for end-of-life care and motivated many doctors to improve the end-of-life care they provide (SUPPORT Principal Investigators, 1995). The Institute of Medicine (IOM) has called for the medical profession to pursue a higher standard for palliative care throughout the life span (Institute of Medicine, 1997).

In January 2000, the Joint Commission on Accreditation of Healthcare Organizations, which accredits most medical facilities in the United States, developed new mandatory standards for the assessment and treatment of pain. Since 2001, the Joint Commission has been scoring pain management programs as part of its accreditation process. Its acknowledgment that pain management programs have an essential role in all medical facilities is an important step toward incorporating palliative care into mainstream medicine. Hopes are that many of the hospitals and nursing homes that are developing pain programs in response to the new pain standards will go beyond pain management and develop programs that incorporate a full range of palliative care services.

CURRENT TRENDS IN PALLIATIVE CARE

Most Americans say they would prefer to die at home. But as *The Dartmouth Atlas of Health Care 1999* (Dartmouth Medical School, 1999) reports, depending on where they live, anywhere from 20 percent to more than 50 percent of Americans die in the hospital. People are more likely to die in hospitals in regions with more hospital beds (Dartmouth Medical School, 1999; Wennberg, 1986). The *Dartmouth Atlas* findings show that:

- Among Medicare enrollees, 15 percent to more than 50 percent will experience at least one stay in an intensive care unit during the last six months of life.
- On average, 11 percent of Medicare enrollees will spend seven or more days in intensive care during the last six months of life.
- As many as 30 percent of Medicare enrollees are likely to be admitted to intensive care during terminal hospitalization.

We do not know what proportion of deaths should occur in the hospital, at home, or elsewhere, and the proportion may vary depending on the numbers of elders living alone, patterns of illness, and financial context. However, since we do know that the majority of American deaths occur in institutions, clinicians must provide good palliative care wherever the patient is. The following situations illustrate why we need positive, realistic end-of-life options outside of the home:

Mrs. P is an eighty-eight-year-old widow dying of colon cancer. Her grown children live in other states and cannot visit for extended periods of time. Mrs. P might find a hospital or subacute unit a more supportive environment than her home. Even if she could afford a full-time paid caregiver at home, it is unlikely that she would have as many different types of social and caregiving contacts at home as she would in a structured caregiving setting such as a nursing home or an in-patient hospice program. Unfortunately, most nursing homes are not equipped to provide the intensive sophisticated palliative care services that a terminal cancer patient requires, and in-patient palliative care services or hospices can serve only patients with short (a few days to a week) life expectancy. In the United States, there is no good option for Mrs. P under the current system.

Mr. S was a ninety-year-old widower with numerous age-related chronic conditions including high blood pressure, Parkinson's disease, severe arthritis, and osteoporosis. He took medication for depression. Two years ago, he was hospitalized for pneumonia, which was treated with antibiotics. After he recovered, he was in a weakened state and required physical therapy in addition to close medical monitoring of his other conditions. Although Mr. S would have preferred to go home, he and his doctors determined that he would receive better care in a nursing home, since he lived alone and

Medicare would not pay for a twenty-four-hour home health aide. As Mr. S's functional ability continued to decline, it became clear that he would not be able to return to his home. When he began to experience organ failure and became eligible for the Medicare hospice benefit, hospice professionals delivered their services in the nursing home, where he eventually died. Mr. S was able to benefit from palliative services throughout his nursing home stay. He was fortunate that the doctors and nurses at his nursing home were trained in palliative medicine and understood the importance of relieving distressing symptoms throughout the span of an illness. Too often, nursing home residents are undertreated for pain; nationally, fewer than 5 percent of people dying in nursing homes are enrolled in the Medicare hospice program (Keay, 1999). The hope is that the Joint Commission's new pain standards will motivate more institutions to improve the way they diagnose and treat pain.

Mrs. M is a sixty-five-year-old woman with late-stage ovarian cancer. She has fought her disease with chemotherapy, but she is losing her battle. She is eligible for hospice, and the comfort care appeals to her, but her seventy-year-old husband cannot care for her physical needs, and she feels uncomfortable having her children see her bloated body and care for her draining wounds, a common complication of late-stage ovarian cancer. Instead, she opted to enter a hospital-based palliative care program to allow professionals to care for her physical needs so that her family would have the time and energy to provide emotional support. The problem with this option is that if life expectancy is greater than one to two weeks, the hospital is not an appropriate or sustainable option.

People with serious illnesses and their families have diverse needs. To accommodate these needs, clinicians are creating new palliative care delivery models in the United States. The following delivery models make palliative care accessible to those consumers whose needs are not met by Medicare's hospice benefit. As these models illustrate, palliative care, including hospice, can be provided in a variety of settings including the hospital, the nursing home, and the patient's own home. To learn more about the extent to which these models have been instituted throughout the United States, the Robert Wood Johnson Foundation funded the Center to Advance Palliative Care, based at the Mount Sinai School of Medicine in New York City, to survey more than two thousand hospitals nationwide, asking them if they had palliative care or pain programs and, if so, what type. The percentages following each model described below represent the breakdown of types of programs within hospitals that had palliative care or pain programs. The percentages do not add up to 100 percent because some hospitals have more than one type of program (Pan and others, 2001):

- Consultation service (43 percent): A team composed of doctors and nurses, typically with a social worker and bereavement counselor, sees patients with palliative care needs anywhere in the hospital.
- Dedicated inpatient unit (23 percent): Palliative care beds are clustered in one area of the hospital, concentrating together patients with similar needs. A dedicated unit, which may be combined with the consultative service, provides visibility and may enhance acceptance of palliative care by hospital staff.
- Combined hospice-palliative care unit (36 percent): An inpatient unit serves both hospice patients and hospital patients with palliative care needs. (The study grouped this and the next category together.)
- Community hospice-hospital contract (36 percent): Through a contractual arrangement with a community hospice program, a hospital provides palliative care in an inpatient unit. This model expands Medicare payment options available to hospitals for these palliative care services, since they are reimbursed (albeit inadequately) through the Medicare hospice benefit.
- Hospital outpatient palliative care clinic (32 percent): The clinic operates in conjunction with a consultative service or inpatient unit to provide continuity of care after discharge from the hospital. This model promotes care continuity and is often linked to home visiting programs.

THE FUTURE OF PALLIATIVE CARE: A FIELD IN TRANSITION AND GROWTH

As these care delivery models illustrate, the field of palliative medicine is evolving into a dynamic and innovative area of medicine. Factors pushing palliative medicine toward growth and transition include changing demographics that will increase the demand for palliative care, increased professional interest in providing quality palliative care, and increased foundation funding aimed at making this professional interest a reality. We are optimistic that palliative medicine has the potential to become an increasingly vibrant field. For this to happen, however, fellowship training programs in palliative medicine must be funded, and reimbursement mechanisms for hospitals and individuals that provide palliative care must be improved.

We are already beginning to make progress in the way undergraduate and graduate medical students are trained in palliative care, but more resources are needed to improve access to palliative care training. In 1995, the American Board of Internal Medicine (ABIM) board of directors asked how many internal medicine residents received end-of-life training. The answer to this question was unknown, and ABIM surveyed all internal medicine residencies to find out. The survey responses were telling: not one internal medicine residency program incorporated end-of-life training into its curriculum.

At around the same time, the IOM's Committee on Care at the End of Life began its two years of study. The IOM's findings supported those of the ABIM: outside the hospice community, there was very little professional interest in studying, teaching, or providing high-quality palliative care (IOM, 1997).

Since that time, the professional mood surrounding palliative care has changed dramatically. Health care professionals are recognizing the importance of providing high-quality care at the end of life. They are remembering that their responsibility to provide high-quality, compassionate care extends to all patients, even those for whom cure is not a viable option.

Why is end-of-life care suddenly seen as an exciting field of medicine? Some of this change is probably the result of increased foundation funding aimed at increasing public and professional awareness of end-of-life issues, particularly from the Robert Wood Johnson Foundation. At Mount Sinai, the foundation is funding the Center to Advance Palliative Care (CAPC) to provide support for the growth of palliative care throughout the country. By all appearances, the ground is fertile in spite of daunting obstacles, including financial constraints and institutional culture. In CAPC's first year, it encountered enthusiastic leaders in every sector who wanted to begin to strengthen palliative care capability in their institution, system, or community.

There has also been a surge of media interest in end-of-life care, perhaps as baby boomers begin to face their own mortality. For instance, Bill Moyers produced an excellent four-part miniseries on death and dying (entitled *On Our Own Terms*) that aired on PBS in September 2000, and *Wit*, the successful off-Broadway play about a woman dying alone in a hospital following a futile, painful course of treatment for her metastatic ovarian cancer, was recently made into an HBO movie.

The most encouraging trend is that much of this increased interest in palliative care is generated by young medical students themselves. Although the road toward practicing palliative care is paved with hurdles and few financial rewards, young doctors are choosing to pursue this challenging yet rewarding career. They are choosing palliative medicine despite its absence of explicit fellowship training, developed career path, and adequate Medicare reimbursements. Young physicians tell me that they chose palliative medicine because they understand that helping people die compassionate deaths is at the core of modern medicine.

In the past, medical professionals cared for the dying as well as they could without the benefits of today's scientific advances. With today's medical technologies, no one should suffer from avoidable physical or emotional pain, and young physicians are beginning to make it their work to ensure that their patients do not. They are beginning their careers in palliative medicine as either their main focus or integrated into their general practices, despite the barriers. If we could eliminate some of these barriers, especially with fellowship training funding in palliative medicine available now from the Veterans Administration, then palliative medicine will become a truly robust area of medicine. The interest in practicing palliative medicine already exists; we now need to find the resources to channel this interest into creating a dynamic and well-recognized field of medicine.

SPECIAL PALLIATIVE CARE NEEDS AND CONCERNS OF OLDER ADULTS

As the baby boomers age, more Americans will require models of end-of-life care aimed at a geriatric population. Since people who die in old age tend to follow a different disease trajectory from those who die young, increasing longevity will change the way palliative care is practiced in many cases. People who die in old age tend to die after a long period of functional decline in which the goals of maintaining function and relieving suffering may require life-prolonging measures (such as cardiac pacemakers or treatment of diabetes and hypertension) as well as symptom-oriented palliation. During this period of decline, numerous chronic conditions are often treated by a primary care physician as well as by various specialists. Palliative care for an older population needs to be sensitive to comorbidities and recognize that treating one condition may exacerbate others. During the often gradual period of physical decline preceding death, older patients can benefit from palliative care while simultaneously receiving curative, preventive, and rehabilitative services.

For example, consider Mary, a ninety-two-year-old woman with congestive heart failure. She is deconditioned (her muscles are weak) following a two-week hospital stay for pneumonia. She can no longer get herself to the toilet or dress herself. Mary, like many other older adults, needs a combination of life-prolonging, preventive, rehabilitative, and palliative care. Life-prolonging measures include the treatment of her heart failure with oxygen, diuretics, and ace inhibitors (drugs to control high blood pressure). Preventive measures include annual mammography and flu vaccination. Rehabilitative measures include physical therapy in her home to restore her ability to move around her home and get out of her bed and into her chair or to the toilet by herself. Simultaneously with these services, Mary is a good candidate for palliative care: she needs help from a social worker to write an advance directive (a document about the type of care that a patient wishes should she or he become incapacitated) and appoint a health care proxy, and she needs treatment for depression and low-dose opiates for breathing difficulties not totally relieved by her cardiac regimen, all of which improve her quality of life and make her feel better even as she is receiving life-prolonging, preventive, and rehabilitative treatments. In addition, Mary is able to stay in her home thanks to her home health aide, who helps manage her care and offers companionship twelve hours each day.

Perhaps because many physicians see practicing palliative medicine as "giving up" on their patients, too few patients of all ages receive good palliative care. Some studies have shown that very old people are undertreated for pain even more than younger patients. In one study of daily pain management for people with cancer in nursing homes, one-fourth of all people over age sixty-five with cancer who reported daily pain were given no pain medication at all, not even acetaminophen. This study showed that older residents received less pain medication than younger patients and were less likely than younger residents to receive acetaminophen or more powerful pain medication, including weak opiates or morphine (Barnabei and others, 1998). This is not an isolated study; it has been estimated that 45 to 80 percent of nursing home residents experience significant levels of untreated pain (American Geriatrics Society [AGS] Panel on Chronic Pain in Older Persons, 1998).

People with cognitive impairments are at an even greater risk of being undertreated for pain because they may be unable to communicate verbally about their level of pain. In one study of eighty-eight patients who recently broke their hips, pain was undertreated in patients with and without cognitive impairment, but nurses gave older patients and patients with cognitive impairment less medication than younger patients and patients without cognitive impairments, despite the fact that doctors had prescribed the same amount of medication to both groups (Feldt, Ryden, and Miles, 1998).

Chronic pain is common in older adults. A recent Harris survey found that one in five older Americans takes analgesic medications several times a week or more. Two-thirds of those who take pain medications regularly had taken prescription pain medications for more than six months. Pain in older adults should be taken seriously and treated; it is not an inevitable aspect of aging, and untreated, it can lead to serious complications and functional decline. Some consequences of chronic pain are depression, decreased socialization, sleep disturbance, and the inability to move around the home or community. All of these health and social problems can lead to even more serious problems. For example, when older adults are unable to exercise, their muscles become weaker, leading to further risk of immobility. As a result of pain and its consequences, people in chronic pain use more health care services than people without pain (AGS Panel on Chronic Pain in Older Persons, 1998). Medicare needs to support adequate palliative care for all beneficiaries, not just those who are actively dying. By paying for medications and adequately reimbursing institutions and providers who deliver good palliative care, people on Medicare might become generally healthier and require fewer health services in the long run.

PALLIATIVE CARE SPECIALTY STATUS: AN ACTIVE DEBATE

There is currently no palliative care specialty certified by the ABMS. Palliative care specialists are board certified in another specialty, usually internal medicine, and then typically engage in a graduate fellowship program or another form of further study in palliative care. Because palliative care is a necessary part of most medical specialties, there is an active debate among palliative care practitioners about the wisdom and practicality of creating a board-certified specialty for palliative care. On one hand, specialty status would elevate the profession's status in the medical field by indicating to the medical community that palliative medicine is a legitimate form of medicine with its own scientific knowledge base. This elevated specialty status would attract more quality people to the profession. A board-certified specialty organization would also promulgate national standards for good palliative medicine, further improving the specialty's legitimacy while protecting consumers. On the other hand, some fear that a palliative care specialty would result in the marginalization of patients considered "palliative" so that too few patients would continue to receive this care. A better solution might involve creating recognition for a strong board-certified specialty of palliative medicine, and then encouraging existing medical specialties to incorporate relevant aspects of palliative medicine into their specialty certification exams.

Primary care physicians' ability and need to incorporate palliative care into their practices will change as the population ages and the consequent need for palliative medicine increases. The high prevalence of chronic and progressive illness in the aging population requires an ability to begin palliative care earlier in the course of illness, often in conjunction with potentially curative or disease-modifying treatment. Examples of common disease trajectories in older adults include congestive heart failure, chronic obstructive pulmonary disease, Alzheimer's disease, and other major chronic illnesses. While these diseases may cause decline in function, patients with these diagnoses may have a prognosis for survival that is greater than the traditional six months considered terminal under the traditional hospice-based palliative care model. With these common age-related conditions, it is often difficult to determine when a patient is actively dying, and it is difficult for physicians to estimate with accuracy how long the patient will live. In these cases, palliative care should increase gradually as the disease progresses.

Who should provide palliative care to patients with chronic or progressive diseases? In many cases, the primary care provider can and should continue to treat a patient's palliative care needs as they shift throughout the course of the illness, including the end of life. This provides continuity of care and avoids the sometimes difficult decision to go into hospice, but requires a primary care provider who is well trained in clinical palliative medicine. Sometimes the nature of the patient's illness or the primary care provider's skills and preferences make it appropriate to consult a palliative care specialist as the disease progresses toward death.

Some primary physicians for people with chronic conditions are themselves specialists, including cardiologists, pulmonologists, neurologists, and psychiatrists. These specialists may not have the skills to provide end-of-life care as their patients' palliative care needs intensify. They may also be uninterested in providing palliative care. In many cases, by the time a disease has advanced enough to require intense palliative care, most of the patient's care is no longer diagnosis related; now it is related to prognosis and functional decline. At this stage of an illness, patients typically require symptom management, function and quality-of-life enhancement, communication with patient and family, and coordination of care needs. This model is more consistent with that of a primary care geriatrician than with other specialists who might be a patient's primary physician earlier in the disease course.

Primary care physicians can incorporate palliative care into their practice when a patient's disease progresses to the point of requiring palliative care. In most cases, a specialist or internist acting as a primary physician can, with adequate training in symptom management and end-of-life communication, provide satisfactory palliative care. As more medical schools incorporate palliative care into their curricula, more specialists and primary care doctors will have the necessary skills to provide whatever palliative care is needed by most of their patients in most situations. However, patients can benefit from the skills of a palliative care specialist in the following two situations, both of which will become increasingly common as the population ages: when a patient has very difficult-to-manage symptoms that require the skills of a trained specialist, or when a patient is actively dying in the hospital and the family requires help with complex, interwoven end-of-life issues. These psychosocial and medical issues are extremely time-consuming to manage and are outside many physicians' expertise and interest.

Palliative Care Specialists

Sometimes seriously ill patients with complex needs are hospitalized with unmet physical needs or difficult-to-diagnose symptomatic distress. These people could benefit from the skills of a palliative care specialist. Consider a seventy-five-year-old patient with chronic atrial fibrillation, mild congestive heart failure, mild hypertension, and glucose intolerance who is doing reasonably well and is cared for by a generalist primary care physician. He develops metastatic prostate cancer and is treated with mitoxantrone chemotherapy and prednisone. The treatment for metastatic cancer worsens his hypertension and provokes flagrant out-of-control diabetes, worsening the congestive heart failure. At this point, the palliative care challenges are as demanding as the internal medicine challenges. How does one use opioid medications to treat bone pain while simultaneously evaluating and modulating the patient's level of consciousness and sedation? Would stimulants be a medically sound treatment option for a person with atrial fibrillation? A palliative care expert is more familiar with this type of situation and regularly uses these medications and treatments. At this point, a palliative care specialist could step in to help the primary generalist or principal care specialist who might be less familiar with how to treat end-of-life patients requiring complex care of this magnitude.

In other situations, the traditional primary care specialist may simply be unable to spare the time (or may not have the skills or the interest) to spend the hours needed in family meetings and planning sessions discussing what are often very emotional and highly charged clarifications, communications, and decisions. In a hospital situation, a palliative care consultant is often called when the referring physician reaches a situation in which he or she is unable to provide the time required for these kinds of counseling and planning sessions. Such activities could be performed well by nurse practitioners as consultants to palliative care interdisciplinary team.

Continuum of Care

Patients with serious illnesses require an evolving continuum of care as their illnesses progress. When a patient with chronic conditions responds well to standard treatment, a primary physician can frequently provide adequate palliative care. However, as complications arise or as the patient approaches the end of life, palliative care needs intensify and become more complicated. At this point, the patient may benefit from a comanaging relationship between the primary physician and a palliative care specialist. At the end of life, when symptom management becomes the only viable goal, it may be appropriate for the palliative care specialist to become the patient's primary doctor.

The following three care models help conceptualize the continuum of care required by patients with serious illnesses. Each patient's case is unique, and different physicians, even within the same specialty, have different interests and skills. Therefore, not all patients and their physicians will, or should, experience all three of these care models as they approach the end of life. However, these models are intended to function as a flexible blueprint for care management throughout the course of a serious illness:

- *Palliative care specialist as consultant.* While a patient with age-related chronic conditions may respond well to the palliative care provided by a primary physician or specialist, this physician may have questions about how to manage certain complicated symptoms. Symptom management becomes more complicated in older patients who tend to have comorbidities, since treating one condition may exacerbate another. In these cases, a primary physician may consult with a palliative care specialist as needed. This allows the patient to benefit from maintained continuity of care with a primary physician while also benefiting from the knowledge and skills of a palliative care specialist.
- *Comanagement between primary physician and palliative care specialist.* As a disease progresses, symptom management may become as important and complex as treatment and management of the disease itself. At this stage of an illness, when palliative care is practiced alongside life-prolonging, preventive, and rehabilitative care, it may make sense for a primary physician and a palliative care specialist to comanage a patient's care, each acting as a primary physician for certain aspects of the patient's care. As long as both physicians accept the patient-centered mission of this care strategy and avoid turf conflict, this model can work well.

If both comanaging physicians are certified in the same specialty, then they must be vigilant about using a distinctly different diagnosis code when submitting claims to Medicare. Medicare has a concurrent care policy for hospital inpatients that prohibits a Medicare carrier from paying for more than one consultation or visit on the same date of service by physicians of the same specialty, unless the concurrent service is for a distinctly different problem. This policy puts palliative care specialists at a disadvantage, since there is no ABMS board-certified palliative care specialty and they are often certified in internal medicine, the same specialty as the primary physician.

• *Palliative care specialist as primary physician.* At the end of life, when symptom management and end-of-life counseling frequently become the most critical needs for patient and family, it may make sense for the palliative care specialist to become the patient's primary physician. For this model to work, the original primary physician must make an effort to assure the patient and family that they are not being abandoned. While a palliative care specialist may have the best skills and expertise for managing the patient's care at this stage of illness, patients and their families benefit in knowing that the primary physician still takes an interest in the patient's care and the family's well-being.

PALLIATIVE CARE IN A CRITICAL CARE SETTING

In critical care units, comprehensive care is managed by a single hospital team. In these settings, generalists may encounter situations in which they would benefit from the skills and knowledge of a palliative care specialist. Critical care physicians are becoming increasingly aware of the high number of deaths that occur within critical care settings and the degree to which principles of palliative care can improve the quality of the dying experience for patients and their families. The critical care specialty boards are even adding palliative care as a special critical care expertise for certification purposes, and the ABIM Subspecialty Board on Pulmonary and Critical Care Medicine has added an optional module on palliative care to its recertification process.

Changing Role of Nurses

Because palliative care is both time-consuming and multidimensional, many palliative care delivery models are structured around a multidisciplinary care team of doctors, nurses, social workers, and other health, mental health, and social service professionals. In some cases, advanced practice nurses may successfully take the lead in coordinating palliative care services and identifying transitional points in a patient's care that might require further physician services.

Mount Sinai School of Medicine is currently partnering with Franklin Health, a community-based complex case management organization, and Blue Cross–Blue Shield to coordinate palliative care for seriously ill, community-dwelling patients. In this project, nurses coordinate palliative care services under the medical direction of a physician manager. Most of the patients' care remains coordinated by their primary physician, who is in direct contact with the team care coordinator. Through direct contact with the patient and the primary physician, nurse coordinators act as specialist consultants who help the primary physician coordinate patients' care. Preliminary findings on the program's impact appear to be positive and show an increased number of deaths at home, more new medications for symptom control, and more advanced directives being followed.

In some ways, excellent end-of-life care is more compatible with the nursing model of care (starting with what the patient needs) than with the traditional medical model (starting with a diagnosis). At the end of life, symptom management is often more critical than diagnosis. For instance, patients with end-stage cancer with pulmonary involvement and end-stage cardiac disease have very similar care needs once life-prolonging efforts have proven futile or inappropriate.

Making This Work

Ideally, palliative care can be incorporated into primary care in most cases. In this model, primary care physicians would consult palliative care specialists in complicated or extreme situations in which the clinical or psychosocial-medical expertise of a specialist is required. For this model to become a reality in hospitals and health systems across the country, the following systemic changes need to occur:

- All generalists and specialists who are the primary physicians of dying patients need training in the basic medical, pharmacological, and psychosocial aspects of palliative care. Physicians need to be trained in prescribing and managing opiates and other pain medications and managing nonpain symptoms of distress and discomfort. And although not all physicians will have the aptitude or interest in providing intense end-of-life counseling, all physicians should be trained in the basic communication skills required for discussing difficult choices with their patients.
- All physicians need training in how to recognize the transition points during a disease course that require palliative care evaluation and treatment. All patients should be continuously evaluated for changing palliative care needs, whether they are actively dying, stabilized, or recovering. All physicians should be able to identify the need

for palliative care, regardless of whether the physician provides palliative care personally or consults with a palliative care specialist when the need for such care arises. Improved undergraduate and graduate medical training in assessing palliative care needs would help generalists determine when a patient requires the skills of a palliative care specialist.

- Because continuity of care is important to seriously ill patients and because generalists do not want to abandon their patients, a patient's primary doctor and a palliative care specialist might choose to comanage the patient's care at the end of life. At Mount Sinai, where the palliative care consult team is designed to assist attending physicians in crisis situations, this model of fifty-fifty joint management frequently occurs in the last month of life. This is a clinically excellent model but requires training on the part of both the generalist and the palliative care specialist. If the generalist cannot recognize the need for palliative care, then she or he will not know when to call for a palliative care consult.
- Adequate resources must be invested in the training of palliative care specialists. As the baby boomers age, there is no doubt that situations will increasingly occur in which patients will benefit from the expert skills, knowledge, and experience of palliative care specialists, both as consultants and as primary doctors at the end of life. Dedicated funding for palliative care fellowship programs would be a strong first step toward achieving this goal. Without adequate training opportunities, we can expect a shortage of palliative care specialists as the baby boomers face old age and death.

CONCLUSION

Palliative care represents a set of clinical competencies that have not been included in the training of most physicians or in the context of most practices—either specialist or generalist. Recent growth in awareness of these knowledge and skill gaps may well lead to greater ability of generalists to provide palliative care to their patients, allowing continuity of the physician-patient relationship and, more important, the family-physician relationship.

There are limits, however, to the capability of generalists to provide this care. One limit is the specialty knowledge base in symptom management of especially difficult or complex patients. Another limit is the time and interdisciplinary staff capability required for patients who need extensive or prolonged counseling. In either of these situations, a palliative care specialist can contribute valuable skills, knowledge, and experience in a comanagement model or in transfer of care. Where the emphasis will move in decades ahead depends in great part on the changes in our health care system and concurrent growth or decline in the continuity-of-care primary care model. Regardless of whether palliative care is delivered by a primary care provider or a specialist, the demand from patients and families for high-quality palliative care will continue to grow.

References

American Geriatrics Society Panel on Chronic Pain in Older Persons. "The Management of Chronic Pain in Older Persons." *Journal of the American Geriatrics Society,* 1998, *46,* 635–651.

Barnabei, R., and others. "Management of Pain in Elderly Patients with Cancer." *Journal of the American Medical Association,* 1998, *279*(23), 1877–1882.

Bosanquet, N. "Patterns of Use of Service." In N. Bosanquet and C. Salisbury (eds.), *Providing a Palliative Care Service: Towards an Evidence Base.* New York: Oxford University Press, 1999.

Dartmouth Medical School. Center for Evaluative Study. *The Dartmouth Atlas of Health Care 1999.* Washington, D.C.: AHA Press, 1999.

Feldt, K. S., Ryden, M. B., and Miles, S. "Treatment of Pain in Cognitively Impaired Compared with Cognitively Intact Older Patients with Hip-Fractures." *Journal of the American Geriatrics Society,* 1998, *46,* 1079–1085.

Institute of Medicine. *Approaching Death: Improving Care at the End of Life.* Washington, D.C.: National Academy Press, 1997.

Keay, T. J. "Palliative Care in Nursing Homes." *Generations,* Spring 1999, pp. 96–98.

National Center for Health Statistics. *National Mortality Followback Study.* [http://www.cdc.gov/nchs/releases/98facts/93nmfs]. 1999.

National Hospice Organization. Fact Sheet, 1999.

Pan, C. X., and others. "How Prevalent Are Hospital-Based Palliative Care Programs?: Status Report and Future Directions." *Journal of Palliative Medicine,* 2001, *4*(3), 315–324.

Robert Wood Johnson Foundation and Milbank Memorial Fund. *Pioneer Programs in Palliative Care: Nine Case Studies.* New York: Milbank Memorial Fund, 2000.

Rowe, J., and Kahn, R. L. *Successful Aging.* New York: Pantheon Books, 1998.

SUPPORT Principal Investigators. "A Controlled Trial to Improve Care for Seriously Ill Hospitalized Patients: The Study to Understand Prognoses and Preferences for Outcomes and Risks of Treatments (SUPPORT)." *Journal of the American Medical Association,* 1995, *274,* 1591–1598.

Wennberg, J. "Which Rate Is Right?" *New England Journal of Medicine,* 1986, *314*(5), 310–311.

CHAPTER THIRTEEN

Alcohol, Drug, and Mental Disorders, Psychosocial Problems, and Behavioral Interventions in Primary Care

Harold A. Pincus

It is impossible to practice effective primary medical care without attention to the range of psychological and social issues embedded in the lives of all human beings. While most thinkers, practitioners, patients, and others involved in health care would tend to agree with this axiom, the separation between the mental and the physical has persisted at least since René Descartes in the seventeenth century; in fact, by means of current organizational and financing strategies, it is actually increasing. Moreover, the failure to integrate mind and body effectively persists in the face of:

- Massive epidemiological evidence on the prevalence of mental disorders in primary care and their personal, family, and societal impact (Goldman, Rye, and Sirovatka, 2000)

Portions of this chapter have been adapted from Watkins, Pincus, and Tanelian (2001), Pincus, Pechura, Elinson, and Pettit (2001), and Pincus (2003).

- Promulgation of powerful conceptual models, such as Engel's biopsychosocial model (1977), and treatment frameworks, such as behavioral medicine and health psychology (Baum, Revenson, and Singer, 2001) and consultation and liaison psychiatry (Schwabb, 1989), that integrate these concepts
- Enormous growth in the basic and clinical research documenting the linkage—actually, indivisibility—of mental and physical processes and the effectiveness of new treatments for mental conditions (Goldman, Rye, and Sirovatka, 2000)
- Exhortations by major governmental leaders, such as the *Surgeon General's Report on Mental Health* (Goldman, Rye, and Sirovatka, 2000), and other national leaders, such as reports by the Institute of Medicine and National Academy of Sciences (deGruy, 1996)

In preparing this chapter, I am assuming that readers are reasonably knowledgeable regarding each of these points. I am also assuming awareness of the persistent problems that have been documented with regard to the adequacy of primary care providers' recognition and treatment of mental and behavioral disorders (deGruy, 1996; Hirschfeld and others, 1997; Kamerow, Pincus, and Macdonald, 1986). In addition, I assume that the rationale for and effectiveness of longitudinal collaborative care models for these conditions are well accepted (Katon and others, 1997; Wagner, Austin, and Von Korff, 1996). Nonetheless, it may be useful to illustrate these points using the examples of problematic alcohol use (Watkins, Pincus, and Tanielian, 2001) and depression (Pincus, Pechura, Elinson, and Pettit, 2001).

PROBLEMATIC ALCOHOL USE

Alcohol-related problems are a significant public health concern in the United States. Alcohol dependence, abuse, and problem drinking increase morbidity and mortality (McGinnis and Foege, 1993) and raise economic, social, and health care costs (Manning and others, 1989; Rice, Kelman, and Miller, 1991). A recent study estimated that the total economic cost of alcohol-related problems was $148 billion in 1992 (Harwood, Fountain, and Fountain, 1999).

Alcohol use disorders are widespread in the U.S. population. The 1992 national Longitudinal Alcohol Epidemiologic Survey interviewed nearly forty-three thousand individuals to determine the prevalence of these disorders among U.S. adults. Forty-five percent were defined as current drinkers (twelve or more drinks in the past year), 17 percent were defined as moderate drinkers (three to thirteen drinks per week), and about 8 percent were defined as heavy drinkers (two or more drinks per day). About 7 percent of current drinkers met criteria for alcohol abuse; about 10 percent met criteria for alcohol dependence. Using data from the 1988 National Health Interview Survey, a population-based study of more than forty thousand adults, Archer and Grant found that 54 percent reported current consumption, 9 percent met criteria for abuse or dependence, and 24 percent reported hazardous drinking (Archer and Grant, 1995).

Alcohol use disorders are common among primary care patients. Fleming, Manwell, Barry, and Johnston (1998) looked at the frequency of at-risk drinking among 19,372 adults attending several primary care clinics in rural and urban Wisconsin. Most were part of a staff model health maintenance organization (HMO). Twenty percent of both men and women met the NIAAA criteria for at-risk drinking. Among patients older than age sixty, 15 percent of men and 12 percent of women regularly reported drinking in excess of these limits (Adams, Barry, and Fleming, 1996). Fourteen percent of males aged sixty-one to sixty-five reported regularly drinking more than six drinks per occasion, as did 3 percent of the women.

While effective treatments exist for the entire spectrum of alcohol-related problems (Fleming, Cotter, and Talboy, 1997; National Institute on Alcohol Abuse and Alcoholism, 1995), fewer than half of those individuals who need treatment actually receive it (Institute of Medicine, 1990). One in five men and one in ten women who visit their primary care providers meet the criteria for at-risk drinking, problem drinking, or alcohol dependence (Manwell, Fleming, Johnson, and Barry, 1998). Primary care providers (PCPs) are in an ideal position to screen for alcohol problems, begin treatment, and monitor progress. However, primary care practices generally are not set up to support PCPs in recognizing and treating alcohol use disorders. Since many of these patients do not consult an alcohol treatment specialist on their own, important opportunities for identification and treatment are being missed. A recent national survey of primary care physicians and patients noted that more than nine in ten physicians fail to identify substance abuse in adults. The majority of patients with substance abuse say that their primary care physician did nothing to assess or treat their substance abuse (Center for Alcohol and Substance

Abuse, 2000). A recent study of primary care physicians in Ohio in which 4,454 patient visits were observed revealed that screening for alcohol problems took place during 8 percent of the visits and only 1 percent of the patients received counseling on alcohol problems (Stange and Jaen, 1998). Other research suggests that many physicians are unaware of patients' substance abuse and do not participate in their patients' recovery (Saitz, Mulvey, and Plough, 1997).

DEPRESSION

An estimated 5 to 25 percent of individuals in the United States will experience major depressive disorder (MDD) in their lifetime, with women suffering at rates two to three times those of men (American Psychiatric Association, 2000). Furthermore, since many depressive episodes do not fully remit and symptoms may last for years, and with recurrence rates estimated at 60 percent or higher, depression is a chronic illness for most individuals suffering from the condition.

The societal costs of depression, which have been discussed in detail elsewhere, consist of morbidity and mortality from suicide and accidents due to impaired concentration, failure to advance in career and school, loss of employment, and increased risk of substance abuse. Furthermore, the United States loses between $30 and $53 billion in productivity and direct medical costs related to depression each year (Greenberg, Finkelstein, and Berndt, 1995; Rice and Miller, 1998). The Global Burden of Disease Study, conducted by the World Bank and the World Health Organization, found unipolar major depression to be the second leading source of disease burden in established market economies, with alcohol use fourth (Murray and Lopez, 1996).

As in alcohol problems, there are strong arguments for identifying and treating depression in a primary care setting. Major depression is two to three times more common in general medical settings than in community samples and is one of the most common health problems seen in primary care (Coyne, Fechner-Bates, and Schwenk, 1994; Kessler and others, 1994; Regier and others, 1993; Zung, Broadhead, and Roth, 1993). Furthermore, persons who are depressed are likely to seek or be receiving care from a primary care physician for other reasons (Katon and others, 1990), visit the emergency room seven times more frequently (Johnson, Weissman, and Klerman, 1992), and have twice the overall medical costs, even after controlling for severity of comorbid general medical conditions (Simon, Ormel, Von Korff, and Barlow, 1995).

A proliferation of effective treatments for depression, including both proven psychotherapeutic approaches and an arsenal of improved (though highly expensive) pharmacological interventions, has been developed, tested, and incorporated into widely accepted evidence-based guidelines for primary care treatment of depression (Agency for Health Care Policy and Research Depression Guideline Panel, 1993; Schulberg, Katon, Simon, and Rush, 1998). In addition, chronic care models of effective treatment in primary care have been developed and tested (Katon and others, 1995, 1999; Wells, 1999; Wells and others, 2000).

As depicted in Figure 13.1, most patients with depression are initially seen (although not necessarily recognized and properly treated) by primary care professionals (Goldberg and Huxley, 1980). Furthermore, even for those whose depression is recognized, treatment in the primary care sector is often suboptimal (Lin and others, 1995; Wells, 1994), and inadequate follow-up and long-term monitoring are also a problem (Katon and others, 1996; Schulberg, Katon, Simon, and Rush, 1998).

Direct pharmaceutical company marketing to consumers and aggressive marketing to nonpsychiatric physicians risk the serious complication of overtreatment with medication. As many as 40 percent of the population may manifest subsyndromal symptoms of depression, and there is little evidence to support, and some evidence against, the use of medications, rather than watchful waiting, in this population (Pincus, Davis, and McQueen, 1999; Williams and others, 2000).

SPECIAL FEATURES OF MENTAL AND BEHAVIORAL CONDITIONS

What makes mental disorders and psychosocial problems different from the other kinds of issues that primary care providers routinely encounter? A few particulars stand out in this regard, although they are not exclusive to these kinds of problems:

- *They are ubiquitous.* All humans at some point in their lives encounter stress, have problems with or lose friends and relatives, have difficulty concentrating, feel despair or sadness or anxiety, or may

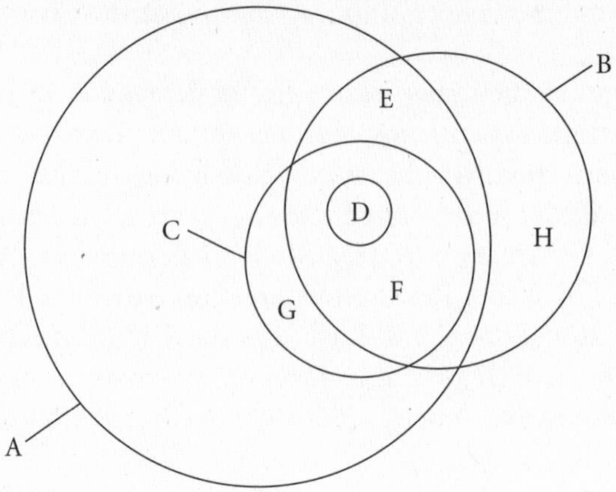

Legend

A See a primary care physician
B Have major depressive disorder (MDD)
C MDD recognized
D MDD appropriately recognized and treated
E MDD not recognized, not treated
F MDD recognized, not appropriately treated
G Recognized but not MDD (false positive)
H Have MDD but do not see a primary care physician

Figure 13.1. Scope of the Problem: Recognition and Treatment of Depression in Primary Care Settings

Source: Adapted from Goldberg and Huxley (1980).

directly or indirectly feel the hazardous effects of alcohol, tobacco, or illegal drugs.

• *They are difficult to define.* Not all individuals who encounter these issues consider them problems or illnesses (or are considered by others to have a problem or illness) or have evidence of impairment as a result. Most of these phenomena lie on a continuum where objective means for making distinctions are rare (which is not all that different from other medical conditions).

• *They are stigmatized.* Whether viewed from the popular media portrayal of a Woody Allenesque New Yorker cartoon or grade B slasher movie, these types of problems are often caricatured by the general public (and by primary care providers). On a more serious and insidious note, there remains extensive bias in insurance, hiring, and other financial and administrative practices. Moreover, perhaps because of their ambiguity and multidimensional nature, there is often an expectation that individuals ought to "bootstrap" themselves up and that failure to do so represents a personal or moral weakness.

- *The role of primary care, medicine, and health care is ambiguous.* By their very nature, these types of problems lie at the intersection of multiple social institutions or systems: education, social welfare, criminal justice, and occupational. The precise boundaries and responsibilities of the various sectors are generally not well specified, and even within a given system, such as health care, the precise roles of generalists and the various subspecialists (for example, psychiatrists and psychologists) are often more subject to local, financial, and organizational factors than to clearly specified, empirically based algorithms.

Perhaps more than with any other interface of primary care, these types of problems call into question the foundations and boundaries of all of medicine, as well as our concepts of health and disease. At the same time, and probably in more ways than not, these types of conditions are very much like the other types of conditions that are the focus of primary care. In fact, the main theme of this chapter reflects the view that the conceptual, financial, organizational, and educational approaches to mental and behavioral conditions should not be different from those of other body systems. As deGruy put it in his superb and comprehensive review of mental health and primary care for the 1996 Institute of Medicine report on primary care, "Systems of care that force the separation of 'mental' from 'physical' problems consign the clinicians in each area of this dichotomy to a misconceived and incomplete clinical reality that produces duplications of effort, data, and ensures that the patient cannot be completely understood" (p. 286).

Thus, in this chapter, I provide some initial concepts and definitions, describe the issues and barriers present at multiple levels in trying to integrate care of these conditions into primary care, and then portray the future, laying out assumptions, population-specific scenarios, and potential risks.

CONCEPTS AND DEFINITIONS: LAYING OUT THE TERRAIN

One of the major problems in discussing the subject of this chapter is the difficulty in defining it. Table 13.1 describes some of the many terms used to characterize this topic. For the purposes of this chapter,

Adjectives	Nouns
Mental	Diseases
Behavioral	Illnesses
Emotional	Disorders
Social	Conditions
Psychological	Problems
Psychosocial	Factors
Biopsychosocial	Issues
Addictive, substance related	Treatments
Cognitive	Interventions
Stress related	Health
Maladaptive	
Brain	
Nervous	

Table 13.1. Selected Terms Used to Describe Behaviorial Health Components in Primary Care.

I am incorporating three main foci (each with its own definitional issues):

- Treatment of alcohol, drug, and mental disorders and psychosocial problems in primary care (ADM/PS)
- Behavioral and psychosocial interventions (B/P/S) in primary care
- Primary care for individuals with mental disorders

Treatment of Mental Disorders and Psychosocial Problems in Primary Care

In many ways the anchor point for defining this group of conditions is the *Diagnostic and Statistical Manual of Mental Diseases,* Fourth Edition (DSM-IV; American Psychiatric Association, 1994). The DSM-IV, which is fully linked to the International Classification of Disease, Ninth Revision, Clinical Modification (the official U.S. classification and coding system) and the International Statistical Classification of Diseases and Related Health Problems, Tenth Revision (used in other countries), is essentially a descriptive system attempting to define relatively homogeneous categories on the basis of their phenomenological presentation, that is, specific signs and symptoms. A core conceptual feature of DSM-IV is the definition of a mental disorder, which essentially requires that the manifestations meet the specific criteria in DSM-IV (for example, for major depressive episode, schizophrenia, alcohol abuse) and have "clinically significant distress or impairment (in major social roles)" (p. xxi). In addition, in situations where specific criteria are not met, as in atypical or subthreshold cases, but the clinical significance criterion is met, a condition is classified as a disorder using a Not Otherwise Specified category (for example, "Depression, NOS").

Unfortunately, the DSM-IV is quite inadequate for primary care (deGruy and Pincus, 1996). Its focus on specialty care and derivation primarily from data gathered in psychiatric tertiary care settings, its length, its complexity, its emphasis on "splitting" into finer categories rather than "lumping," and particularly its focus on mental disorders as compared to psychosocial problems or other subthreshold (but not subclinical) conditions (Pincus, Davis, and McQueen, 1999) have made it less useful to and less used in primary care.

The DSM-IV does actually attend to nondisorders, that is, psychosocial problems, through the "Other Conditions That May Require Clinical Attention" section and its multiaxial system (Axis IV Psychosocial/Environmental Problem checklist), as depicted in Table 13.2. These components, however, are generally given little attention in clinical or academic use, and as a result, there is a disconnect between primary care providers' and mental health specialists' perspectives on diagnosis, as depicted in Figure 13.2 (Pincus, Davis, and McQueen, 1999). Although both may agree on diagnosis of certain conditions manifested by individuals as needing or not needing attention to their disorder or problem, there are also huge discrepancies, as represented in the off-diagonal boxes (boxes 2 and 4 in Figure 13.2).

Numerous studies have documented the low rate of primary care recognition of mental disorders, as defined by standard psychiatric research diagnostic tools. At the same time, mental health specialists and the psychiatric academic and research leadership tend to be uninterested in primary care practice patients with various forms of psychosocial problems or who are distressed or impaired but may not meet formal DSM criteria. Furthermore, even individuals without any disorder or problem may benefit from one or more forms of behavioral or psychosocial intervention. Thus, for the purpose of this chapter, we are including in our purview individuals represented in all four boxes of Figure 13.2.

	Depressive disorders	Substance use problems	Panic disorder	Somatization	Other—anxiety disorders (e.g., social, specific phobias)	Substance abuse	Bipolar disorder	Substance dependence	Severe personality disorder	Schizophrenia
Longitudinal follow-up and monitoring	Pr	Pr	Pr	Pr	Pr/Ps	Pr/B/Ps	Pr/Ps	Pr/B/Ps	B2Ps	PsB2
Extended complex B/P/S interventions	B1	B1	B	B	B	B	B2	B2	B2	B2
Second-level or higher medications	Pr	Ps	Ps	Ps	Ps	Ps	Ps	Ps	Ps	Ps
Brief B/P/S interventions	Pr/B1	Pr/B1	Pr/B1	Pr/B1	B1/pr	B/pr	B/Ps	B/Ps	B/Ps	B/Ps
Initial medication	Pr	Pr	Pr	Pr/Ps	Pr/Ps	Ps/Pr	Ps	Ps/Pr	Ps	Ps
Diagnosis and comprehensive P/S assessment	Pr	Pr	Pr	Pr/B1	B1/Pr	B1/Pr	B/Ps	B/Ps	B/Ps	Ps
Counseling and psychoeducation	Pr	Pr	Pr	Pr/B1	B1/Pr	B1/Pr	B/Ps	B	B	B
Recognition or limited P/S assessment	Pr	Pr	Pr	Pr	Pr	Pr	Pr	Pr	Pr	Pr
Primary care for general medical conditions	Pr	Pr	Pr	Pr	Pr	Pr	Pr	Pr	Pr	Pr

Table 13.2. Potential Provider Roles and Functions in Relation to Specific Conditions.

Note: This table does not include child conditions and populations and geriatric conditions. Pr: primary care provider in a specialty setting. B1: behavioral health specialist in a primary care provider setting. B2: behavioral health specialist in a specialty setting. Ps: psychiatrist.

Primary Care–Identified Mental Health Condition

Psychiatry-DSM-Identified Mental Disorder		+	−
	+	1	2
	−	4	3

Figure 13.2. Relation of Primary Care Providers' Perspectives on Diagnosis to Those of Mental Health Specialists

Note: Boxes 1 and 3 represent agreement regarding diagnosis. Boxes 2 and 4 represent disagreement.

Behavioral and Psychosocial Interventions in Primary Care

While the advances in psychopharmacology have been exceptionally dramatic, a more subtle, but in some ways equally important, revolution has been occurring within the domain of nondrug interventions. Highly specific, manualized, short-term-evidence-based behavioral technologies have been developed and tested to treat a wide range of conditions (Krupnick and Pincus, 1992)—some for specific mental disorders, such as cognitive behavioral therapy or interpersonal therapy for depression, dialectical behavioral therapy for borderline personality disorder, and cognitive rehabilitation for schizophrenia, with others aimed specifically at behavioral factors associated with general medical conditions. Still others may involve psychoeducation or cognitive behavioral techniques that might best be considered as preventive health interventions, some of which should be available to all individuals in a population, such as education about safer sexual practices and tobacco use prevention activities. Many interventions that are categorized as complementary or alternative medicine (CAM) are behavioral in nature. Inasmuch as I will be recommending broader integration of behavioral health specialists into primary care, the skills many of these individuals will possess will apply to interventions across the range of conditions depicted in Figure 13.2, as well as those that apply to preventive interventions and general medical conditions. In addition, many of these interventions can be implemented by PCPs.

Primary Care for Individuals with Mental Illness

Individuals with mental disorders, especially severe conditions such as schizophrenia and Alzheimer's disease, are more likely to suffer from general medical conditions as well as inadequate primary medical care (Koran and others, 1989). Many factors contribute to these findings. The nature of their mental disorder may make it difficult for individuals to seek out and trust in care. Reimbursement mechanisms and the organization of services are incredibly confusing, with separate systems, personnel, and rules and reduced communication and collaboration. Anyone would be challenged to navigate through that level of complexity, let alone individuals with severe mental illness.

BARRIERS TO EFFECTIVE CARE

Effective attention to each of the issues noted is hampered by longstanding barriers that are both historical and structural. These barriers also exist at the patient provider, practice organization, plan or insurer, and purchaser levels.

Historical and Structural Barriers

For centuries, mental and physical disorders have been perceived differently from each other, and this is reflected in how institutions for providing care have been constructed. The mental health system, especially for care of individuals for more severe disorders, has long been largely based in the public sector, generally a responsibility of states. The substance abuse treatment system is even more entrenched and separated from mental health in an underresourced public auspice, generally more closely linked to criminal justice and social welfare than to medicine.

The providers also grew up in largely different worlds; only a minority of mental health specialists are psychiatrists, and even they have had mixed connections with the rest of medicine (for example, in the 1970s, psychiatry briefly did away with the medical internship requirement). Various forms of psychologists, social workers, substance abuse counselors, and therapists often have little, if any, exposure to primary care except for their own personal medical care. They are just as likely to be linked to or placed within social services systems, educational systems, and criminal justice systems as primary care.

The separation between the two systems is perhaps most palpable in the lack of parity in insurance coverage provided for mental illness and substance abuse disorders. Various trends in financing and care have further supported this separation: the community mental health movement, psychoanalysis, the 1980s growth of private psychiatric hospitals, and behavioral health carveout arrangements.

Important links between mental and behavioral health and general medicine, including neuroscience research, consultation liaison psychiatry, and health psychology, do exist. Unfortunately, each has limitations in overcoming these barriers. Neurobiological paradigms have tended to replace psychoanalytical concepts in mainstream psychiatry. Despite the linkages to medicine from a physiological perspective, this "preoccupation with brain biology and psychopharmacology has evolved in a way that is rather unhelpful to generalists. . . . Primary care clinicians have lost a theoretical framework for understanding the human condition and giving meaning to symptoms" (deGruy, 1996, p. 299). Similarly, health psychology and behavioral medicine and psychiatric consultation liaison services have developed outside the realm of primary care. Connections to medicine or to medical concepts in biology or frameworks developed in the context of specialty care will not work: "the view from within primary care practice is an absolute prerequisite" (deGruy, 1996, p. 305).

An important optimistic trend is the increasing placement of mental health specialists in primary care settings. Mostly incorporating psychiatric nurses and social workers, these arrangements pave the way for important future shifts to restructure the relationship between primary care and mental and behavioral health.

Patient Barriers

Societal stigma is a barrier to treatment of mental health problems and often has an impact on the health care decisions of affected individuals (Katz, Kessler, Lin, and Wells, 1998; Williams and others, 1999) and their PCPs (National Depressive and Manic-Depressive Association,

2000). Surveys of primary care physicians have indicated that many of their patients with depression were reluctant to accept such a diagnosis, and even more were hesitant to see a mental health specialist (Williams and others, 1999). Concerns about confidentiality deter individuals from seeking or receiving help, particularly when using employer-based health plans to pay for services. Some patients worry that awareness of their psychiatric condition will have a detrimental effect on their relationships with family or friends, and others are simply unaware of modern conceptions of mental illnesses as medical conditions with highly effective treatments. In many cases, the illness itself causes feelings of pessimism, nihilism, and low energy that interfere with help-seeking behaviors or results in unemployment and loss of insurance coverage.

Provider Barriers

Primary care providers have a unique opportunity to detect depressive symptoms early and provide adequate care or timely referral for their patients (Williams and others, 1999). However, limited time, as well as the primary care physician's own interests, background, and training, may also act as barriers to appropriate depression treatment in primary care settings (Williams and others, 1999). Patient resistance to diagnosis, as well as somatic presentations, act as barriers to recognition and treatment of depression in the primary care setting.

With regard to training, there is no clear consensus concerning what primary care providers should know about depression or how this information should be taught. The content and level of specificity among primary care specialties (family practice, internal medicine, pediatrics, and obstetrics/gynecology) with regard to training certification and accreditation requirements is also highly variable. Also, while various program models for mental health training of primary care physicians have been identified and implemented (Cole and others, 2000; Pincus, Strain, Houpt, and Gise, 1983), there remains significant variation across different primary care specialties in the content of these training programs, the focus on specific diagnostic and treatment issues at various levels of complexity, and the degree to which the curriculum is structured (for example, whether the structure is formal and specified versus informal and case based). In addition, physicians obtain considerable information on new medications from pharmaceutical company promotional activities and their representatives (Bero, Galbraith, and Rennie, 1992; Orlowski and Wateska, 1992), and this information may not be optimally balanced.

Practice Barriers

There is wide variation in how primary care practices are organized to care for people with behavioral health problems and how clinical practices are linked to mental health specialty care (Figure 13.3). These arrangements can theoretically range from a fully integrated team approach (*A* in the figure) in which there is frequent communication

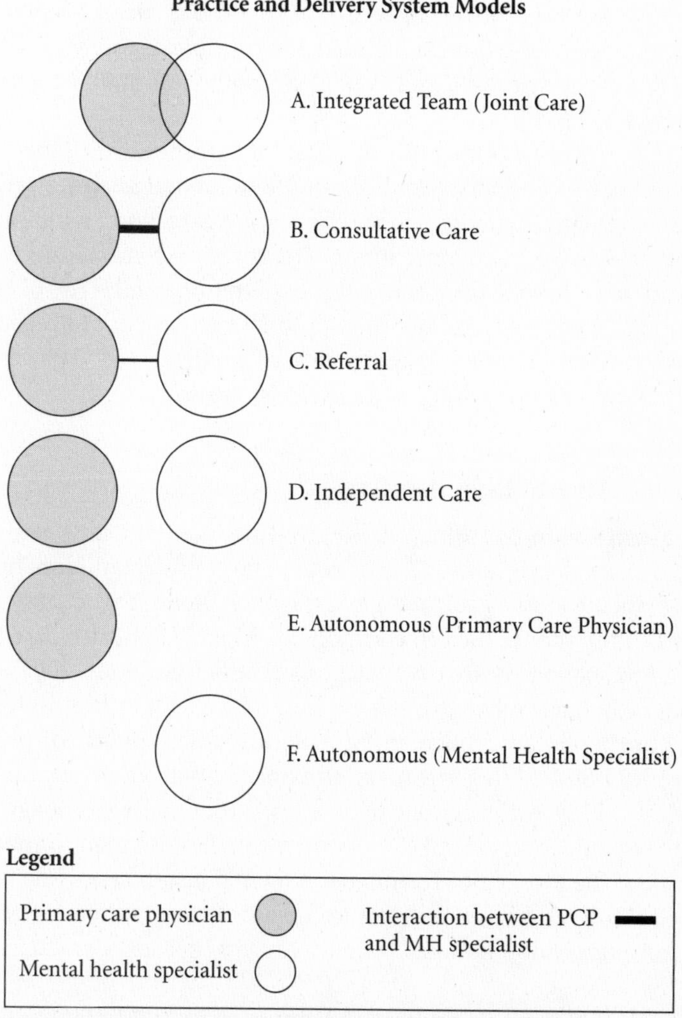

Figure 13.3. Practice and Delivery System Models
Source: Pincus (1987).

between the primary care physician and mental health specialist to a totally autonomous approach of primary care providers (*E*) or mental health specialists (*F*). In the real world, however, there is often ambiguity about who is responsible for care, primary care or mental health practice, and limited communication and teamwork between primary care and mental health practices, with a tendency for typical practice arrangements to be like those toward the lower half of Figure 13.3 (Pincus, 1987; Tanielian and others, 2000). Moreover, these practice arrangements are mostly focused on acute assessment, management, and referral. Chronic or recurrent conditions such as depression and panic disorder require a planned, longitudinal framework (Bickman, Lambert, Andrade, and Penaloza, 2000; Goldman, Morrissey, and Ridgely, 1994).

Ambiguity of responsibility and lack of communication between specialists and generalists are not unique to mental health. Furthermore, systematic structures for orchestrating care along a longitudinal perspective of a chronic illness are as rare for such illnesses as depression as they are for asthma. It is hard to find regular use of components of a chronic care treatment model such as patient registries and chronic care managers, application of sophisticated yet available information system technology, and decision support.

Health Plan Barriers

Infrequent use of coordinated, longitudinal mental health and primary care models is not surprising when one considers modern health care financing and organization in the United States, particularly with regard to the mental health component. Most U.S. health care is financed by managed care organizations (Dudley and Luft, 2001), and managed behavioral health has evolved into a $4.4 billion industry, with approximately 78 percent of Americans with public or private insurance enrolled in some form of managed behavioral health care (Findlay, 1999). Although it can be argued that managed behavioral health organizations (MBHOs) were originally intended to manage the risk of the most resource-intensive mental health cases, one unintended result has been a shift in incentive structures for coordination and communication between primary care and specialty practices and providers.

For example, in the idealized indemnity model (*A* in Figure 13.4), both sets of providers generally have established professional rela-

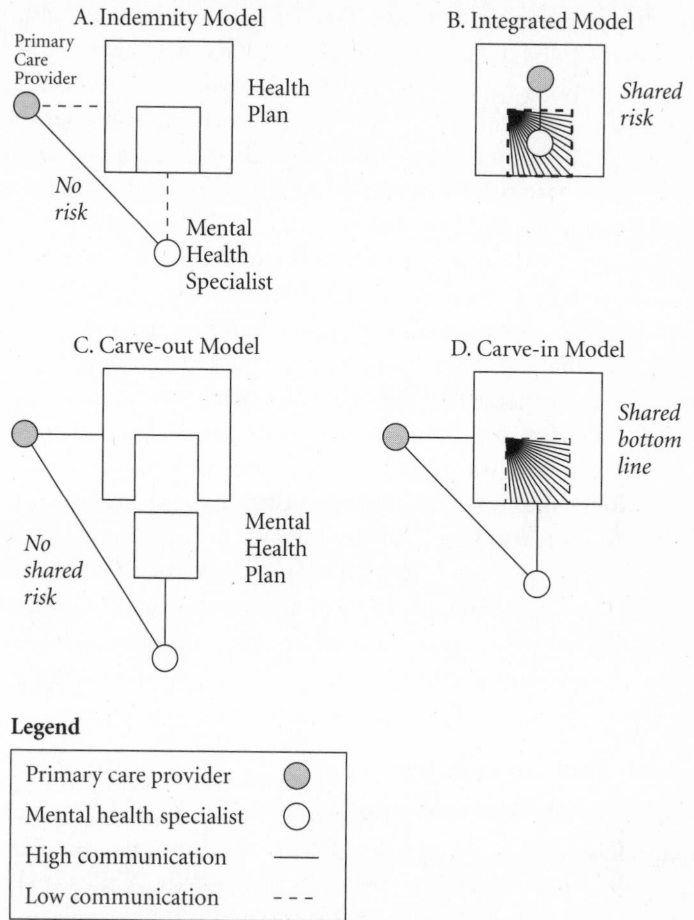

Figure 13.4. Health Plan Structure, Risk, and Communication

tionships with each other and have little connection to the financing system, and there is no intrinsic contractual or financial relationship between providers, except that both can benefit from mutual referral. The integrated managed care system model (*B* in the figure), predominantly in staff model HMOs, is able to establish collaborative relationships among providers and can generally link clinical information. Financial incentives for coordination and communication between primary and specialty care are more likely to be shared across medical and surgical, behavioral, and pharmacy costs.

When behavioral health is carved out (*D* in Figure 13.4) and also, generally, when carved in (*C* in Figure 13.4), the primary care and behavioral health networks are entirely separate. To make a referral to a mental health specialist, a primary care physician may be able to offer the patient only a toll-free telephone number to the MBHO triage center in another state. Particularly in carve-out structures, collaboration and communication are not only limited but also discouraged with financial and structural disincentives. The primary care sector has a financial incentive to shift responsibility for direct care to the MBHO. The MBHO typically does not share in any rewards or risks for more efficient management and reduced costs associated with more appropriate pharmacy or medical or surgical utilization.

Approaches for improving primary care for depression and anxiety disorders in both integrated and network managed care plans have been developed and tested (Katon and others, 1997; Meredith and others, 1999; Simon, Von Korff, Rutter, and Wagner, 2000), but these collaborative arrangements are unlikely to remain in place after a demonstration is concluded. The Robert Wood Johnson Foundation national program, Depression in Primary Care, is intended to develop strategies to realign these incentives.

Purchaser Barriers

Ultimately, public purchasers such as Medicare or Medicaid and private purchasers such as employers wield enormous, though often indirect, power in the design of the health care system. While purchasing decisions are amenable to systematic and quantitative analysis, there is little evidence that such analysis takes place. Furthermore, despite the publication of data on the increasing value of mental health care (Frank, McGuire, Normand, and Goldman, 1999; Kessler and others, 1999; Wells and others, 1999), a persisting general view that such costs are continually rising also has a negative influence on purchaser decisions (Frank, McGuire, Normand, and Goldman, 1999). Purchasers may also be uninformed about the substantial indirect costs of mental illness such as depression due to absenteeism and disability.

While substantial efforts have been made to expand purchaser capacity to monitor the performance of health plans in nonfinancial areas such as quality, implementation has been variable. For example, the National Committee for Quality Assurance (NCQA) has developed accreditation standards for MBHOs that include elements for coordinating with primary care, as well as behavioral health and consumer satisfaction reporting elements (as in the Health Plan Employer Data Information Set). Unfortunately, accreditation elements are fairly nonspecific and easily met and may not capture crucial elements of the evidence-based chronic care model. Moreover, there is little evidence that purchasers have moved aggressively to incorporate mental health quality measures in their purchasing decisions (Findlay, 1999).

THE FUTURE

Trends and Assumptions

These barriers are quite formidable, and it is unlikely that they will crumble in the near future. Nonetheless, important current trends with regard to the health care system and its evidence base portend immense changes in the relationship between primary care and mental and behavioral health. These trends (and their associated assumptions) are likely to result in several changes:

- *More effective and targeted medications with fewer side effects and risks.* The development of selective serotonin reuptake inhibitors has already revolutionized the treatment of depression in primary care (Pincus and others, 1998). Since the door has already been opened quite widely in getting PCPs to feel comfortable in prescribing pharmacological agents, future drug development may be less revolutionary in shifting PCP practice. However, the clear trend is toward developing more compounds tied to more specific indications that are so safe and easy to dose that the threshold for PCP prescribing will be quite low.
- *More targeted, effective, and efficient psychosocial and behavioral treatments for specific mental illnesses and substance use disorders and for prevention and treatment of general medical conditions.* Parallel to the development of medications, new psychosocial technologies will be developed, refined, and formally tested. Far different from our current conceptions (even now outmoded) of psychotherapy as forty-five- to fifty-minute face-to-face weekly or more frequent sessions, these approaches will be targeted to specific clinical and practical needs. They will be time limited from one session to twelve, of variable length (from five minutes to ninety minutes), administered face-to-face, through

broadband video, the Internet, or DVD in the PCP's or behavioral health specialist's office or in the patient's home or work environment. More important, these technologies will be packaged for specific target situations (for example, panic disorder with or without agoraphobia, marital discord, and nonadherent adolescent diabetes).

- *Diagnostic categorization schemes with more relevance for primary care.* There is a significant disconnect between the mental health specialty diagnostic system (DSM-IV) and the needs of primary care providers. Moreover, the existing instruments and screening tools have largely not been geared toward primary care practice. Primary care-oriented screening and assessment tools such as the PRIME-MD (Spitzer and others, 1994) have been important steps toward linking the two perspectives, but they remain somewhat cumbersome and tied to specialist concepts. New conceptual approaches will be needed to better bridge psychiatry, primary care, and other behavioral sciences such as psychology, especially with regard to classifying and studying the psychological problems that PCPs identify but do not fit into the DSM/IMD framework (box 4 in Figure 13.2). Ultimately, better and more relevant diagnostic systems and tools will enhance the identification of problems and the targeting of specific management strategies.

- *Clinical information systems that enable effective tracking and provide decision support.* The electronic medical record is fast approaching, but there remain significant potential technical and financial impediments to its widespread implementation. While it is assumed that the field will find effective ways to maintain needed record keeping and communication in the face of the Health Insurance Portability and Accountability Act of 1996 and its children, maintaining an effective bridge between general medical and mental health and substance abuse information will remain complex and controversial. Although lessened stigma and broader acceptance of understanding of mental health issues will help, society and the field are likely to expect a different standard with regard to privacy, confidentiality, and sharing of behavioral health records. With greater PCP involvement in mental health and broader presence of behavioral health specialists in primary care, mechanisms will need to be established that balance these concerns.

- *Integrated financing and practice arrangements for primary care and behavioral health.* This may be the most problematic assumption, since it envisions the elimination (or drastic reinvention) of carve-out arrangements, which thus far have been quite attractive to purchasers. It would also require full parity for mental health and substance-related conditions, another assumption with significant political hurdles. An alternative scenario might be an even more isolated (perhaps even autistic) behavioral health system that operates separately from primary care much as the criminal justice or educational systems do now. I view this scenario as less likely for several reasons: more resources for behavioral health are likely to be available under the health care umbrella than as a totally independent system (and acceptance of that strategy as parity is moving forward); PCPs will demand a closer connection because their needs are increasingly not being met; purchasers will see more value of such integration; patients will increasingly demand behavioral health services (including complementary or alternative medicine); and the low-hanging fruit of cost savings from carve-outs has already been harvested.

Population-Specific Scenarios

A somewhat simplistic and outmoded notion of the potential pathway of primary care involvement in behavioral health and psychosocial care has PCPs' screening and either treating or referring individuals with specific mental disorders. A more variegated list of functions is presented in the vertical axis of Table 13.2, which demonstrates the broad potential roles and capacities of primary care. Implicit in this broader notion of primary care involvement is an expanding role of behavioral health specialists located in primary care settings, as also displayed in Figure 13.5, providing a picture of the relative roles of PCPs and behavioral health specialists for different subgroups.

Table 13.2 is a matrix providing a sample description of the underlying assumptions regarding relevant roles of primary care providers and behavioral specialists (psychiatrists and nonpsychiatrists) for particular conditions. With respect to each condition, the roles and functions are arrayed, and the specific provider and location (both in primary care and specialty settings) are listed in each cell. This type of analysis forms the basis for pictorial descriptions in Figures 13.5 and 13.6. Figure 13.6 depicts the overall framework for care delivery in which specific populations (circles *A* to *E*) are linked to particular service providers and settings (as depicted by various levels of shading):

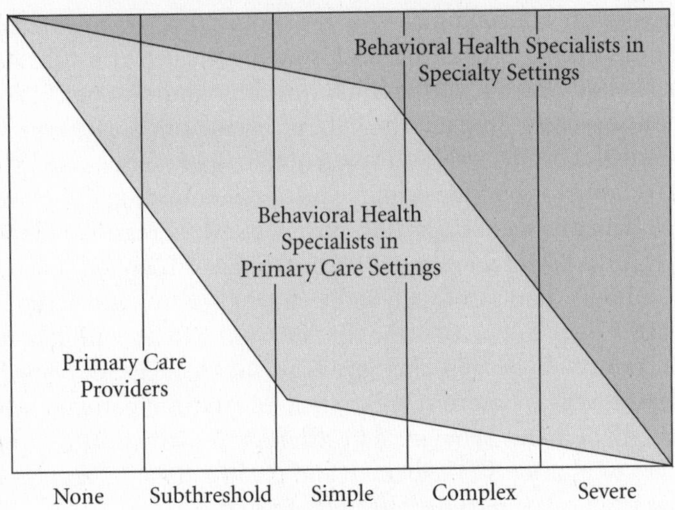

Figure 13.5. Relative Degree of Involvement of Primary Care Providers and Behavioral Health Specialists

- Care for individuals with severe to complex mental illnesses or substance use disorders (circle *A* in Figure 13.6).

Most of the time, we think of primary care and mental health integration from the perspective of integrating behavioral health care into primary care; however, there is a compelling need to consider a reversed perspective. Individuals with severe mental and addictive disorders (schizophrenia, substance dependence, bipolar disorder, and more debilitating forms of chronic anxiety, depressive, and personality disorders) are known to have higher mortality rates than the general population. Although some of the excess mortality is due to direct mental health outcomes (suicide), a substantial proportion is due to general medical conditions, such as cardiovascular, infectious disease, or respiratory problems. These individuals are also likely to have less access to care due to the barriers described above. It has also been well documented that the general medical conditions are often unrecognized and inadequately treated in this population. For many of these individuals, especially those treated in the public sector, community mental health centers, addiction treatment programs, and other specialty clinics are likely to be the principal or only points of contact with the health care system (Druss, Rohrbaugh, Levinson, and Rosen-

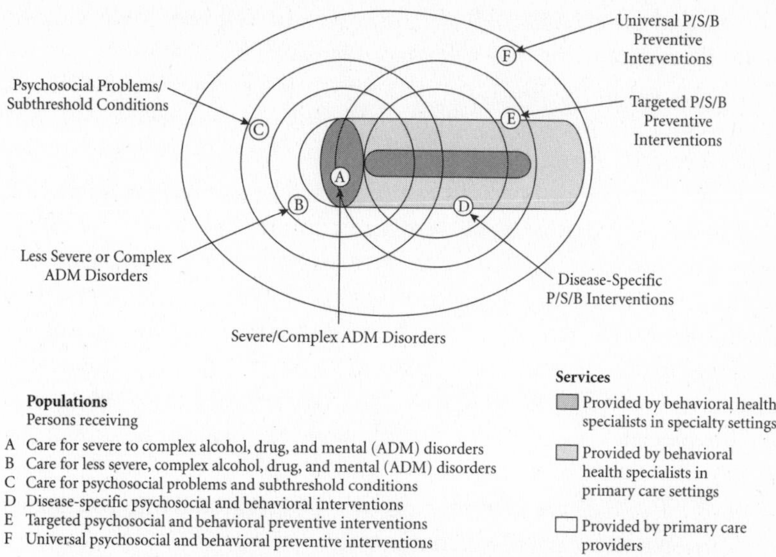

Figure 13.6. Overall Framework of Mental Health Care Delivery

Note: P/S/B: Psychosocial and behavioral interventions.

heck, 2001). Although there have been exhortations over the past several decades for psychiatrists to take on responsibility for the primary care of individuals with severe mental disorders, primary activities are a tiny portion of psychiatrists' focus.

Thus, to improve primary care for these individuals, it will be necessary to go where they go (the specialty mental health system) and bring in primary care providers rather than rely on psychiatrists and other mental health specialists. Such an approach would also allow for better integration across other levels of specialty behavioral care, which these patients often require, and other systems (for example, vocational, welfare, criminal justice), since these connections are better established on the mental health side than primary care. Although the barriers to integrating primary care into specialty behavioral health settings treating these populations are formidable, on-site, integrated models providing primary care and case management that incorporate preventive care, patient education, and close collaboration with mental health professionals have been tested and found effective. Using a nurse practitioner and a part-time family practitioner, one randomized controlled study documented significant improvement in the quality and outcomes of care without any increase in costs

(Bover and others, 2000). It will, however, be essential to develop financing mechanisms that will encourage such integration.

• Care for individuals with less severe or complex alcohol, drug, and mental disorders or psychosocial problems or subthreshold conditions (circles *B* and *C* in Figure 13.6).

I am referring not only to the common presentations of mental and behavioral disorders currently in primary care, that is, individuals with undifferentiated depressive and anxiety disorders, as well as those with varieties of psychosocial problems including problem drinking and tobacco use. I also believe that there will be an important role for the primary care sector in some of the more complicated and severe conditions that are currently treated in the behavioral health specialty sector. Thus, the following are likely to be present:

- Longitudinal care management will be integrated into primary care in a strategic, planned manner.
- PCPs and care managers will have enhanced skills in psychopharmacological and psychosocial intervention techniques.
- Behavioral health specialists will be on site for more complex treatments (both psychosocial and pharmacological).
- Psychiatrists will be more accessible, primarily for informal and formal (primarily—but not exclusively—psychopharmacological) consultation.

As Table 13.2 indicates, for both sets of conditions, PCPs will continue to have responsibility for the primary general medical care, but they would also be expected to have in place a systematic capacity for limited assessment of psychosocial problems and strengths and conduct screening for both lesser and more severe disorders. In addition, for all psychiatric conditions initially detected or encountered in primary care settings, the PCP would be expected to maintain an ongoing monitoring capacity, determining whether the patient is still taking prescribed medication, and following through with any referral. The PCP would also maintain ongoing communication links, even using an electronic medical record, with any behavioral specialist involved.

In most cases, for lower-severity or uncomplicated conditions, such as initial treatment of major depression or early nonadherence to hypertension regimens, the PCP would have responsibility for a more extensive assessment and initial treatment (both medications and limited psychosocial interventions such as psychoeducation).

Perhaps most important, for a large proportion of cases that are currently treated in the behavioral health specialty area (more complex cases of depressive and anxiety disorders, substance-related problems and abuse), behavioral health specialists located in primary care settings will be the mainstay of care. There are many advantages to such arrangements. The dropoff from referral to a separate, more distant (and stigmatized) consultant will be reduced. Communication will be enhanced between primary care and behavioral health with regard to individual patients and, more important, on a general level. Propinquity will allow easy, informal consultation and an ongoing educational presence that will raise PCPs' skills in and awareness of these issues. Also, the presence of behavioral health specialists establishes a more effective behavioral health quality improvement capacity in the practice. Furthermore, the new short-term, more targeted psychosocial interventions are well suited for primary care environments. In any case, the behavioral health specialists will be there anyway because they will be providing care for individuals needing some form of psychosocial and behavioral intervention (circles *D, E,* and *F* in Figure 13.6).

New behavioral technologies will be developed and be applicable to populations well beyond those traditionally considered to have mental disorders. Specific interventions to promote healthy habits and prevent illness (both physical and mental) will be widely available and applied universally (circle *F*), as well as to targeted populations profiled to be at higher risk for specific conditions (circle *E*). While many of the universal interventions will be applied by community organizations or broad population initiatives such as advertising or the Internet, primary care settings will be an important site, especially for targeted interventions.

The standard of care for virtually all chronic medical conditions (both "physical" and "mental") will include the application of disease-specific psychosocial behavioral interventions, ranging from psychoeducation to adherence enhancement to specific cognitive rehabilitation techniques that alter the course of the disease. Primary care settings, with responsibility for the bulk of longitudinal chronic illness care, will also have the responsibility for implementing these interventions and maintaining the necessary staff and expertise to do so. Thus, disease-specific psychosocial behavioral interventions will be routinely incorporated in chronic disease management systems within primary care by primary care providers, care managers, and in many cases for more complex or technical interventions, by behavioral health specialists in primary care settings. The training and personnel implications for primary care are profound.

RISKS, DANGERS, AND CAVEATS

Prognostication has uncertainties and risks, and the assumptions and picture of the future presented could have untoward outcomes—for example:

- Segregation of individuals with severe to complex alcohol, drug, and mental disorders. To the extent that these conditions are seen as separate from the rest of medicine, with different organizational and financing arrangements, as we have seen for centuries, mental disorders are likely to be increasingly stigmatized and underfunded. Moreover, while access to quality primary care may increase, more specialized medical or surgical services may become less accessible. This would be especially damaging if the future role of primary care is diminished relative to specialty care overall.
- Limited attention of PCPs to alcohol, drug, and mental disorders and psychosocial and behavioral problems. PCPs are overwhelmed by the exponentially rising set of expectations and responsibilities placed on them. The human capacity to attend to the myriad conditions and attendant protocols and guidelines is limited. Unless PCPs' accrediting and credentialing organizations recognize the importance of these conditions and place them at high priority, history again suggests they will be ignored. This means that mental health and behavioral care will need to be in the forefront of accreditation and credentialing requirements, the development of quality monitoring systems, electronic medical record, and decision support technologies. There will also be pressures for imperfect or partial integration of mental health and behavioral issues. The growth of newer medications along with the enormous power of industry marketing may result in hypertrophy of pharmacological approaches and a stunting of the behavioral components.
- Failure of financing mechanisms to facilitate integrated care. Ultimately, dollars drive the health care system. The historic separation, organizationally and financially, of primary care and behavioral health creates enormous financial barriers and disincentives for effective coordinated care. Overall, the level of health care resources devoted to behavioral health (with the exception of pharmacy costs) has signifi-

cantly dropped over the past decade. Thus, not only will there need to be clever approaches developed to realign these incentives, but there will need to be an enhancement of resources targeted toward behavioral conditions, especially substance abuse.

• A return to a narrow definition of medicine, health, and health care. It may be that the challenges presented are too overwhelming and the scope of health care envisioned too broad. Conceivably, given the conceptual, financial, and practical complexities, as well as the costs and scope, society (and medicine) may choose to conform to the pressures of stigma and historical antecedents and narrow the scope of health care to treatment of physical diseases. Such a reaction, while unlikely, would be extremely unfortunate.

CONCLUSION

The definitions and issues pertaining to the subject of this chapter are quite complex. Enhanced, comprehensive primary care for individuals that incorporates attention to alcohol, drug, and mental disorders, psychosocial problems, and behavioral interventions will require overcoming an array of barriers at multiple levels. Nonetheless, the future is likely to see better integration of primary care providers into specialty mental health and of behavioral health into primary care. A major strategy will be the incorporation of behavioral health specialists within primary care settings. Although there are potential risks in such a future scenario, the quality of care and health outcomes for individuals should improve substantially. Of course, all of this is dependent on ensuring adequate access to and financing of health care (primary, specialty, and mental health) for all Americans.

References

Adams, W. L., Barry, K., and Fleming, M. "Screening for Problem Drinking in Older Primary Care Patients." *Journal of the American Medical Association,* 1996, *276*(24), 1964–1967.

Agency for Health Care Policy and Research Depression Guideline Panel. *Clinical Practice Guideline 5. Depression in Primary Care: Treatment of Major Depression.* Rockville, Md.: U.S. Department of Health and Human Services, 1993.

American Psychiatric Association. *Diagnostic and Statistical Manual of Mental Disorders.* (4th ed.) Washington, D.C.: American Psychiatric Association Press, 1994.

American Psychiatric Association. *Diagnostic and Statistical Manual of Mental Disorders.* (4th ed., text revision) Washington, D.C.: American Psychiatric Association, 2000.

Archer, L., and Grant, B. "What Happens If Americans Drank Less: The Potential Effect on the Prevalence of Alcohol Abuse and Dependence." *American Journal of Public Health,* 1995, *85*(1), 61–66.

Baum, A., Revenson, T., and Singer, J. (eds.). *Handbook of Health Psychology.* Mahwah, N.J.: Erlbaum, 2001.

Bero, L., Galbraith, A., and Rennie, D. "The Publication of Sponsored Symposiums in Medical Journals." *New England Journal of Medicine,* 1992, *327*(16), 1135–1140.

Bickman, L. E., Lambert, W., Andrade, A. R., and Penaloza, R. V. "The Fort Bragg Continuum of Care for Children and Adolescents: Mental Health Outcomes over Five Years." *Journal of Consulting and Clinical Psychology,* 2000, *68*(4), 710–716.

Bover, P., and others. "Randomised Controlled Trial of Non-Directive Counselling, Cognitive-Behaviour Therapy, and Usual General Practitioner Care for Patients with Depression. II: Cost Effectiveness." *British Medical Journal,* 2000, *321,* 1389–1392.

Center for Alcohol and Substance Abuse. *Missed Opportunity: National Survey of Primary Care Physicians and Patients on Substance Abuse.* Chicago: Survey Research Laboratory, University of Illinois at Chicago, 2000.

Cole, S., and others. "The MacArthur Foundation Depression Education Program for Primary Care Physicians: Background Participant's Workbook, and Facilitator's Guide." *General Hospital Psychiatry,* 2000, *22*(5), 299–358.

Coyne, J. C., Fechner-Bates, S., and Schwenk, T. L. "Prevalence, Nature, and Comorbidity of Depressive Disorders in Primary Care." *General Hospital Psychiatry,* 1994, *16*(4), 267–276.

deGruy, F. "Mental Health Care in the Primary Care Setting." In M. S. Donaldson, K. D. Yordy, K. N. Lohr, and N. A. Vanselow (eds.), *Primary Care: America's Health in a New Era.* Washington, D.C.: National Academy Press, 1996.

deGruy, F., and Pincus, H. A. "The DSM-IV-PC: A Manual for Diagnosing Mental Disorders in the Primary Care Setting." *Journal of the American Board of Family Practice,* 1996, *9*(4), 274–281.

Druss, B. G., Rohrbaugh, R. M., Levinson, C. M., and Rosenheck, R. A. "Integrated Medical Care for Patients with Serious Psychiatric Illness." *Archives of General Psychiatry,* 2001, *58,* 861–868.

Dudley, R. A., and Luft, H. "Health Policy 2001: Managed Care in Transition." *New England Journal of Medicine,* 2001, *344*(14), 1087–1091.

Engel, G. "The Need for a New Medical Model: A Challenge for Biomedicine." *Science,* 1977, *196*(4286), 129–136.

Findlay, S. "Managed Behavioral Health Care in 1999: An Industry at a Crossroads." *Health Affairs,* 1999, *18*(5), 116–124.

Fleming, M., Cotter, F., and Talboy, E. *Training Physicians in Techniques for Alcohol Screening and Brief Intervention.* Washington, D.C.: U.S. Department of Health and Human Services, Public Health Service, National Institutes of Health, and the National Institute on Alcohol Abuse and Alcoholism, 1997.

Fleming, M., Manwell, L., Barry, K., and Johnston, K. "At Risk Drinking in an HMO Primary Care Sample: Prevalence and Health Policy Implications." *American Journal of Public Health,* 1998, *88*(1), 90–93.

Frank, R. G., McGuire, T. G., Normand, S.-L., and Goldman, H. H. "The Value of Mental Health Care at the System Level: The Case of Treating Depression." *Health Affairs,* 1999, *18*(5), 71–88.

Goldberg, D., and Huxley, P. *Mental Illness in the Community.* London: Tavistock, 1980.

Goldman, H. H., Morrissey, J. P., and Ridgely, M. "Evaluating the Robert Wood Johnson Foundation Program on Chronic Mental Illness." *Milbank Quarterly,* 1994, *72*(1), 39–47.

Goldman, H. H., Rye, P., and Sirovatka, P. *A Report of the Surgeon General.* Washington, D.C.: Department of Health and Human Services, 2000.

Greenberg, P. E., Finkelstein, S. N., and Berndt, E. R. "Calculating the Workplace Cost of Chronic Disease." *Business and Health,* 1995, *13*(9), 27–28.

Harwood, H., Fountain, D., and Fountain, G. "Economic Cost of Alcohol and Drug Abuse in the United States, 1992: A Report." *Addiction,* 1999, *94*(5), 631–635.

Hirschfeld, R., and others. "The National Depressive and Manic-Depressive Association Consensus Statement on the Undertreatment of Depression." *Journal of the American Medical Association,* 1997, *277*(4), 333–340.

Institute of Medicine. *Broadening of the Base of Treatment for Alcohol Problems: Report of a Study by a Committee of the Institute of Medicine, Division of Mental Health and Behavioral Medicine.* Washington, D.C.: National Academy Press, 1990.

Johnson, J., Weissman, M. M., and Klerman, G. L. "Service Utilization and

Social Morbidity Associated with Depressive Symptoms in the Community." *Journal of the American Medical Association,* 1992, *267*(11), 1478–1483.

Kamerow, D. B., Pincus, H. A., and Macdonald, D. I. "Alcohol Abuse, Other Drug Abuse, and Mental Disorders in Medical Practice: Prevalence, Costs, Recognition and Treatment." *Journal of the American Medical Association,* 1986, *255*(15), 2054–2057.

Katon, W. J., and others. "Distressed High Utilizers of Medical Care." *General Hospital Psychiatry,* 1990, *12*(6), 355–362.

Katon, W. J., and others. "Collaborative Management to Achieve Treatment Guidelines: Impact on Depression in Primary Care." *Journal of the American Medical Association,* 1995, *273*(13), 1026–1031.

Katon, W. J., and others. "A Multifaceted Intervention to Improve Treatment of Depression in Primary Care." *Archives of General Psychiatry,* 1996, *53,* 924–932.

Katon, W. J., and others. "Collaborative Management to Achieve Depression Treatment Guidelines." *Journal of Clinical Psychiatry,* 1997, *58*(suppl.), 20–23.

Katon, W. J., and others. "Stepped Collaborative Care for Primary Care Patients with Persistent Symptoms of Depression." *Archives of General Psychiatry,* 1999, *56,* 1109–1115.

Katz, S. J., Kessler, R. C., Lin, E., and Wells, K. B. "Appropriate Medication Management of Depression in the United States and Ontario." *Journal of General Internal Medicine,* 1998, *13*(2), 77–85.

Kessler, R. C., and others. "Lifetime and Twelve-Month Prevalence of DSM-III-R Psychiatric Disorders in the United States." *Archives of General Psychiatry,* 1994, *51*(1), 8–19.

Kessler, R. C., and others. "Depression in the Workplace: Effects on Short-Term Disability." *Health Affairs,* 1999, *18*(5), 163–171.

Koran, L., and others. "Medical Evaluation of Psychiatric Patients, I: Results in a State Mental Health System." *Archives of General Psychiatry,* 1989, *46,* 733–740.

Krupnick, J. L., and Pincus, H. A. "The Cost-Effectiveness of Psychotherapy: A Plan for Research." *American Journal of Psychiatry,* 1992, *149*(10), 1295–1305.

Lin, E. H., and others. "The Role of the Primary Care Physician in Patients' Adherence to Antidepressant Therapy." *Medical Care,* 1995, *33*(1), 67–74.

Manning, W. G., and others. "The Taxes of Sin: Do Smokers and Drinkers Pay Their Way?" *Journal of the American Medical Association,* 1989, *261*(11), 1604–1609.

Manwell, L., Fleming, M., Johnson, K., and Barry, K. "Tobacco, Alcohol and Drug Use in a Primary Care Sample: Ninety-Day Prevalence and Associated Factors." *Journal of Addictive Diseases,* 1998, *17*(1), 67–81.

McGinnis, J., and Foege, W. H. "Actual Causes of Death in the United States." *Journal of the American Medical Association,* 1993, *270,* 2207–2212.

Meredith, L., and others. "Treating Depression in Staff-Model Versus Network-Model Managed Care Organizations." *Journal of General Internal Medicine,* 1999, *14*(1), 39–48.

Murray, C.J.L., and Lopez, A. D. (eds.). *The Global Burden of Disease.* Cambridge, Mass.: Harvard School of Public Health, 1996.

National Depressive and Manic-Depressive Association. *Beyond Diagnosis: A Landmark Survey of Patients, Partners, and Health Professionals on Depression and Treatment.* Chicago: National Depressive and Manic-Depressive Association, 2000.

National Institute on Alcohol Abuse and Alcoholism. *A Physicians' Guide to Helping Patients with Alcohol Problems.* Washington, D.C.: National Institute on Alcohol Abuse and Alcoholism, 1995.

Orlowski, J., and Wateska, L. "The Effects of Pharmaceutical Firm Enticements on Physician Prescribing Patterns: There's No Such Thing as a Free Lunch." *Chest,* 1992, *102*(1), 270–275.

Pincus, H. A. "Patient-Oriented Models for Linking Primary Care and Mental Health Care." *General Hospital Psychiatry,* 1987, *9*(2), 95–101.

Pincus, H. A. "The Future of Behavioral Health and Primary Care: Drowning in the Mainstream or Left on the Banks?" *Psychosomatics,* 2003, *44,* 1–11.

Pincus, H. A., Davis, W. W., and McQueen, L. E. "'Subthreshold' Mental Disorders: A Review and Synthesis of Studies on Minor Depression and Other 'Brand Names.'" *British Journal of Psychiatry,* 1999, *174,* 288–296.

Pincus, H. A., Pechura, C. M., Elinson, L., and Pettit, A. R. "Depression in Primary Care: Linking Clinical and System Strategies." *General Hospital Psychiatry,* 2001, *23,* 311–318. © 2001 Elsevier Inc. Used by permission.

Pincus, H. A., Strain, J. J., Houpt, J. L., and Gise, L. "Models of Mental Health Training in Primary Care." *Journal of the American Medical Association,* 1983, *249*(22), 3065–3068.

Pincus, H. A., and others. "Prescribing Trends in Psychotropic Medications: Primary Care, Psychiatry, and Other Medical Specialties." *Journal of the American Medical Association,* 1998, *279*(7), 526–531.

Regier, D., and others. "The De Facto US Mental and Addictive Disorders Service System." *Archives of General Psychiatry,* 1993, *50*(2), 85–94.

Rice, D., Kelman, S., and Miller, L. "Estimates of Economic Costs of Alcohol and Drug Abuse and Mental Illness, 1985 and 1988." *Public Health Reports,* 1991, *106,* 280–292.

Rice, D., and Miller, L. "Health Economics and Cost Implications of Anxiety and Other Mental Disorders in the United States." *British Journal of Psychiatry,* 1998, *34*(suppl.), 4–9.

Saitz, R., Mulvey, K., and Plough, A. "Physician Unawareness of Serious Substance Abuse." *American Journal of Drug and Alcohol Abuse,* 1997, *23*(2), 343–354.

Schulberg, H. C., Katon, W. J., Simon, G. E., and Rush, A. "Treating Major Depression in Primary Care Practice: An Update of the Agency for Health Care Policy and Research Practice Guidelines." *Archives of General Psychiatry,* 1998, *55*(12), 1121–1127.

Schwabb, J. "Consultation-Liaison Psychiatry: A Historical Overview." *Psychosomatics,* 1989, *30,* 245–254.

Simon, G. E., Ormel, J., Von Korff, M., and Barlow, W. "Health Care Costs Associated with Depressive and Anxiety Disorders in Primary Care." *American Journal of Psychiatry,* 1995, *152*(3), 352–357.

Simon, G. E., Von Korff, M., Rutter, C. M., and Wagner, E. "Randomised Trial of Monitoring, Feedback, and Management of Care by Telephone to Improve Treatment of Depression in Primary Care." *British Medical Journal,* 2000, *320,* 550–554.

Spitzer, R., and others. "Utility of a New Procedure for Diagnosing Mental Disorders in Primary Care: The PRIME-MD 1000 Study." *Journal of the American Medical Association,* 1994, *272*(22), 1749–1756.

Stange, K., and Jaen, C. "Illuminating the 'Black Box': A Description of 4454 Patient Visits to 138 Family Physicians." *Journal of Family Practice,* 1998, *46*(5), 377–389.

Substance Abuse and Mental Health Services Administration. *Naltrexone and Alcoholism Treatment, BKD268: Treatment Improvement Protocol.* Washington, D.C.: U.S. Department of Health and Human Services, 1998.

Tanielian, T., and others. "Referrals to Psychiatrists. Assessing the Communication Interface Between Psychiatry and Primary Care." *Psychosomatics,* 2000, *41*(3), 245–252.

Wagner, E. H., Austin, B. T., and Von Korff, M. "Organizing Care for Patients with Chronic Illness." *Milbank Quarterly,* 1996, *74*(4), 511–544.

Watkins, K., Pincus, H. A., and Tanielian, T. *Evidence Based Care Models for Recognizing and Treating Alcohol Problems in Primary Care Settings.* Pittsburgh, Pa.: RAND, 2001.

Wells, K. B. "Depression in General Medical Settings. Implications of Three Health Policy Studies for Consultation-Liaison Psychiatry." *Psychomatics,* 1994, *35*(3), 279–296.

Wells, K. "The Design of Partners in Care: Evaluating the Cost-Effectiveness of Improving Care for Depression in Primary Care." *Social Psychiatry and Psychiatric Epidemiology,* 1999, *34,* 20–29.

Wells, K. B., and others. "Quality of Care for Primary Care Patients with Depression in Managed Care." *Archives of Family Medicine,* 1999, *8*(6), 529–536.

Wells, K. B., and others. "Impact of Disseminating Quality Improvement Programs for Depression in Managed Primary Care." *Journal of the American Medical Association,* 2000, *283*(2), 212–220.

Williams, J. W., and others. "Primary Care Physicians' Approach to Depressive Disorders." *Archives of Family Medicine,* 1999, *8*(1), 58–67.

Williams, J. W., and others. "Treatment of Dysthymia and Minor Depression in Primary Care." *Journal of the American Medical Association,* 2000, *284*(12), 1519–1526.

Zung, W., Broadhead, W., and Roth, M. "Prevalence of Depressive Symptoms in Primary Care." *Journal of Family Practice,* 1993, *37*(4), 337–344.

CHAPTER FOURTEEN

Primary Care for Children and Adolescents

Michael Weitzman
Jonathan D. Klein
Tina L. Cheng

Eighty-five million people in the United States are below the age of twenty-one years—31 percent of the population. Children's health services are different from those used or needed by adults. In part, children's health care is different because children require health care professionals to have relationships with families and with community institutions, such as schools and day care, in addition to the relationship with the patient. These differences go beyond these advocacy and community roles to encompass and acknowledge developmental transitions—from birth through childhood, adolescence, and the transition to adult care. Primary care for children and youth is based on the fact that the majority of patients are basically healthy or have benign self-limited disease. Thus, the emphasis in primary care is on physical, psychological, and social health promotion and disease prevention. The system of primary care for children and youth, as for all other groups in the United States, is in the midst of profound change (Lewin, 1995; Nazarian, 1995).

The state of health of America's children is mixed. In 1998, the U.S. infant mortality rate was 7.2 deaths per 1,000 births. And although this was the lowest rate ever, this ranks only twenty-sixth among industrialized nations. Although immunization rates have improved, 22 percent of children were still missing immunizations in 1998. As many as 16 percent of children, or over 11 million children, do not have health insurance, and while the implementation of the State Children's Health Insurance Program has improved access to care for 2 million previously uninsured children and adolescents, tremendous variation in insurance and access remains. The majority of the mortality and morbidity of adolescents and young adults is preventable, yet many adolescents continue to suffer adverse consequences of injuries, violence, tobacco, alcohol and substance use, sexually transmitted diseases, and early, unintended pregnancy. Adolescents are among those least likely to have access to health care, and they have the lowest rate of primary care use of any age group in the United States (U.S. Congress, Office of Technology Assessment, 1991). Adolescents and young adults, especially those in poverty, are more likely to be uninsured than any other age group (Newacheck and McManus, 1988b; Children's Defense Fund, 1992; Carnegie Corporation, 1989; Brindis, 1993).

The major marketplace-driven change in health care in the late 1990s and early 2000s was focused on cost containment. Associated with this growth of managed care and managed costs was a shift from fee-for-service medicine to capitated and other arrangements and the development of large, integrated service delivery systems designed to meet the majority of medical service needs. For children and youth, this may have resulted in less freedom in the choice of primary care provider, less access to subspecialists, and fragmentation of some services, such as social services, mental health or substance abuse services, early intervention programs, or home visiting services (Weitzman, Doniger, and Partner, 1994; Weitzman, 1997). Recently, the cost control pendulum has begun to swing back toward greater concern about quality. Other significant forces reshaping health services for children include social and demographic changes, changes in government policy and support of child and family-related human services, changes in health insurance and entitlements, and scientific and technological advances.

In this chapter, we explore the basic mission of child and adolescent health services in the United States. As Haggerty (1995) stated, "The core . . . continue[s] to be providing technically competent, empathic care for children in families and communities . . . to help all children achieve their optimal function physically, mentally and socially" (p. 805). We examine the implications of current trends in health personnel and service availability for children and adolescents, utilization and quality-of-care issues, and the impact that emerging scientific and social trends may have on the care system for children and youth.

WHO PROVIDES CHILDREN'S HEALTH CARE?

The National Ambulatory Medical Care Survey data for 1997 shows that pediatricians provided 57 percent of all office-based visits for patients younger than eighteen years of age, and family or general practitioners provided 22 percent of all visits (American Academy of Family Physicians, 2001c). The proportion of all primary care office visits provided by pediatricians was 69 percent, up from 60 percent in 1979 (Ferris and others, 1998). Visits by type of physician vary by age. In 1997, pediatricians provided 81 percent of primary care visits for U.S. children from birth to two years and 62 percent for those aged three to seventeen years (Ferris and others, 1998). For those aged ten to nineteen years, the proportion of office visits provided by pediatricians was 24 percent. From 1980 to 1997, there was a doubling in the number of pediatricians and a 235 percent increase in family practitioners ("The Future of Pediatric Education II," 2000).

The percentage of U.S. medical school graduates entering pediatric residency positions increased from 10 percent of medical school seniors in 1992 to 13 percent in 2001 (Association of American Medical Colleges, 2001). In 2001, 1,755 graduates from U.S. medical schools matched to pediatric training programs, up from 1,315 in 1991. Approximately 97 percent of the 2,290 first-year pediatric residency positions available were filled through the National Resident Matching Program in 2001 (77 percent filled by U.S. graduates), the highest rate ever for pediatrics (American Academy of Family Physicians, 2001a).

In 1991, 66 percent of pediatricians were generalists, 15 percent were board-certified subspecialists, 11 percent were trained in a subspecialty but were not board certified, and 7 percent were trained in a subspecialty for which there is no formal board certification. Although the major professional activity of 95 percent of all pediatricians in 1997 was patient care in office- and hospital-based settings, 19 percent of general pediatricians were involved in subspecialty-related clinical activities, and 13 percent of those with subspecialty training exclusively practice general pediatrics (Brotherton, 1994).

In 2001, there were 71,716 general pediatricians and 13,047 pediatric subspecialists certified by the American Board of Pediatrics (2001). The relationship between and roles of primary care providers and subspecialists will likely evolve in the changing health care environment. There are few data comparing quality of care provided by primary care providers and subspecialists in pediatrics, and data in internal medicine are not conclusive ("The Future of Pediatric Education II," 2000). There has been a decline in interest in pediatric subspecialties due to multiple factors ("The Future of Pediatric Education II," 2000). It is likely that fewer pediatric trainees will enter subspecialties, primary care pediatricians will be asked to assume more responsibility for problems previously referred to subspecialists, and some pediatric subspecialists will increase their involvement in primary care. Each of these potential changes has implications for the quality of care for children. In some situations, efforts to contain costs may lead managed care programs to rely on nonpediatric subspecialists to meet the needs of children with subspecialty needs. No empirical data are available to monitor the effects of these changes on the quality of care children receive or their health status.

Family practitioners also provide primary health care for children and adolescents. There was a large increase in medical students entering family practice in the mid-1990s, followed by a steep decline (American Academy of Family Physicians, 2001b). Approximately 76 percent (49 percent U.S. graduates) of the 3,096 first-year family practice residency positions available were filled through the National Resident Matching Program in 2001, compared with 65 percent (56 percent U.S. graduates) of 2,467 positions in 1991 (American Academy of Family Physicians, 2001b).

Twenty-nine percent of all pediatricians are international medical graduates, compared with 22 percent of all physicians. Both the Third Report of the Pew Health Professions Commission and the Institute of Medicine's report, *The Nation's Physician Workforce: Options for Balancing Supply and Requirements* (Lohr, Vanselow, and Detmer, 1996), and key medical organizations ("The Future of Pediatric Education II," 2000) have recommended that the total number of first-year residency slots be reduced to reflect the current number of graduates of U.S. medical schools more closely. International medical graduates, however, disproportionately enter pediatrics and family practice and are an important part of the pediatric workforce. Moreover, a disproportionate number enter residency programs that provide ambulatory and inpatient services for the urban poor and uninsured and remain in these underserved communities as a source of pediatric care. Proposed decreases in international medical graduates allowed into U.S. training programs may further reduce access to health care for these children, with profound implications for different geographical areas (Health Resources and Services Administration, 2000).

There are approximately ten thousand pediatric nurse practitioners in the United States, the majority of whom are involved in the delivery of primary care services. More than 60 percent of the six thousand members of the National Association of Pediatric Nurse Associates and Practitioners work in urban areas with populations of more than 100,000, and many serve poor, underserved families (Dunn, 1993). Although some care settings were initially reluctant to use pediatric nurse practitioners or physician assistants to provide pediatric primary care services because of a concern that these practitioners would be perceived as providing inferior care (Stone, 1995), it has been shown that these providers can meet the majority of children's primary care needs (Brown and Grames, 1993; DeAngelis, 1994; Sox, 1979; U.S. Congress, Office of Technology Assessment, 1986).

Geographical maldistribution of child health clinicians continues to be a challenge. It is estimated that two-thirds of the twenty-nine hundred physician-shortage areas in the United States are in rural areas (North Carolina Rural Health Research Program, 1997). Despite legislative efforts to influence the distribution of health care providers, the "Future of Pediatric Education II" (2000) stated that in 1999 there were an estimated 7 million children in health professional shortage areas and that an additional two thousand to thirty-five hundred clinicians would be needed to care appropriately for these children (Health Resources Administration, 1980). Technological advances, through telemedicine support of practices in remote and underserved areas, offer some promise; however, continued support for primary care training and effective strategies to promote workforce distribution are still needed.

One significant change in the pediatric workforce is the trend toward an increasing number of women primary care clinicians. In 1997, 46 percent of practicing pediatricians and over 64 percent of first-year pediatric residents were women ("The Future of Pediatric Education II," 2000). In 1998, 43 percent of family practice residency graduates were women compared to 9 percent in 1978. The predominance of women affects workforce projections because women tend to work fewer hours than men. Women are also more likely to enter primary care practice (Fletcher and Fletcher, 1993; Warde, Allen, and Gelberg, 1996).

SYSTEMS OF CARE FOR CHILDREN AND YOUTH

One of the special issues for children's health is that of access to care for adolescents. We use adolescent health care in this section as an example of many of the unique characteristics of pediatric health care needs (Klein, Kotelchuck, and DeFriese, 1990). Access to care for adolescents encompasses the following issues (Klein and others 1992):

- Availability: Age-appropriate services and trained health care providers must be present.
- Visibility: Health services for adolescents must be recognizable and convenient and should not require complex planning by adolescents or their parents.
- Quality: A basic level of service must be provided to all youth, and adolescents should be satisfied with the care they receive.
- Confidentiality: Adolescents should be encouraged to involve their families in health decisions, but confidentiality must be assured.
- Affordability: Public and private insurance programs must provide adolescents with both preventive and other services designed to promote health behaviors and decrease morbidity and mortality.
- Flexibility: Services, providers, and delivery sites must consider the developmental, cultural, ethnic, and social diversity among adolescents.
- Coordination: Service providers must ensure that comprehensive services are available.

The developmental characteristics of adolescents make these issues critical for adolescents' health. Similarly, the preventable health problems of adolescents make the availability and visibility of specific preventive services—including family planning and reproductive health services, diagnosis and treatment of sexually transmitted disease and human immunodeficiency virus (HIV), mental health counseling and treatment, and substance abuse counseling and treatment—critically important for this age group. Services must be available in a wide range of health care settings, including community-based adolescent health, family planning and public health clinics, school-based and school-linked health clinics, physicians' offices, health maintenance organizations (HMOs), and hospitals. Without multiple entry points and a diversity of care resources, adolescents are less likely to connect with appropriate care resources.

Confidentiality, cost, and convenience are key determinants of adolescents' use of and satisfaction with care (Resnick, Blum, and Hedin, 1980; Klerman, Kovar, and Brown, 1981). Although most physicians support providing confidential care to adolescents, many are uncomfortable with negotiating independent care and decision making with families, and few routinely arrange alternative billing or other systems to ensure adolescents' confidentiality.

THE CONTENT OF CHILDREN'S HEALTH SERVICES

The American Academy of Pediatrics and the Maternal and Child Health Bureau recommend that children and youth receive, at a minimum, the following preventive health care (American Academy of Pediatrics, 2001):

- One prenatal visit
- Seven visits before one year of age (one immediately after birth, one within the first week of life, and at one, two, four, six, and nine months of age)
- Visits at twelve, fifteen, and eighteen months
- Yearly visits between two and six years of age
- Visits at eight and ten years of age
- Yearly visits between eleven and twenty-one years

These visits serve as the core events of children's preventive care visits in primary care, providing opportunities for health promotion and disease prevention activities—for example:

- Health guidance for behavioral, developmental, and social issues (for example, injury prevention, diet, exercise)
- Screening and counseling for biological and psychosocial problems, such as lead poisoning, anemia, tuberculosis, malnutrition (both under- and overnutrition), developmental delays, and vision and hearing problems; and for immunizations
- For adolescents, prevention based on the American Medical Association/Centers for Disease Control evidence- and consensus based-guidelines, the Guidelines for Adolescent Preventive Services (Klerman, Kovar, and Brown, 1981)
- Health guidance for parents about adolescent development and behaviors, parental monitoring, parents as role models, and signs of problems or concerns
- Annual health guidance (health promotion counseling) addressing injury reduction, healthy diet, physical activity and exercise, responsible sexual behavior, and avoidance of tobacco, alcohol, and other substances
- Targeted screening or counseling interventions for adolescents at risk for or with concerns about hypertension, hyperlipidemia, obesity, eating disorders, substance abuse, sexual orientation, pregnancy, sexually transmitted diseases, HIV, cervical cancer, school performance, depression, suicidality, abuse, and tuberculosis

It is during these visits that the basis for primary care—longitudinality, comprehensiveness, coordination, and continuity—and the relationship and therapeutic linkage between family and primary care provider are established (Starfield, 1985). Health supervision or preventive visits also allow for the development of linkages between families and other services and follow-up for chronic health conditions. It seems apparent that a specially trained professional workforce, with interest and competence in a wide range of health promotion and disease prevention activities, is needed to provide this array of services.

In 1990, children in prepaid care had four to five preventive health care visits per year compared to three per year for children in fee-for-service care (Smoller, 1992; Valdez and others 1989). Uninsured children made fewer visits than those who were insured (Holl and others, 1995). However, even children who receive health care often do not receive adequate preventive counseling, health promotion, or screening (Igra and Millstein, 1993; Brindis, 1993). Most physicians perform recommended preventive services at low rates (Igra and Millstein, 1993; Lewis, 1990; Russell and others, 1992).

If health insurance plans attempt to control costs by supporting preventive services, utilization of preventive services by children may increase. Yet some insurers question the content or frequency of currently recommended well-child visits and have tried to eliminate some of these visits and activities. The evidence base for pediatric and adolescent clinical guidelines, especially for counseling and anticipatory guidance, has been criticized (Berg, 1996; Elster and Kuznets, 1993). A few studies have demonstrated the effectiveness of screening and brief counseling interventions in adults, but fewer still have documented this in children and adolescents, except for immunizations and injury prevention counseling (Bass and others, 1993). However, the absence of evidence should not be construed as evidence of absence of efficacy (Perrin, Guyer, and Lawrence, 1992; Starfield, 1985). Many of the studies that have tried to assess the effectiveness of brief counseling interventions have not had sufficient power and did not document whether the clinical services were delivered (Gans, McManus, and Newacheck, 1991; Agency for Health Care Policy and Research, 1998). In addition, there remains substantial professional and consumer consensus about the importance of the primary care visits to patients (Agency for Health Care Policy and Research, 1998). Similarly, consumer and health insurance groups interested in the quality of care have begun to recognize the importance of effective pediatric preventive care services (Lansky, 1988).

The issue of how much can be accomplished in a fifteen-or thirty-minute visit cannot be ignored. Pediatricians are asked to provide anticipatory guidance or therapeutic interventions for a growing number of behavioral problems, school difficulties, risk-taking behaviors, and environmental threats. Trigger or screening questionnaires can streamline these clinical interactions, and coordination with other health promotion activities in school and communities is also necessary. Other strategies that have been proposed include expanded roles for nonphysician primary care providers, development and utilization of alternatives to primary care services, and greater coordination and use of family resource centers for health education and anticipatory guidance of parents and families, both individually and in groups.

QUALITY OF CHILDREN'S HEALTH CARE

Assessing and improving health care quality is a national priority. Access, immunization rates, and the rates at which children and adolescents have well-child visits are HEDIS (the Health Employee Data and Information Set) measures, used by the National Committee for Quality Assurance (NCQA) as indicators of quality for managed care organizations. But these measures provide no information about the provision of preventive counseling and screening.

In response to the limitations of current measures, the Child and Adolescent Health Measurement Initiative (CAHMI), a collaborative of more than fifty organizations, was established in 1998 by the Foundation for Accountability and NCQA to provide leadership and resources for measuring and communicating information about the quality of health care for children and adolescents. The CAHMI has developed three measurement sets for children: Early Childhood Development (Promoting Health Development) for children from birth to forty-eight months; Children with Chronic Conditions or Special Health Care Needs for children from birth to thirteen years old; and Adolescent Preventive Care (Young Adult Health Care Survey) for fourteen to eighteen year olds. These measures were developed with a wide array of stakeholders, including families, and are applicable to consumer information, quality improvement, public health monitoring, and policy needs. They have proven feasible, reliable, and valid, and they are working their way through the process of consideration as new HEDIS measures.

SPECIAL POPULATIONS

Children in Poverty

Substantial disparities persist in children's health and in their access to and use of health care services. Significant differences in the percentage of children who have a regular source of primary care and who are up-to-date in having their well-child needs met are linked to region, family income, insurance status, source of care, and child health status. Variations in provider, site of care, and number of ambulatory care visits are similarly linked (Holl and others, 1995; National Center for Health Statistics, 1993).

Increasing numbers of children and adolescents are in poverty or near poverty. In 1999, 17 percent of children under age eighteen, or 12.1 million U.S. children, were living in poverty compared to 16 percent of children, or 10.4 million in 1979 (U.S. Bureau of the Census, 2000a). In 1999, 14 percent, or 10.8 million children and adolescents in the United States, were uninsured (American Academy of Pediatrics, 2001), and 29 percent of those eighteen to twenty-four years old did not have insurance (U.S. Bureau of the Census, 2000b). Those without insurance are three times more likely than the privately insured to go without needed medical care (Newacheck and others, 2000).

Thirty-five percent of poor and 27 percent of near-poor children in the largest U.S. cities (those with populations over 1 million) rely on hospital-based clinics and community health centers for care (Weitzman, Byrd, and Auinger, 1996). Children using these sources of care are five times more likely to be at risk for physical, mental health, educational, or social problems than children who use private physicians (Weitzman, Byrd, and Auinger, 1996). Recently, there have been significant reductions in spending on public hospitals and clinics, and those associated with academic medical centers have been especially vulnerable. Changes that endanger hospital-based clinics or community health centers, on which poor, near-poor, and uninsured children disproportionately rely, may result in significant negative effects on the quality of care they receive and their health status.

Medicaid managed care programs have been growing. However, we do not know the impact of Medicaid managed care on the quality of primary care services for poor and near-poor children, both for those who continue to use hospital clinics and health centers and those who use private sources of care. On one hand, many who had used public sources of care may be able to access the private sector. On the other hand, the failure of managed care plans to adequately cover screening, counseling, referrals, case management, care coordination, social work, or mental health services could have detrimental effects on the most socially and economically disadvantaged children and families. Also of great importance is that as the child population becomes more diverse, a lack of culturally appropriate services limits the ability of some minorities to use existing health services, both within and outside managed care programs.

Children with Special Health Care Needs

Who should provide which aspects of care for children with special health care needs in the United States remains a profoundly important question. The number of children with chronic health conditions that limit their daily functional activities has nearly doubled in recent decades (Newacheck, Budetti, and McManus, 1984; Newacheck, Budetti, and Halfon, 1986). The National Health Interview Survey on Disability (1994–1995) identified 15 to 18 percent of children as having an ongoing developmental, physical, or mental chronic health condition affecting their functioning or requiring services to maintain a functional level (Newacheck and others, 1998).

How children with chronic health conditions and their families fare under managed care arrangements is likely to depend on many factors, including the effectiveness of advocacy efforts; the financial rates and carve-outs negotiated by managed care groups, primary care, and subspecialty providers, hospitals, and academic departments of pediatrics with third-party payers for the care of children with relatively rare but complicated and costly medical problems; and the comprehensiveness of the benefit packages for these children. Many chronic conditions among children in the United States are mild and have little impact on their daily functioning or utilization of health services. But some groups of children (such as premature infants who have been discharged from special care nurseries) have extensive use of inpatient and ambulatory services under fee-for-service medicine and continue to have high rates of utilization for hospital and outpatient services under managed care arrangements (Cavalier and others, 1996). Approximately 10 percent of children with chronic conditions, an estimated 2 million children, have severe conditions that result in extensive use of health services. It is estimated that 2 percent of children with severe health conditions account for approximately 25 percent of all child health expenditures (Butler and others, 1985) and that 10 percent of children are responsible for 60 percent of expenditures (Newacheck and McManus, 1988a). The National Health Interview Survey indicated that 3.8 percent of children with chronic health problems account for 9 percent of outpatient visits and 30 percent of inpatient days (Newacheck, Halfon, and Budetti, 1986).

It is estimated that about 70 percent of all childhood hospital admissions are now for chronic health conditions (Homer and others, 1992). This growth in care for chronic conditions is due both to the increased survival rate of low-birthweight infants and to children with a wide range of chronic medical and surgical conditions (including cystic fibrosis, sickle cell anemia, and congenital heart defects). In addition, there has been an increasing incidence of chronic conditions such as asthma, HIV infection, and injury-related sequelae. While advances in the understanding of the genetic, environmental, and nutritional basis of many chronic health conditions ultimately will translate into a reduction in many of these conditions, improved therapies and technologies will continue to result in prolonged survival for these children.

The health care of many children with chronic conditions is extremely expensive, and the quality of care they receive may be greatly influenced by the changing health care environment. There is likely to be an increase in referrals to pediatric subspecialists and child health professionals in related fields, such as physical therapy, occupational therapy, social services, early intervention, and mental health. At the same time, there will be many developments that facilitate the provision of services away from the hospital, in the home or community.

With changes in child health financing, there are many areas for concern for these children and their families. They include the potential for restricted access to needed medical and nonmedical services, such as limited visits to subspecialists or hospitalizations, restrictions on needed ancillary services and medications, and referrals to nonpediatric rather than pediatric subspecialists. There also is the danger of shifting coverage and restrictions in choice of primary care, subspecialty, and ancillary providers, thus disrupting relationships between children and families and their health care providers. These relationships often are central to the quality of care provided and the quality of life of children and families.

Children from Diverse Family Backgrounds

Ethnic minority and new immigrant families are likely to become the majority of the U.S. population by 2020 (Day, 1993). The number of Latino children in the United States has surpassed other minority groups, growing from 9 percent of the child population in 1980 to 15 percent in 1999. By the year 2020, one in five U.S. children will be Latino (Council of Economic Advisors for the President's Initiative on

Race, 1998). Racial and ethnic differences in access to care, morbidity, and mortality are clear (National Center for Health Statistics, 1999). Black and Hispanic children are also substantially less likely than majority children to have a usual source of care or to be insured (Weinick and Krauss, 2000).

Pachter (1994) has described clinical encounters as an interaction between two cultures—the culture of medicine and the culture of patients. These different groups often have different perceptions, attitudes, knowledge, communication styles, and approaches to health-related issues. Different values, belief systems, priorities, and life stresses may influence perceptions of health and illness and interactions with the health care system. Child health clinicians of the future must be aware of the diversity of patients. Addressing cultural competence will be increasingly important in patient care (Weinick and Krauss, 2000). Clearly, efforts to provide and promote access to primary care are critical, as is the need to ameliorate language barriers through interpreters, bilingual staff, and bilingual educational materials and outreach.

Diversity in family structures will also affect primary care. The proportion of children living in a traditional nuclear family with their biological mother and father was 56 percent in 1996 (U.S. Bureau of the Census, 2001). Just as continuing immigration requires an understanding of ethnic and cultural diversity, changes in family structure will require familiarity in handling issues of single parents, divorce, blended families, and gay and lesbian couples.

OPPORTUNITIES AND CHALLENGES FOR CHILDREN'S PRIMARY CARE

Changing patterns in the organization of health care have the potential both to improve and hinder the care received by children and adolescents. Similarly, changes in the science of medicine, as well as in technology both in and out of health care, may have significant implications for health care delivery to children and their families. What follows is not meant to be a comprehensive compendium of opportunities and challenges, but rather a listing of several key issues in the future of children's primary care services:

- The growth of large, integrated service delivery systems, if such growth in fact continues, may lead to improved community orientation for primary care and to a more explicit mandate to consider the well-being of large numbers of children and families in local policy decisions. These delivery systems may result in consolidation of services to reduce duplication and fragmentation and opportunities to monitor the patterns of and quality of care delivered.

• Large systems also may threaten the quality of health care for children and adolescents. If child health providers are not involved in the design of integrated service delivery systems and utilization review programs, so that they are appropriate for children and adolescents, child health services may suffer. The focus on cost containment may erode support for many of the most vital child health services. Primary care providers seeing increasing numbers of children may have less opportunity to provide anticipatory guidance, behavioral assessment and interventions, and counseling regarding health promotion and disease prevention. Some insurers limit availability or coverage of mental health or social services and referrals for subspecialty evaluation or care or ancillary services such as occupational or physical therapy.

• Creation of integrated health service delivery systems and Medicaid managed care plans may have a negative effect on the quality of care for children and families who rely on safety net providers, such as some hospital-based clinics or community health centers. These market-driven changes are designed primarily to cut costs and serve those who already are insured, and there are few data about their effects on those living in or near poverty.

• The focus on primary care, cost containment, and gatekeeping may result in increased coordination of care and a greater role for child health providers in the care of children with chronic health impairments. This will result in improved care if needed services that primary care providers cannot provide themselves are available to children and families.

• Alternatively, the development of competing health service delivery systems could significantly disrupt doctor-patient and doctor-doctor relationships. Employers' decisions may require families to change the sources of their care, disrupting referral patterns and professional support networks. Pressure to see an increasing volume of patients may limit the involvement of community-based primary care providers in clinical training (Weitzman, Garfunkel, and Connaughton, 1996). It may also serve as a disincentive for involvement in community activities.

• Computer technology and the Internet have affected the method and speed of access to information and the nature of communication among physicians, patients, and other members of the health care team. These technological advances have also provided opportunities for distance education and support for patients in remote and underserved areas. But the media and Internet also have generated an explosion of misinformation available to physicians and their patients. Many consumers have difficulty critically appraising health related information. The education of primary care clinicians must include training in the informatics of health care and the potential promise and problems inherent in technological change. Clinicians also should acquire skills on how to access, assess, and use medical information, both for continuing medical education and as effective adjuncts in support of clinical health promotion efforts.

• There is an urgent need to develop a workforce for the interface of information technology and child health care. There is a great opportunity to improve child health and health care through the development and implementation of electronic records; systems to reduce medical errors; means to enhance communication, coordination, and quality of care for children with chronic health conditions; tracking and monitoring systems for preventive health service needs; and continuing medical education.

• The incidence of infectious diseases is likely to decrease as new vaccines continue to be developed. Although it is likely that pediatric primary care providers will continue to play a critical role in the identification and transfer of children requiring hospitalization, continued advances in the ability to manage conditions in outpatient settings may also mean that less time will be spent in the care of hospitalized children. There is a trend for many hospital inpatient services to have pediatric hospitalists who care for hospitalized patients and less involvement of primary care physicians in the care of their patients who are hospitalized. There also appears to be a trend for primary care practitioners to see their newborn patients while in the hospital after delivery less often. Thus, there is the danger of many missed opportunities at the time of birth for family assessment; breast-feeding promotion; and counseling on injury prevention, tobacco-related exposure, and sudden infant death. There also is the danger of discontinuity of care and miscommunication when children are acutely ill and hospitalized across the pediatric age range.

• Advances in molecular biology and genetics have been prominent in recent years and will continue to have an impact on our understanding of diseases and their diagnosis and treatment. Prenatal diagnosis and identification of individuals predisposed to physical and mental health problems offer great opportunity for prevention and intervention. Along with this new knowledge will be ethical implications and challenges. Primary care clinicians for children are at the forefront of these advances and will have a major role in assisting families in understanding and interpreting information and in advocacy against discrimination or adverse selection in access to care or to insurance.

CONCLUSION

How can we ensure that primary care for children and adolescents provides comprehensive service packages and sufficient support to allow health care providers to identify and coordinate services for the common biomedical, behavioral, and educational problems of children? Could the private sector accommodate an influx of low-income children with high levels of social, mental health, and educational needs if all children had health insurance? Alternatively, how should we protect or enhance the capacity of safety net hospital clinics and community health centers? And how can we enhance integration of services across service sectors?

These questions raise still others—about how best to change medical education so that sufficient numbers of appropriately trained primary care providers are available to work in underserved urban and rural areas and how best to recruit, retain, and support professionals in these areas. How best to care for children with chronic health impairments and how to facilitate the development of new pediatric primary care roles to address issues that disproportionately contribute to a large burden of suffering in children and adults, such as maternal depression, domestic violence, parental smoking, and children's unmet oral health needs, are all questions of great importance to the health of our nation.

To answer these questions, it is necessary to recognize the unique and often multiple needs of a very large percentage of children, the central role that primary care can play in the early identification of children at risk, and the importance of forcefully and effectively articulating the needs of children and families in the midst of health services changes affecting the entire U.S. population.

Child and adolescent primary care services, like all other primary care services, are at a crossroad. Efforts to balance cost, quality, and accountability and a variety of social influences on morbidity and mortality continue to change the practice of medicine and progress on improving the health status of our nation's children. In seeking a clear vision about the future of primary care in the United States, the basic premise of children's health care systems and services separate and distinct from those for adults remains valid. Only by strengthening these systems can we hope to provide the care necessary to help all children and adolescents to achieve their optimal physical, mental, and social potential.

References

Agency for Health Care Policy and Research. "Translating Evidence into Practice 1998, Conference Summary." [http://www.ahcpr.gov/clinic/trip1998/]. 1998.

American Academy of Family Physicians. "2001 NRMP Results: Pediatrics." [http://www.aafp.org/match/table02.htm]. 2001a.

American Academy of Family Physicians. "2001 NRMP Results: Family Practice." [http://www.aafp.org/match/table01.htm]. 2001b.

American Academy of Family Physicians. "National Ambulatory Medical Care Survey." 2001c. Unpublished data.

American Academy of Pediatrics. "Implementation Principles and Strategies for the State Children's Health Insurance Program." *Pediatrics,* 2001, *107,* 1214.

American Academy of Pediatrics. "Recommendations for Preventive Pediatric Health Care. Committee on Practice and Ambulatory Medicine." [http://www.aap.org/policy/re9939.html]. 2001.

American Board of Pediatrics. "Number of Diplomates Certified." [http://www.abp.org]. 2001.

Association of American Medical Colleges. "National Residency Matching Program Data Indicate a Rebalancing of Specialty Interests Among U.S. Medical Students." [http://www.aamc.org/newsroom/pressrel/010322.htm]. 2001.

Bass, J. L., and others. "Childhood Injury Prevention Counseling in Primary Care Settings: A Critical Review of the Literature." *Pediatrics,* 1993, *92,* 544–550.

Berg, A. O. "Clinical Practice Guidelines Panels: Personal Experience." *Journal of the American Board of Family Practitioners,* 1996, *9,* 366–370.

Brindis, C. D. "What It Will Take: Placing Adolescents on the American National Agenda for the 1990s." *Journal of Adolescent Health,* 1993, *14,* 527–530.

Brotherton, S. E. "Pediatric Subspecialty Training, Certification, and Practice: Who's Doing What." *Pediatrics,* 1994, *94,* 83–89.

Brown, S. A., and Grames, D. E. *Nurse Practitioners and Certified Nurse Midwives: A Meta-Analysis of Studies on Nurses in Primary Care Roles.* Washington, D.C.: American Nursing Association, 1993.

Butler, J. A., and others. "Health Care Expenditures for Children with Chronic Illness. In N. Hobbs and T. M. Merrin (eds.), *Issues in the Care of Children with Chronic Illnesses.* San Francisco: Jossey-Bass, 1985.

Carnegie Corporation. *Turning Points: Preparing American Youth for the Twenty-First Century.* New York: Carnegie Corporation, 1989.

Cavalier, S., and others. "Postdischarge Utilization of Medical Services by High-Risk Infants: Experiences in a Large Managed Care Organization." *Pediatrics,* 1996, *97,* 693–699.

Children's Defense Fund. *The State of America's Children, 1992.* Washington, D.C.: Children's Defense Fund, 1992.

Council of Economic Advisors for the President's Initiative on Race. *Changing America: Indicators of Social and Economic Well-Being by Race and Hispanic Origin.* Washington, D.C.: Council of Economic Advisors for the President's Initiative on Race, 1998.

Day, J. C. *Population Projections of the United States, by Age, Sex, Race, and Hispanic Origin: 1993–2005.* Washington, D.C.: U.S. Bureau of the Census, 1993.

DeAngelis, C. D. "Nurse Practitioner Redux." *Journal of the American Medical Association,* 1994, *271,* 868–871.

Dunn, A. M. "1992 NAPNAP Membership Survey, Part II. Practice Characteristics of Pediatric Nurse Practitioners Indicate Greater Autonomy for PNPs." *Journal of Pediatric Health Care,* 1993, *7,* 296–302.

Elster, A. B., and Kuznets, M. J. *Guidelines for Adolescent Preventive Services.* Baltimore, Md.: Williams & Wilkins, 1993.

Ferris, T. G., and others. "Changes in the Daily Practice of Primary Care for Children." *Archives of Pediatric and Adolescent Medicine,* 1998, *152,* 227–233.

Fletcher, R. H., and Fletcher, S. W. "Here Come the Couples." *Annals of Internal Medicine,* 1993, *119,* 628–630.

"The Future of Pediatric Education II: Organizing Pediatric Education to Meet the Needs of Infants, Children, Adolescents, and Young Adults in the Twenty-First Century." *Pediatrics,* 2000, *105,* S161–212.

Gans, J. E., McManus, M. A., and Newacheck, P. W. *Adolescent Health Care: Use, Costs, and Problems of Access.* Chicago: American Medical Association, 1991.

Haggerty, R. J. "Child Health 2000: New Pediatrics in the Changing Environment of Children's Needs in the Twenty-First Century." *Pediatrics,* 1995, *96,* 804–811.

Health Resources Administration. *Summary Report of the Graduate Medical Education: National Advisory Committee.* Washington, D.C.: National Advisory Committee to the Secretary, Department of Health and Human Services, 1980.

Health Resources and Services Administration. *HRSA State Health Workforce Profile, New York. December 2000.* Rockville, Md.: U.S. Department of Health and Human Services, 2000.

Holl, J. L., and others. "Profile of Uninsured Children in the United States." *Archives of Pediatric and Adolescent Medicine,* 1995, *149,* 398–406.

Homer, C. J., and others. *Hospital Use by Children with Chronic Illness.* Washington, D.C.: Ambulatory Pediatric Association, 1992.

Igra, V., and Millstein, S. "Current Status and Approaches to Improving Preventive Services for Adolescents." *Journal of the American Medical Association,* 1993, *269,* 1408–1413.

Klein, J. D., Kotelchuck, M., and DeFriese, G. H. *Comprehensive Multi-Service Delivery Systems for Adolescents.* Washington, D.C.: Office of Technology Assessment and the Carnegie Council on Adolescent Development, 1990.

Klein, J. D., and others. "Access to Health Care for Adolescents." *Journal of Adolescent Health,* 1992, *13,* 162–170.

Klerman, L. V., Kovar, M. G., and Brown, S. S. *Adolescents: Health Status and Needed Services: Report of the Select Panel for the Promotion of Child Health.* Washington, D.C.: Department of Health and Human Services, 1981.

Lansky, D. "Measuring What Matters to the Public." *Health Affairs,* 1988, *17,* 40–41.

Lewin, L. S. "Adapting Your Pediatric Practice to the Changing Health Care System." *Pediatrics,* 1995, *96,* 799–803.

Lewis, C. E. *Health Services Research in Prevention: Primary Care Research: An Agenda for the 90s.* Rockville, Md.: U.S. Department of Health and Human Services, 1990.

Lohr, K. N., Vanselow, N. A., and Detmer, D. E. *The Nation's Physician Work Force: Options for Balancing Supply and Requirements.* Washington, D.C.: Institute of Medicine, 1996.

National Center for Health Statistics. *Health, United States, 1992 and Healthy People 2000 Review.* Washington, D.C.: U.S. Department of Health and Human Services, 1993.

National Center for Health Statistics. *Health, United States, 1999, Health and Aging Chartbook.* Hyattsville, Md.: U.S. Department of Health and Human Services, 1999.

Nazarian, L. F. "A Look at the Private Practice of the Future." *Pediatrics,* 1995, *96,* 811–812.

Newacheck, P., Budetti, P., and McManus, P. "Trends in Childhood Disability." *American Journal of Public Health,* 1984, *74,* 232.

Newacheck, P., Budetti, P., and Halfon, N. "Trends in Activity Limiting Chronic Conditions Among Children." *American Journal of Public Health,* 1986, *76,* 178–184.

Newacheck, P., Halfon, N., and Budetti, P. "Prevalence of Activity Limiting Chronic Conditions Among Children Based on Household Interviews." *Journal of Chronic Disease,* 1986, *39,* 63–69.

Newacheck, P., and McManus, P. "Financing Health Care for Disabled Children." *Pediatrics,* 1988a, *81,* 385–394.

Newacheck, P. W., and McManus, M. A. "Health Insurance Status of Children in the US." Pediatrics, 1988b, 82, 462–468.

Newacheck, P. W., and others. "An Epidemiologic Profile of Children with Special Health Care Needs." *Pediatrics,* 1998, *102,* 117–123.

Newacheck, P. W., and others. "The Unmet Health Needs of America's Children." *Pediatrics,* 2000, *105,* 989–997.

North Carolina Rural Health Research Program, University of North Carolina at Chapel Hill Cecil G. Sheps Center for Health Services Research. *Facts About Rural Physicians.* Washington, D.C.: U.S. Department of Health and Human Services, 1997.

Pachter, L. M. "Culture and Clinical Care." *Journal of the American Medical Association,* 1994, *271,* 690–694.

Perrin, J., Guyer, B., and Lawrence, J. M. "Health Care Services for Children and Adolescents." *Future of Children,* 1992, *2,* 58–77.

Resnick, M. D., Blum, R. W., and Hedin, D. "The Appropriateness of Health Services for Adolescents: Youth Opinions and Attitudes." *Journal of Adolescent Health Care,* 1980, *1,* 137–145.

Russell, N. K., and others. "Unannounced Simulated Patients' Observations of Physicians' STD/HIV Prevention Activities." *American Journal of Preventive Medicine,* 1992, *8,* 235–240.

Smoller, M. "Telephone Calls and Appointment Requests: Predictability in an Unpredictable World." *HMO Practitioner,* 1992, *6,* 25–29.

Sox, H. C. "Quality of Patient Care by Nurse Practitioners and Physician's Assistants: A Ten-Year Perspective." *Annals of Internal Medicine,* 1979, *91,* 459–468.

Starfield, B. *The Effectiveness of Medical Care: Validating Clinical Wisdom.* Baltimore, Md.: Johns Hopkins University Press, 1985.

Stone, E. L. "Nurse Practitioners and Physician Assistants: Do They Have a Role in Your Practice?" *Pediatrics,* 1995, *96,* 844–850.

U.S. Bureau of the Census. "Historical Poverty Tables." [http://www.census.gov/hhes/poverty/histpov/hstpov3.html]. 2000a.

U.S. Bureau of the Census. *Health Insurance Coverage 1999.* Washington, D.C.: U.S. Department of Commerce, 2000b.

U.S. Bureau of the Census. "The 'Nuclear Family' Rebounds." *Department of Commerce News,* Apr. 13, 2001.

U.S. Congress, Office of Technology Assessment. *Nurse Practitioners, Physician Assistants and Certified Nurse-Midwives: Policy Analysis.* Washington, D.C.: U.S. Government Printing Office, 1986.

U.S. Congress, Office of Technology Assessment. *Adolescent Health, Vol. 1: Summary and Policy Options.* Washington, D.C.: U.S. Government Printing Office, 1991.

Valdez, R. B., and others. "Prepaid Group Practice Effects on the Utilization of Medical Services and Health Outcomes for Children: Results from a Controlled Trial." *Pediatrics,* 1989, *6,* 25–29.

Warde, C., Allen, W., and Gelberg, L. "Physician Role Conflict and Resulting Career Changes: Gender and Generational Differences." *Journal of General Internal Medicine,* 1996, *11,* 729–735.

Weinick, R. M., and Krauss, N. A. "Racial/Ethnic Differences in Children's Access to Care." *American Journal of Public Health,* 2000, *90,* 1771–1774.

Weitzman, M. "The Role of the Health Care Practitioner." In R.E.K. Stein (ed.), *Health Care for Children: What's Right, What's Wrong, What's Next.* New York: United Hospital Fund, 1997.

Weitzman, M., Byrd, R. S., and Auinger, P. "Children in Big Cities in the United States: Health and Related Needs and Services." *Ambulatory Child Health,* 1996, *1,* 347–346.

Weitzman, M., Doniger, A. S., and Partner, S. F. "Seeking Pathways to a Coordinated System of Health and Human Services for High-Risk Urban Children and Families: The Rochester, New York Experience." *Bulletin of the New York Academy of Medicine,* 1994, *71,* 267–280.

Weitzman, M., Garfunkel, L., and Connaughton, S. "The Funding of Pediatric Education in Community Settings." *Pediatrics,* 1996, *88,* 284–285.

PART FOUR

Recommendations for the Future

This final chapter presents ideas and suggestions about how to address current dilemmas in primary care.

CHAPTER FIFTEEN

Primary Care

The Next Renaissance

Jonathan Showstack
Nicole Lurie
Eric B. Larson
Arlyss Anderson Rothman
Susan B. Hassmiller

Three decades ago, there was a renaissance in primary care that helped create the foundations of the field as we know it today. Although primary care has developed as a vital intellectual and applied concept, there have not been the hoped-for changes in the medical care system to support the goals of comprehensive, continuous, patient-centered, and outcomes-oriented care. In fact, it appears that the dominance of specialty care is increasing and interest in primary care as a career has waned, and changes in reimbursement and health care organization, such as the advent of managed care, have been relatively negative for primary care.

The current state and direction of primary care are described in this book and elsewhere (Moore and Showstack, 2003; Safran, 2003;

A version of this chapter was originally published in *The Annals of Internal Medicine,* 2003, *138,* 268–272.

1. Health care must be organized to serve the needs of patients.
2. The goal of primary care systems should be the delivery of the highest-quality care as documented by measurable outcomes.
3. Information and information systems are the backbone of the primary care process.
4. Current health care systems must be reconstructed.
5. The health care financing system must support excellent primary care practice.
6. Primary care education must be revitalized, with an emphasis on new delivery models and training at sites that deliver excellent primary care.
7. The value of primary care practice must be continually improved, documented, and communicated.

Exhibit 15.1. Seven Core Principles in Support of a Renaissance of Primary Care.

Anderson Rothman and Wagner, 2003; Sandy and Schroeder, 2003). In this chapter, we suggest seven core principles, set out in Exhibit 15.1, to support a renaissance in primary care and a set of actions, identified in Exhibit 15.2, to address this crisis and enable primary care to play a significant role in achieving the goals of high-quality, patient-centered, efficient, and user-friendly care for individuals and populations. We offer these thoughts as persons who believe passionately in the basic principles of primary care and are deeply concerned about its future.

CORE PRINCIPLES

Seven core principles should guide the next renaissance of primary care:

1. Health care must be organized to serve the needs of patients.
2. The goal of primary care systems should be the delivery of the highest-quality care as documented by measurable outcomes.
3. Information and information systems are the backbone of the primary care process.
4. Current health care systems must be reconstructed.
5. The health care financing system must support excellent primary care practice.
6. Primary care education must be revitalized, with an emphasis on new delivery models and training at sites that deliver excellent primary care.

Redesign Primary Care Organization and Finance
- Undertake a national five- to ten-year effort to create new and innovative patient-centered primary care systems.
- Design, implement, and evaluate a personal health information and choice system that is patient centered and outcomes oriented.
- Create new health care financing systems to support and encourage patient-centered primary care services and systems.

Reform Primary Care Education
- Require that primary care providers receive their clinical training in patient-centered, outcomes-oriented, primary care settings that include state-of-the-art information systems.
- Revise graduate medical education funding to provide adequate support and incentives for training in high-quality primary care settings.
- Develop a common core curriculum, and integrate training experiences across different primary care specialties and practices.

Expand and Disseminate Knowledge About Primary Care
- Create a primary care institute within the National Institutes of Health to perform, fund, and disseminate the results of research on primary care organization and delivery and establish centers of excellence in primary care practice to facilitate the development and evaluation of new models of primary care practice and teaching.
- Establish a clearinghouse to aggregate and disseminate the results of primary care research and demonstration projects to the public, providers, administrators, academicians, and policymakers.
- Provide recognition to exemplary primary care practice.

Exhibit 15.2. Reconstructing Primary Care.

7. The value of primary care practice must be continually improved, documented, and communicated.

Principle 1: Health Care Must Be Organized to Serve the Needs of Patients

Health care should achieve optimal health and medical outcomes within available resources and be respectful of and responsive to a person's needs, values, and preferences. Patient-centered care (Gerteis, Edgman-Levitan, Daley, and Delbanco, 2002) includes the patient as an active participant in the clinical decision-making process and incorporates into the care process an understanding of the individual patient's preferences and needs. Such care is user friendly to both patients and providers, with everything from the design of information systems to the hours of operation structured to create a partnership between patient and provider.

Patient-centered care is a core principle of primary care and is supported by the goals of comprehensiveness and continuity. Yet much of the current organization of medical care is structured to accommodate incentives in the reimbursement system and the preferences of providers, often with patients' needs included only as an afterthought. Responding to patients' needs and desires must be a fundamental objective of future health care systems.

Principle 2: The Goal of Primary Care Systems Should Be the Delivery of the Highest-Quality Care as Documented by Measurable Outcomes

The central goal of primary care systems should be the delivery of high-quality care that leads to the best possible outcomes. We agree with the conclusions of the Institute of Medicine's recent analysis (2001) of the quality of health care: it is time to create systems that are safe and effective. The definition of *quality* could, and should, be based in large part on definable outcomes. Accomplishing this goal will require research to establish appropriate indicators of primary care quality and the development of methods to identify, collect, and evaluate the most relevant information. Although a true outcomes-based system may be some years away, enough is known today about processes and practices that lead to good outcomes that these processes and practices should guide the redesign of primary care systems.

Systems of care need to be accountable to consumers, providers, and payers, and this accountability must include the measurement of individual and population outcomes. The concept of accountability has yet to evolve fully, and today's systems of oversight, such as Health Plan Employer Data and Information Set (HEDIS) measures (National Committee for Quality Assurance, 1990), are more oriented to overall system outcomes than to ensuring individual outcomes. As accountability becomes more clearly defined and operationalized, it should become part of and assist in routine quality improvement efforts. This will require patient- and outcomes-oriented information systems with adequate mechanisms to protect confidentiality.

Principle 3: Information and Information Systems Are the Backbone of the Primary Care Process

Information and the exchange of information are key to the primary care process in assisting in the clinical decision-making process, tracking the preventive and acute care provided, educating patients, assessing outcomes, and providing patients with the information they need to manage their health and make decisions about their care. The effective provision of primary care requires the processing of large amounts of knowledge, ranging from an individual's risk factors and health status to the likelihood that a particular diagnostic procedure or therapy will be optimal for a particular patient. More so than for procedure-based specialists, information is at the core of the primary care process, and information systems are primary care's technology.

Today's health care information systems were designed primarily in response to administrative needs, with reimbursement at the top of the list (Singer, Enthoven, and Garber, 2001). While these encounter-based systems may serve their narrow administrative purposes well, they rarely collect information that allows management of a patient's needs over time or an assessment of the effects of clinical processes on patient outcomes. Encounter-based systems encourage discontinuity for patients, poor communications among providers, and underuse of the information that is available, and they often produce less than optimal care. Even in academic medical centers, where the most advanced clinical technologies are developed and used, patients often cannot be tracked from the inpatient to the outpatient setting or among different types of providers, nor can patients and providers access and share information.

What is needed is a personal health information and choice system. Such an imagined (but possible) system is an essential component of patient-centered and accountable health care and would, almost by definition, enhance the role of primary care providers. Containing information about a person's health, her risk profile, and her recent preventive and clinical care, this system would be patient centered in both the information that it contains and the ability to access that information. Persons, whether they are active patients or not, would be able to interact with the system, communicate with their provider, review their medical records (a recently established requirement; Pear, 2002a), view results of tests and therapies, and add information about their current health status. Decision support tools would assist both patients and providers in identifying clinical choices and probable outcomes in a manner that is both understandable and useful, and the system would include links with community resources and key Internet sites to enhance the short amount of time available for patient education in a routine visit. The system would also link closely with emerging efforts to rebuild the information technology components of the public health infrastructure and maximize the opportunities to develop robust connections between the personal health services delivery system and public health.

The knowledge and technology needed to create and implement such systems are available today. What is needed now is the political will to devote the necessary resources to this effort. We believe that the development and implementation of patient-centered health information systems should be among the highest priorities for the future use of resources in health and health care.

Principle 4: Current Health Care Systems Must Be Reconstructed

Health care organization is an oxymoron. In reality, we have an extremely complex and fragmented set of providers, facilities, and services that have been created based on requirements for reimbursement and the needs of providers. Patient needs and outcomes and provider accountability usually have been only secondary considerations when designing systems of care. Although it is not necessarily the worst offender in this regard, primary care has generally played a very passive role in the design and implementation of health care systems. Rather than taking the lead, for example, in the development of organizations that are devoted to health maintenance and in which primary care has a central role, primary care providers were relatively passive when assigned the role of gatekeeper by managed care organizations.

We can imagine a new and better type of health care system designed to address patient and population needs and preferences. Such a system would be participant controlled, outcomes oriented, structured to address the particular needs of the system's population, and focused on the ongoing relationship between a patient and his or her primary provider. Care models would be developed based on the functions that are necessary to achieve desired outcomes. Quality of care would be measured through active and ongoing assessment, ideally by an independent evaluator. The organization's integrated information systems would provide a real-time assessment of processes and outcomes so that quality issues could be resolved quickly, with key indicators of quality and outcomes published regularly. Such a system would be much closer to the ideal of a true health maintenance organization than is the bastardization of that term by today's managed care.

Health care systems need to be both flexible and agile, with a capacity for rapid change in response to new circumstances. In the future, systems should be allowed to use resources that in that setting produce the desired outcomes. For example, some (perhaps most) patients may prefer a physician as their primary provider, and others may choose a nurse practitioner; some may want multiple providers functioning in a team, with others preferring an individual. The organizing principle should be achieving the best outcomes possible within the creative use of available resources, while allowing patient choices and preferences to help guide the use of those resources.

Principle 5: The Health Care Financing System Must Support Excellent Primary Care Practice

Patient-oriented and accountable health systems cannot survive unless current payment practices are changed radically. Such changes must, at a minimum, include adequate reimbursement for basic primary care services such as performing a history and physical examination, counseling patients about their health behaviors, and, possibly most important, being an advocate for and helping to guide patients through the health care system. The current financing system is also often a barrier to continuous and comprehensive care and contributes to quality-of-care problems associated with both over- and underuse of services (Institute of Medicine, 2001).

The negative effects of current financial systems on patients and their clinical outcomes have been ignored for far too long by government and private payers. There is little doubt that the current financing system is adverse to the goals of primary care. In many communities, primary care practitioners have had to abandon practice because of inadequate reimbursement, and hospitals have abandoned their sponsored primary care clinics due to continued losses (Larson, 2001). The recent reduction in Medicare reimbursement for physicians has arguably hurt primary care more than other specialties (Pear, 2002b).

Despite some movement over time toward prospective payment systems, the financial disincentives toward primary care have changed little in recent decades. These adverse incentives were described and quantified over two decades ago (Schroeder and Showstack, 1978), and they still influence how medicine is practiced. Primary care services remain undervalued in comparison to surgery and other specialty services, with so-called cognitive services (that is, most services other than surgery and the application of technology) receiving relatively low reimbursement. The large difference in reimbursement between cognitive and technological services produces strong incentives to perform procedures that may or may not be in the best interests of patients. The use of office-based technologies such as chest X rays and simple laboratory tests, for example, can increase the reimbursement for a typical office visit significantly (Schroeder and Showstack, 1978). These same adverse incentives also affect services provided in institutions. At the University of Washington Medical Center, for example, the primary care clinics would appear to be in significant financial deficit except for the fact that revenues generated from computerized tomography and magnetic resonance imaging scanners in the same building are listed on the same balance sheet.

The financial structure of health care and the current reimbursement system cannot be changed overnight. We believe that the best way to change the economic incentives in health care is to design new financing systems in parallel with the creation of new patient-centered systems of care. Although there may be winners and losers among providers in a redesigned reimbursement system, the design should be a win for patients, with the reimbursement system designed to support core primary care functions. At a minimum, the current financial disincentives toward adequate primary care should be eliminated; optimally, the reimbursement system should support and encourage continuity of care and patient-centered and accountable systems of care.

We also believe strongly that while changing the current financing system is absolutely necessary, it is not a sufficient precondition for the reconstruction of primary care. Without substantial changes in the way that health care is organized and delivered, changing reimbursement for primary care services would be a stopgap measure at best.

Principle 6: Primary Care Education Must Be Revitalized, with an Emphasis on New Delivery Models and Training in Sites That Deliver Excellent Primary Care

Health professions education has begun to move toward recognition of the changing demographics and needs of the population, with the increasing inclusion of cultural competence, health promotion and disease prevention, and community service as part of the formal curriculum. Most primary care clinical education, however, occurs in settings that are not structured to provide optimal care.

Academic health centers and graduate training programs in primary care should be leaders in testing and implementing new and innovative ways to deliver high-quality care. Yet the clinical experiences of primary care trainees often occur in relatively dysfunctional and user-unfriendly clinics with poor information systems and little or no continuity among different types of providers. Too often the result is discouraged primary care residents, who then opt for subspecialty training and practice. To make matters worse, in these times of economic difficulties, many academic health centers are emphasizing lucrative specialty care and increasing the historic marginalization of primary care.

New models and settings need to be considered for primary care clinical training. Clinical training should occur in settings that provide high-quality, continuous, patient-centered, outcomes-oriented, team-based care. The new delivery models suggested would provide much more appropriate settings for primary care clinical education experiences.

Principle 7: The Value of Primary Care Practice Must Be Continually Improved, Documented, and Communicated

There needs to be a concerted national effort to redesign, implement, and evaluate new forms of primary care delivery. Studies should identify the appropriate functions that are necessary for delivering care to particular patient groups, the strengths and weaknesses of different configurations of primary care providers and systems, and ways to restructure the relationship between primary care providers and medical specialists.

To support the design and evaluation of new models of care, a primary care institute should be established within the National Institutes of Health to perform, fund, and disseminate the results of research on primary care organization and delivery. Some of the work of such a proposed institute has already begun in the Center for Primary Care at the Agency for Healthcare Research and Quality (AHRQ), but the budget to support the level of work truly required for such an enterprise is woefully inadequate. The creation of centers of excellence in primary care practice would also facilitate the development and evaluation of new models of care. Similar to the Centers of Excellence in Patient Safety Research supported by the AHRQ (www.ahcpr.gov/news/press/pr2000/excellpr.htm) and the Cancer

Centers Program of the National Cancer Institute (http://www3.cancer.gov/cancercenters/description.html), centers of excellence in primary care practice would perform innovative multidisciplinary research to improve the organization and delivery of primary care services, develop new training models for primary care, and disseminate the latest research findings about best practices in primary care. The current Primary Care Practice–Based Research Networks could be used as a basis for some of this research (http://www.ahcpr.gov/research/pbrnfact.htm). In addition, the results of evaluations of primary care models and practices need to be aggregated and reviewed in the light of the increasing diversity and changing needs of our population, and a clearinghouse should be developed through which information about primary care education, delivery, and research can be disseminated.

The value of primary care is not understood well by the public or by most providers, administrators, and policymakers. While patients place a high value on primary care, many feel that primary care has failed to live up to its promise (Safran, 2003). Unfortunately, and mistakenly in the eyes of many, primary care has become synonymous with hassles and obstacles to obtaining needed care. The public needs to be educated about how good primary care should work and why it sometimes fails in today's often uncoordinated medical care system. An important step in the direction of improving perceptions about and knowledge of primary care would be a national communications strategy that educates the public, providers, and policymakers about the value and rationale for primary care. Supporters of primary care should identify outstanding innovative primary care practices and then disseminate this information through a variety of means, perhaps including an award for such innovation.

CONCLUSION

At the start of the twenty-first century, a vital, patient-centered primary care system has much to offer a rapidly changing population with increasingly diverse needs and expectations. The potential for a new renaissance of primary care is a great opportunity for patients and health care professionals. The changes suggested here may not be easy to accomplish or acceptable to some, but if we keep the needs of persons and patients clearly in sight and design systems to meet those needs, primary care will thrive and patients will be well served.

References

Anderson Rothman, A., and Wagner, E. "Chronic Illness Management: What Is the Role of Primary Care?" *Annals of Internal Medicine,* 2003, *138*(suppl.), 256–261.

Gerteis, M., Edgman-Levitan, S., Daley, J., and Delbanco, T. L. (eds.). *Through the Patient's Eyes: Understanding and Promoting Patient-Centered Care.* San Francisco: Jossey-Bass, 2002.

Institute of Medicine. Committee on Quality of Health Care in America. *Crossing the Quality Chasm: A New Health System for the Twenty-First Century.* Washington, D.C.: National Academy Press, 2001.

Larson, E. B. "General Internal Medicine at the Crossroads of Prosperity and Despair: Caring for Patients with Chronic Diseases in an Aging Society." *Annals of Internal Medicine,* 2001, *134,* 997–1000.

Moore, G., and Showstack, J. "Primary Care Medicine in Crisis: Toward Reconstruction and Renewal." *Annals of Internal Medicine,* 2003, *138*(suppl.), 244–247.

National Committee for Quality Assurance. *The Health Plan Employer Data and Information Set.* 1990. [http://www.ncqa.org/Programs/HEDIS/].

Pear, R. "Bush Rolls Back Rules on Privacy of Medical Data." *New York Times,* Aug. 9, 2002a, p. A1.

Pear, R. "Many Doctors Say They Are Refusing Medicare Patients." *New York Times,* March 17, 2002b, p. 1.

Safran, D. G. "Defining the Future of Primary Care: What Can We Learn from Patients?" *Annals of Internal Medicine,* 2003, *138*(suppl.), 248–255.

Sandy, L., and Schroeder, S. "Primary Care in a New Era: Disillusion and Dissolution?" *Annals of Internal Medicine,* 2003, *138*(suppl.), 262–267.

Schroeder, S. A., and Showstack, J. A. "Financial Incentives to Perform Medical Procedures and Laboratory Tests: Illustrative Models of Office Practice." *Medical Care,* 1978, *16,* 289–298.

Singer, A. J., Enthoven, A. C., and Garber, A. M. "Health Care and Information Technology: Growing Up Together." In E. H. Shortliffe, L. E. Perreault, G. Wiederhold, and L. M. Fagan (eds.), *Medical Informatics: Computer Applications in Health Care and Biomedicine.* New York: Springer-Verlag, 2001.

Name Index

Subject Index

C